Addictions - Diagnosis and Treatment

Edited by William M. Meil and John A. Mills

Published in London, United Kingdom

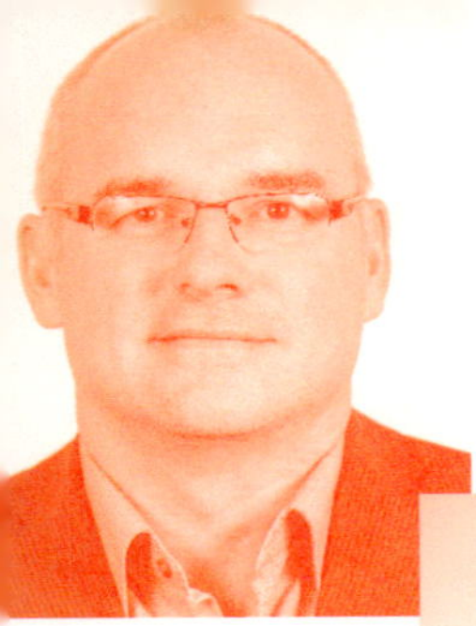
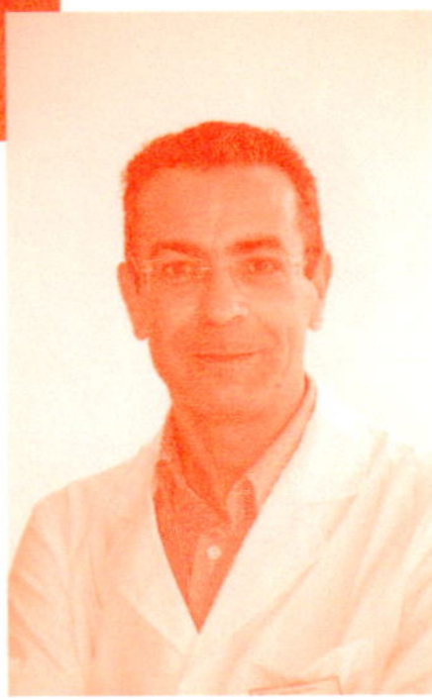
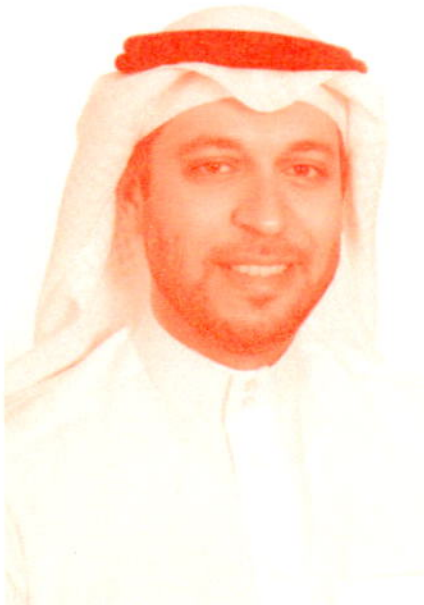
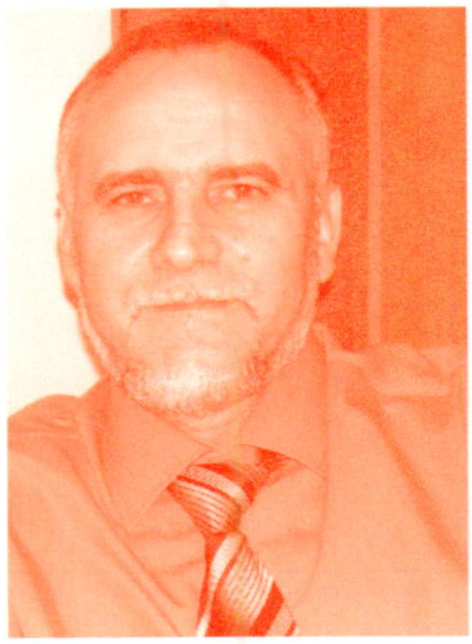
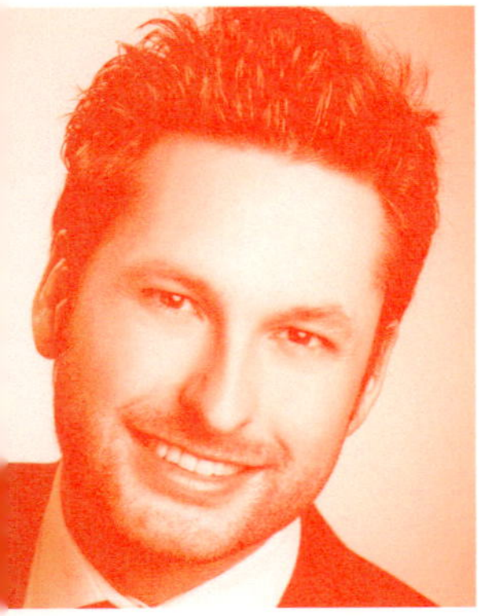
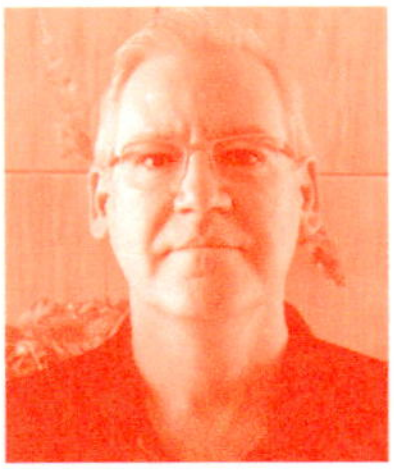
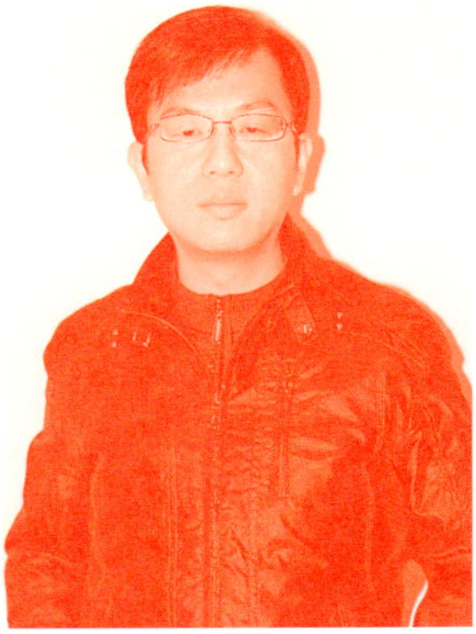

IntechOpen

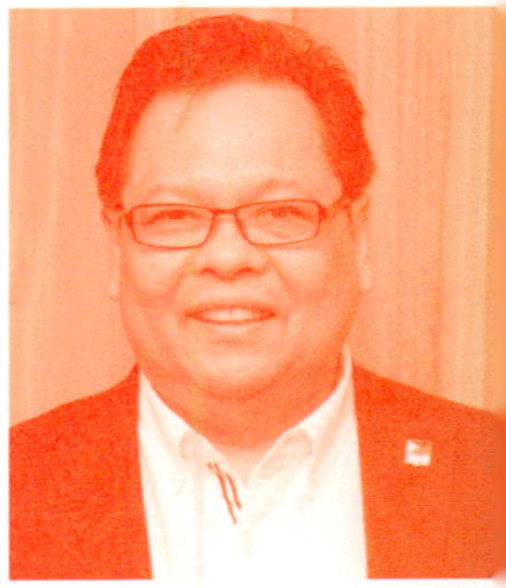
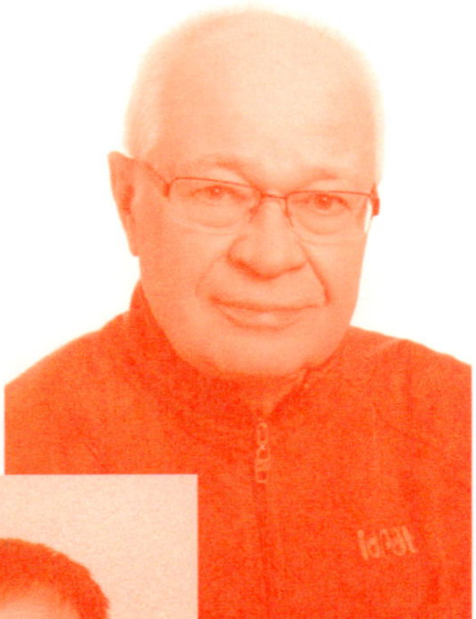
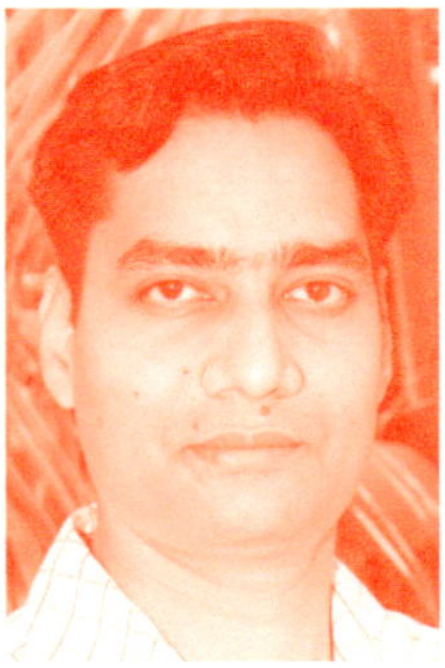
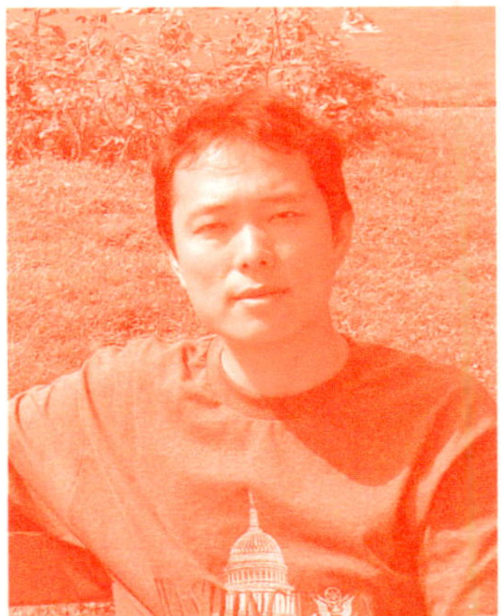
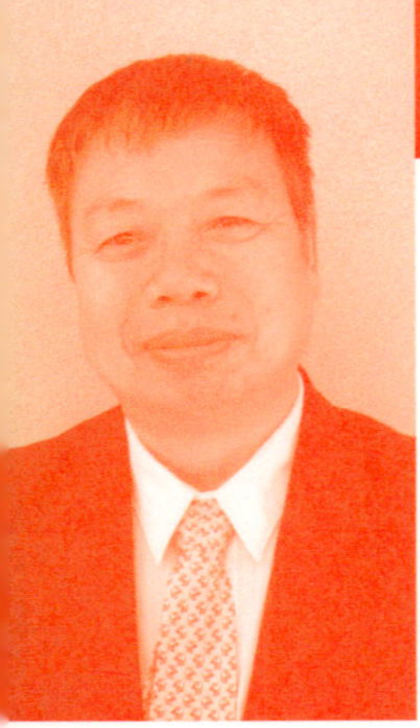
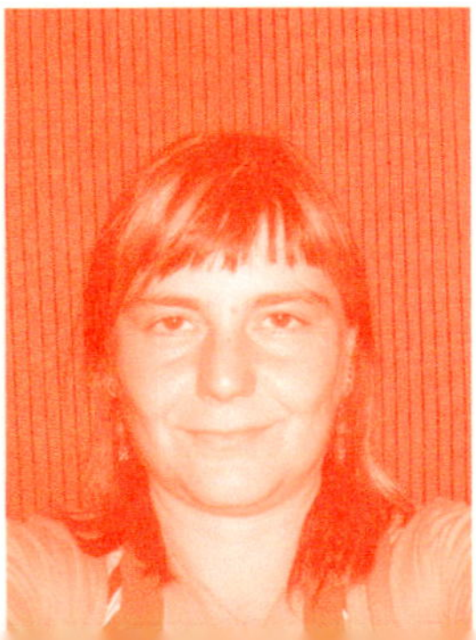

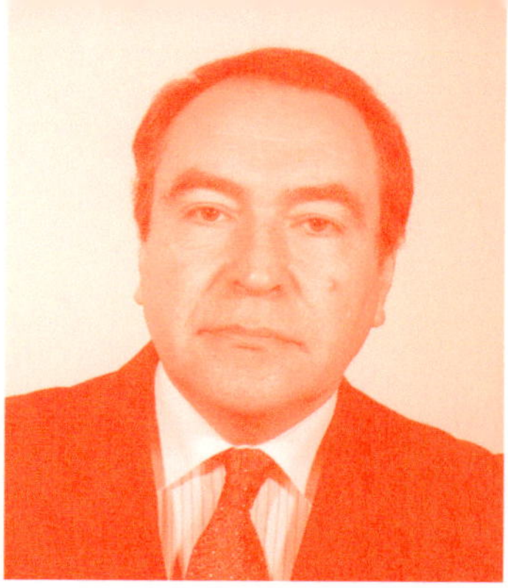
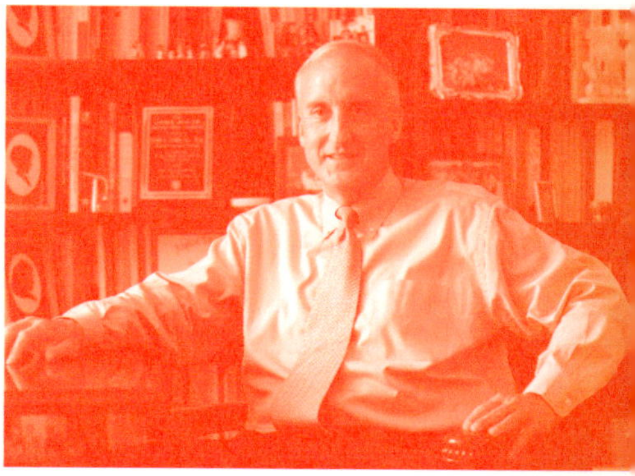
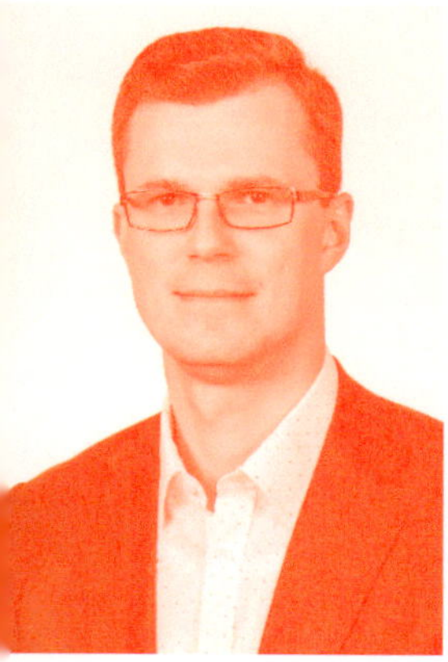
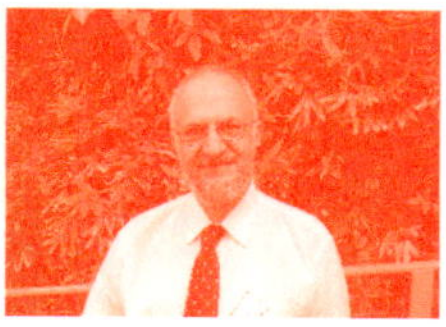
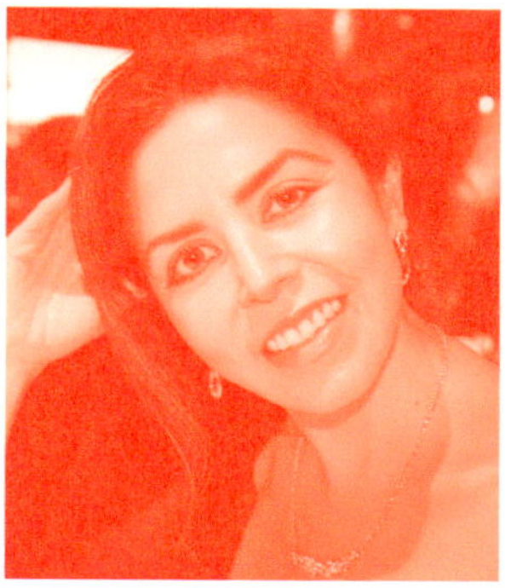

Supporting open minds since 2005

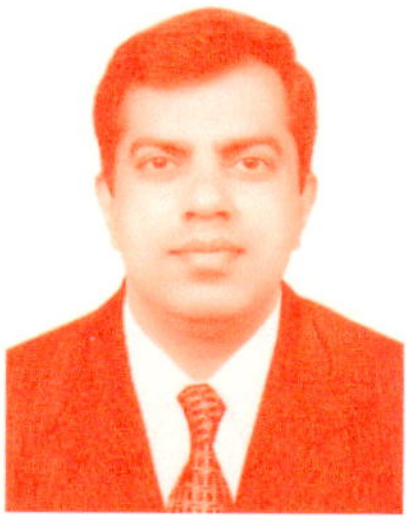
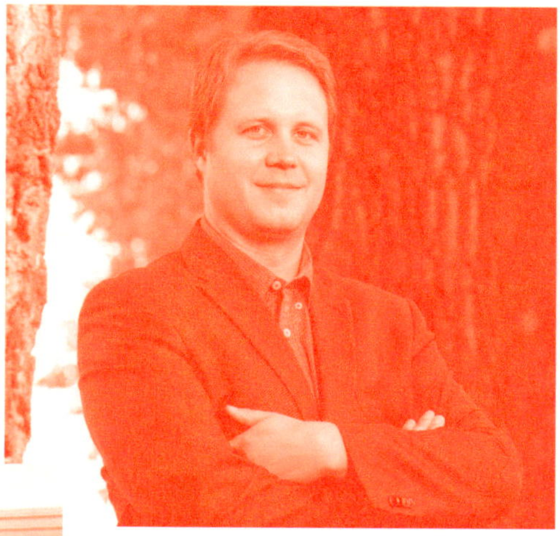
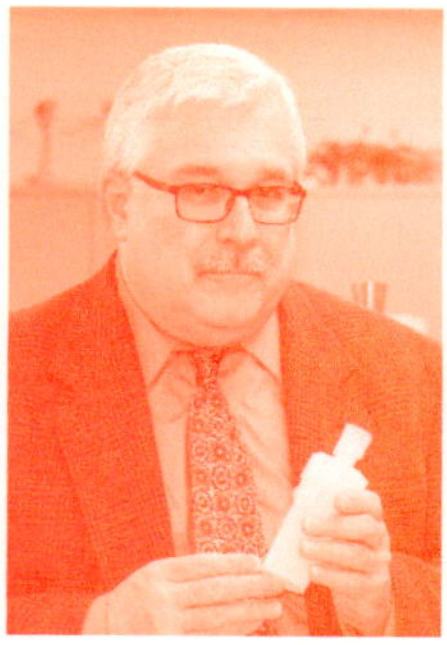
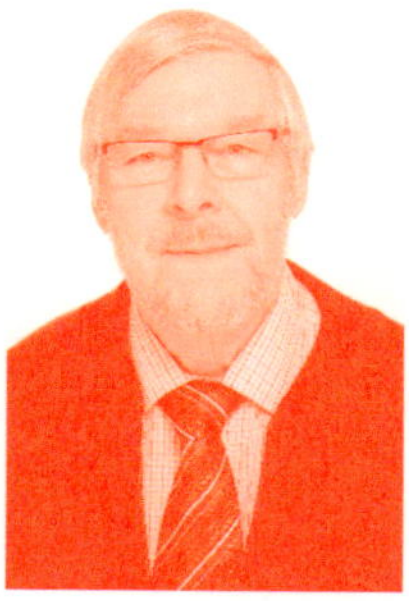
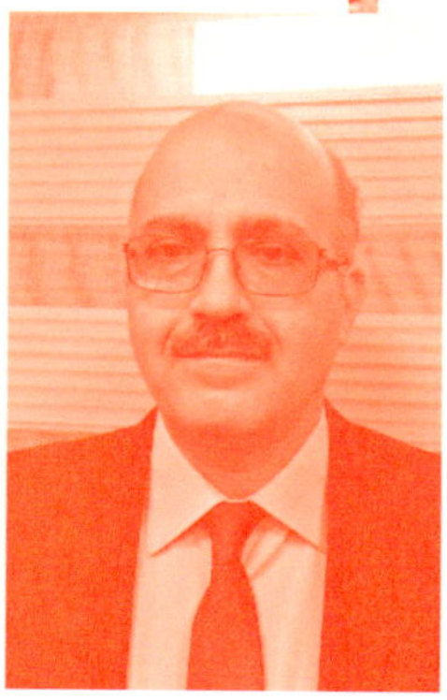
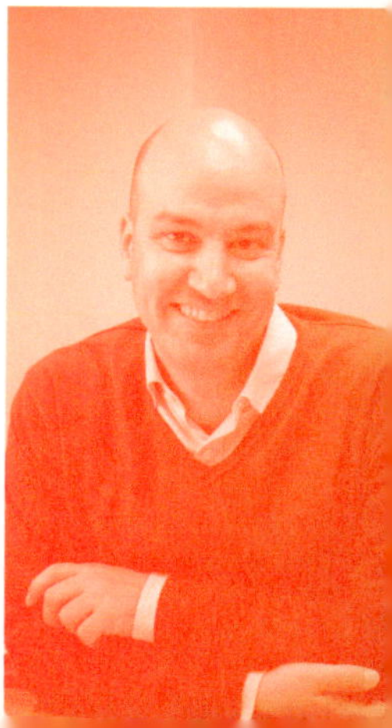
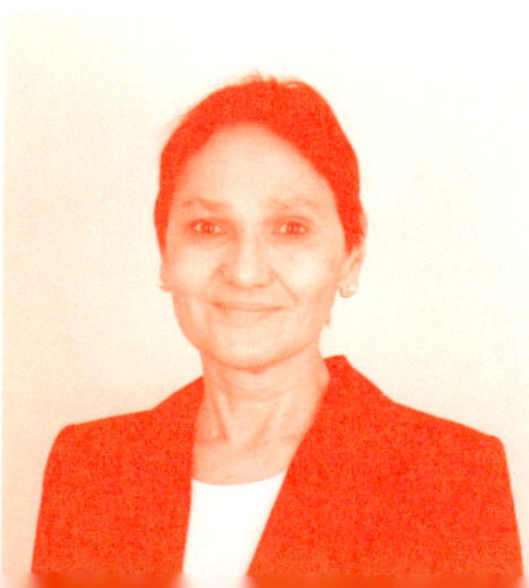

Addictions - Diagnosis and Treatment
http://dx.doi.org/10.5772/intechopen.91534
Edited by William M. Meil and John A. Mills

Contributors
Dorothy Greene, Christina L. Ruby, Zachary S. Harmon, Emily N. Welch, Victor Garcia, Alex Heckert, Emily Lambert, Katherine Fox, William M. Meil, William J. Farrell, Reem Satti, John A. Mills, Maren Krizner, Beata Gavurova, Martin Rigelsky, Viera Ivankova, Samson Duresso, C. Brendan Clark, Jacob D. Armstrong, Amy Bauman, Krystal J. Moroney, Ewa J. J. Kleczyk, Jill Bana, Rishabh Arora

First published in London, United Kingdom, 2021 by IntechOpen
IntechOpen is the global imprint of INTECHOPEN LIMITED, registered in England and Wales, registration number: 11086078, 5 Princes Gate Court, London, SW7 2QJ, United Kingdom
Printed in Croatia

British Library Cataloguing-in-Publication Data
A catalogue record for this book is available from the British Library

Additional hard and PDF copies can be obtained from orders@intechopen.com

Addictions - Diagnosis and Treatment
Edited by William M. Meil and John A. Mills
p. cm.
Print ISBN 978-1-83968-632-0
Online ISBN 978-1-83968-633-7
eBook (PDF) ISBN 978-1-83968-634-4

For EU product safety concerns:
IN TECH d.o.o., Prolaz Marije Krucifikse Kozulić 3, 51000 Rijeka, Croatia, info@intechopen.com or visit our website at intechopen.com.

Meet the editors

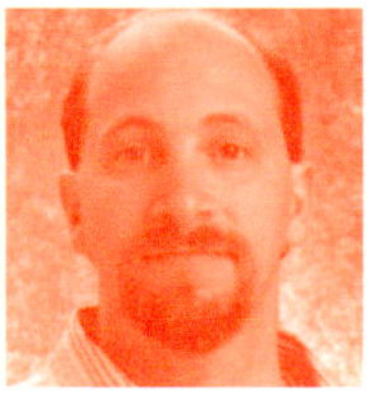

Dr. William M. Meil is a full professor in the Psychology Department, Indiana University of Pennsylvania. Previously, he was a postdoctoral fellow at The Northeastern Ohio Universities Colleges of Medicine and Pharmacy. He received an MA in Psychology from The University of Hartford, Connecticut, and a Ph.D. in Psychology from Washington State University, Pullman, Washington. His research has spanned human and laboratory animal studies investigating the neurobiological basis of substance abuse and addiction. The current focus of his research is the examination of executive function, emotion regulation, and impulsivity as predictors of addictive behavior and recovery from addiction. He is the author of many peer-reviewed journal articles and book chapters.

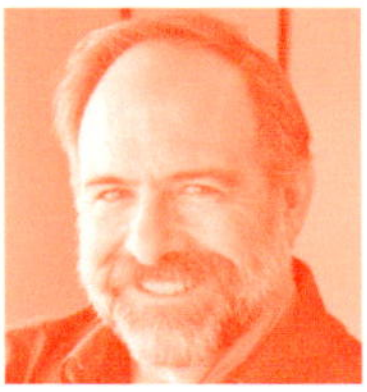

Dr. John Mills completed a BA with distinction in Psychology, an MEd in Counseling, and a Ph.D. in Counseling Psychology. He has since completed an MS in Sports Science and graduated education in music (low brass). He has worked for more than three decades as a clinician and clinician educator in both mental health and substance abuse therapeutics. He currently teaches psychology at the undergraduate and doctoral levels, and he has published and presented in a number of areas that have emphasized ethics, clinical practice, and clinical supervision. He is board-certified in counseling psychology by the American Board of Professional Psychology and is a registrant with the National Register of Health Service Psychologists.

Contents

Preface

Problems with substance use have plagued humanity for centuries. Because of the vast personal and material costs associated with these problems, society looks to public health professionals and managers of public policy for assistance. The art and science of substance abuse therapeutics have also evolved, but there is still a great need for developing our understanding of addictions and techniques to mitigate problems associated with Substance Use Disorders (SUD). As both domains (diagnosis and treatment) evolve, it remains critically important to communicate actively the findings to promote the reciprocal influence between diagnosis and intervention to augment the overall advancement of the field. In developing this book, we asked potential authors for chapters related to the diagnosis and intervention of addictions, and we had certain ideas about the topics that we might receive. As it turned out, we received many works that were unpredicted and represented high-quality contributions from a variety of viewpoints. Not only does the work include different views from the humanities but it also incorporates ideas from the cutting edge of modern science. These chapters represent biological, human, cultural, and health-based perspectives that emphasize meeting people as they really are and bringing real possibilities to the future of addiction treatment. There is an integration of the past, the present, and the likely future directions of both diagnosis and treatment. Thus, the nine chapters in this book are a tribute to the current nature of the field. From the key considerations of human diversity to the cutting-edge examination of trends across large populations, advances in the field are being realized from many perspectives. The chapters are divided into two sections, with four chapters devoted to diagnosis and five chapters that consider intervention.

The book begins with a discussion of the contributions of psychopharmacology in SUD diagnosis. This rapidly expanding area of understanding documents our evolving appreciation of how neuroplastic changes in brain anatomy and chemistry are linked with various stages of the addictive process and provides insight into the diagnosis of SUD. Chapter 2 presents a quite different perspective by examining the benefits of a grassroots religious-based intervention for problematic drinking practiced in Mexico and amongst the Mexican immigrant community in the United States. This qualitative evaluation illustrates the value of understanding how a deeply held set of beliefs within a specific culture can promote insight into the understanding and prevention of alcohol addiction.

In another look from a diverse human perspective, Chapter 3 considers sex differences and the comorbidity of addiction and depression in young adults in the Czech and Slovak Republics. This chapter serves as an important reminder that the predictive variables used to identify those at risk for developing SUD may vary by region and locale. Chapter 4 presents a new line of consideration. While once an obscure and fanciful set of ideas, artificial intelligence and machine learning represent approaches that are advancing rapidly and have demonstrated applicability. Chapter 4 illustrates how these advanced analytic procedures can be leveraged upon large data sets to understand serious health issues in our time. In particular, this chapter examines how the COVID-19 pandemic and diagnosis of SUD are related by assessing a large volume of data obtained from healthcare claims databases and state-level alcohol consumption information.

The second section of the book focuses on treatment. Chapter 5 leads by considering Alcoholics Anonymous, a long-standing approach to intervention, but in the context of modern evidence. We know about such 12-step approaches from innumerable anecdotal reports, but this modern consideration examining the foundational philosophy of the 12 steps, the key elements that support recovery, cultural considerations, empirical evidence, and suggestions for integration of this approach into clinical practice is more than overdue. Chapter 6 presents an integration of systems that commonly interact in the real world. As the law continues to provide considerable regulation of substance-related behavior, the reality of community corrections remains vital to our understanding of approaches to addiction on both system and individual levels. This chapter looks at both assessment and treatment of addictions in the community corrections model of intervention highlighting their effectiveness as well as how various forms of therapy differ in community corrections as compared to other populations.

Continuing in the consideration of multi-faceted and ecologically valid approaches, Chapter 7 adopts the biopsychosocial framework for understanding SUD and chronic pain to inform the treatment of both conditions. The efficacy of several psychotherapeutic approaches to addressing these conditions are covered as is the potential for decreasing the role of opioid analgesics for long-term pain management. Given the considerable economic pressure on any healthcare delivery system, it is important to cultivate mechanisms by which treatment can be made more effective and cost-effective. The role of supervision in promoting high-quality and cost-effective interventions for addictions cannot be underestimated. In many contexts, effective supervision is a mechanism for advancing the skills of practitioners, promoting the well-being of professionals, and increasing treatment efficacy. Chapter 8 addresses the integration of two well-established models of supervision to create a form of supervision that goes beyond business as usual by creating more nuanced and individualized supervisory experiences. Chapter 9 closes the book by profiling three innovative and controversial therapeutic approaches for SUD: the use of classic serotonergic hallucinogenic drugs (LSD and psilocybin), anti-addiction vaccines, and the use of transcranial magnetic stimulation. It reviews the theoretical basis for use, history, status of the literature supporting their use, limitations, and potential applications. It is our hope that the reader will walk away from this book understanding that advances in addiction diagnosis and treatment will come through both scientific breakthroughs and an appreciation of humanity and cultural diversity.

William M. Meil, Ph.D. and John A. Mills, Ph.D., ABPP
Professor of Psychology,
Indiana University of Pennsylvania,
Indiana, Pennsylvania, USA

Section 1

Addiction Diagnosis

Chapter 1

Psychopharmacological Perspectives and Diagnosis of Substance Use Disorder

Samson Duresso

Abstract

A considerable body of research has accumulated over several decades and altered the current understanding of substance use and its effects on the brain. This knowledge has improved the perception of the disease of addiction and has opened the door to new ways of thinking about diagnosis, prevention, and treatment of substance use disorders. The purpose of the current chapter is to briefly outline and summarize the major psychopharmacological framework underlying substance use disorder (SUD) and the factors that involve in the transformation of some people from recreational use or misuse of alcohol or drugs to SUD. The chapter explains the overall neurocircuitry theories of the addiction cycle: binge/intoxication, withdrawal/negative affect, and preoccupation/anticipation. It briefly discusses how psychoactive substances produce changes in brain functioning that facilitate the development of addiction and contribute to craving which eventually leads to relapse. The chapter also deals with similarities and differences among various classes of addictive substances in their effects on the brain and behavior and briefly describes the main risk factors that involve SUD. Finally, an attempt is made to briefly discuss the major DSM 5 based behavioral criteria that involve SUD, corresponding to the most abused substances worldwide.

Keywords: Addiction, Substance use, addiction cycle, substance use disorder, Neurocircuitry, Reward system, Neuroadaptation, Incentive-Sensitization, Incentive-Salience, DSM-5 criteria

1. Introduction

Addiction is the recurrent use of mood-altering substances, such as alcohol and other drugs, despite their adverse health and psychosocial consequences. The interplay among genetic, psychosocial, and environmental factors influences the development and manifestations of the disorder [1]. For some individuals, becoming physiologically dependent on a certain substance is likely to be a developmental process. Individuals may start with a positive attitude towards a substance, begin to practice using it, become regular users, progress to being heavy users and finally become dependent on it. While developing a positive attitude towards a certain substance, for instance, cigarettes and beginning to experiment with it, may be strongly related to exposures to smoking by other family members [2], becoming heavy smoker, on the other hand, is more strongly related to frequent exposures to peer smoking and being able to access cigarettes readily [3].

IntechOpen

Addiction, which was once viewed mainly as a moral failing or character fault, is now considered as a chronic illness of the brain characterized by clinically significant impairments in health, social function, and involuntary control over drug use [4, 5]. Although the mechanisms may be different, addiction, like most physiological disorders, is chronic, subject to relapse, and influenced by genetic, developmental, psychosocial, and environmental factors. Addictive substances exert significant influences on the brain that may affect thoughts, emotions, and behaviors. Substances of abuse have powerful effects on the brain and produce euphoria (extreme pleasure) which provokes users to seek those substances repeatedly despite the risks for significant harms.

As individuals continue to misuse alcohol or other substances, neuroadaptations occur due to progressive changes in the structure and function of the brain. Neuroadaptation compromises brain function and eventually results in the transition of an individual from controlled, occasional substance use to chronic misuse, which can be difficult to control. These brain changes may persist long after an individual stops and produce a continuous or periodic craving for the substance that can lead to relapse: More than 60 percent of people treated for a certain substance use disorder experience relapse within the first year after completion of treatment [6], and some may remain at increased risk of relapse for many years.

Much of our knowledge about the effects of substance use and misuse on the brain as well as the development of addiction comes from the study of laboratory animals. Neurobiological studies in animals have examined both the immediate effects (acute impact) of addictive substance in the brain right after ingestion and the long term or chronic impact of drug use to understand, at the most basic level, the mechanisms through which substance use alters brain structure and function and facilitates the transition from occasional use to misuse, addiction, and relapse. Although the animal models do not fully reflect the human experience, animal studies help researchers investigate addiction and related behavioral changes under highly controlled conditions that may be difficult or unethical to replicate in humans [7].

To supplement the work in animals, a growing body of substance use research has been conducted with humans. The use of brain-imaging technologies, such as magnetic resonance imaging (MRI) and positron emission tomography (PET) scans for studying the effects of alcohol and drugs on the human brain have significantly advanced the current knowledge of SUD by allowing researchers to see inside the living human brain. Using these technologies, researchers can investigate and characterize the biochemical, functional, and structural changes in the brain which result from addictive substances and find out how such changes may ultimately contribute to substance use, misuse, and addiction [8]. Animal and human studies are integrated and inform each other for a more complete picture of the neurobiology of addiction [9].

The structural and functional changes caused by using drugs can be long-lasting and can lead to harmful behaviors seen in individuals who continued to abuse drugs. Although the initial decision to try a drug of choice is mostly voluntary, eventually, as drug abuse takes over or an individual transforms from occasional user to heavy user, his/her ability to exert self-control may become seriously affected. Brain imaging studies conducted on drug-addicted individuals typically revealed that physical changes have been observed in the areas of the brain that are critical to judgment, decision making, learning, memory, and self-control. Scientists believe that these changes alter the way the brain works and may help explain the compulsive and destructive behaviors of addiction [10].

Susceptibility for addiction varies from individual to individual as for any other diseases. This depends on the amount and level of risk factors a person has. The more the risk factors the greater the chance that taking drugs will lead to abuse and addiction. No single factor determines whether a person will become addicted to drugs. The overall risk for addiction is influenced by the biological makeup of the individual including sex or ethnicity, developmental stage, and the surrounding social environment such as home, school, and the neighborhood.

Individuals with mental disorders are at greater risk of drug abuse and addiction than the general population [11]. A growing body of research reveals that SUDs and many psychiatric disorders share comparable neural mechanisms. There are several clinical resemblances and symptom overlaps between SUDs and affective disorders [12]. Epidemiological studies revealed that co-occurring substance abuse and psychiatric problems are common in clinical practice. SUDs and a variety of mental illnesses have similar changes in the dopamine-mediated reward system as well as different neurotransmitter systems such as GABA, and serotonin [10]. According to recent findings from neuroimaging research, similar abnormalities in frontal-limbic brain circuitry are implicated in SUDs and depressive disorders. Individuals with SUDs have been found to have lower frontal metabolism and anterior cingulate activation [13, 14]. Depressive symptoms are typically observed after acute and chronic drug withdrawal due to anomalies in the CRF and HPA axis, as well as alterations in catecholamines, serotonin, GABA, and glutamate systems [15]. Hence, chronic stress-induced neuroadaptations in brain stress system and reward pathways may increase the susceptibility to self-administer the substances of abuse and predispose or reveal a vulnerability to psychiatric conditions, SUDs, or both [16, 17].

The influence of home and family environment is usually most important in childhood. Children who are exposed to parental substance use early in life are more likely to develop SUD in their future life through behavioral modeling [18–20]. It is more likely that parents or older brothers or sisters who abuse alcohol or drugs can increase other children's risks of developing drug problems [21]. In addition, children with poor social skills and poor academic achievement may be at more risk of developing drug problems in school [22].

The route of administration of the substance being used is also a potential factor that may influence the progress of an individual from a regular user to a heavy user or abuse. For instance, as both smoked and injected drugs enter the brain fast and produce a powerful rush of pleasure, smoking a drug or taking it through the vein increases its addictive potential. This intense high feeling of pleasure (euphoria), however, can gradually fade away and a rebound effect of agitation or low feelings may occur. Then, these feelings develop into cravings and drive individuals to recurrent drug abuse to recapture the high pleasurable state which can worsen the risk of developing addiction [23].

The age of the onset of drug use is another potential factor that increases the likelihood of drug abuse by individuals. Although starting drugs at any age can eventually lead to addiction, early substance use is a strong indicator of problems ahead related to substance abuse and addiction [24]. Research findings have shown that people who start taking drugs at an early age are more likely to be at increased risk for adult substance dependence [25]. The part of the brain, the prefrontal cortex, which is responsible for assessing situations, making sound judgment and decisions, and keeping our emotions and desires under control is still maturing during adolescence. The fact that this critical part of an adolescent's brain is still a work-in-progress puts young people at increased risk of making poor decisions regarding trying drugs for the first time and/or continuing drug abuse thereafter. Adolescents at this stage are developing judgment and decision-making skills which may limit their ability to assess risks accurately and make sound decisions about using drugs. Therefore, introducing drugs while the brain is still developing may have profound and long-lasting results concerning drug addiction. Early use of psychoactive substances changes the structure and functions of the brain which can lead to addiction and other serious problems [26]. Thus, preventing early use of alcohol or other drugs may reduce the risk of progressing to later abuse and addiction.

Interindividual differences in addiction risk are mostly determined by genetic variation. The impact of genetic variation on total addiction risk has been estimated to be 50% in studies focusing on variability across identical and nonidentical siblings [27]. The largest study to date on 1.2 million people that looked at common genes in alcohol and nicotine use identified genes involved in dopaminergic and glutamatergic neurotransmission, transcription and translation, and brain development [28]. They also revealed that a crucial genetic component of SUDs appears to impact a vulnerability to disorders with pathological symptoms via a general-purpose underlying mechanism.

Besides these common genetic characteristics, genetic variants that are mainly unique in a particular drug have been found. The most well-known genetic variants are those that code for the alcohol dehydrogenase (ADH) and aldehyde dehydrogenase (ALDH) enzymes, which cause poor alcohol metabolism and protect against alcoholism [28]. Like other complex biobehavioral disorders, addiction is a polygenic disease involving multiple genes and genetic networks [29, 30]. Genetic research has aided our understanding of addiction-related neurobiological processes. Addiction-related gene variations can increase the risk of drug misuse and addiction by altering neurotransmitter systems, drug metabolic pathways, and brain circuitry. For example, genetic polymorphisms in the nicotinic acetylcholine receptor subunits expressed in the medial habenula are linked to development of withdrawal symptoms [31] and are at least partially accountable for the genetic predisposition or vulnerability to tobacco addiction [32, 33]. This has demonstrated that the habenula is involved not just in nicotine addiction, but also in the unpleasant emotional states associated with the long-term use of numerous drugs of abuse [29], such as alcohol [30] and opioids [34].

Epigenetic factors are a diverse set of transcriptional tuning processes that generate and sustain gene expression–mediated physiological outcomes in response to environmental inputs [13]. Plasticity is at work in the transition to compulsive drug use, changing the physiology of the brain to produce addictive states. Physiologically, the rewiring of brain reward circuitries, particularly dopamine neurons in the ventral tegmental area (VTA), is thought to cause vulnerability to relapse after periods of attempted abstinence from drugs of abuse such as cocaine use. The same enzyme that attaches serotonin to Histone 3 can also catalyze the attachment of dopamine to H3 — a process, known as dopaminylation, which may control drug-seeking behavior [35]. Cocaine-induced transcriptional plasticity in the midbrain is mediated by histone H3 glutamine 5 dopaminylation (H3Q5dop). As a result, long-term cocaine use alters neuronal circuits in the brain's reward system, necessitating a consistent intake of the drug for the circuits to function normally. To make the proteins for those changes, certain genes must be turned on and off, and this is an epigenetic mechanism activated by dopamine acting on H3, not a change in DNA sequence. Epigenetic mechanisms provide a convergent regulatory framework within which the plasticity required to produce an addicted state can emerge and then remain long after drug use has stopped [36, 37].

2. The addiction cycle

There are many theories and models of addiction. While some of the theories and models present their theoretical approaches at an individual level, some explain the addictive behavior in terms of population or group interaction and influence. It is also important to note that many theories of addiction are complex and have evolved over time and therefore may overlap across one or more explanatory domains or perspectives.

The learning theory of addiction is relatively a broad category that emphasizes the importance of associations among cues, responses, and positive (pleasant) or negative (noxious) reinforcers. Among the specific models and theories under this category are operant learning, classical conditioning, and drug withdrawal theory [38, 39]. Moreover, the incentive sensitization theory of addiction also incorporates aspects of learning theory as it proposes that repeated exposure to drugs and drug-associated cues capitalizes on neuroplastic changes in mesocorticolimbic circuits and classical conditioning to make drugs and drug paired stimuli more motivationally salient [40, 41] .

The drive theories of addiction explain that addiction involves the development of powerful drives reinforced by homeostatic mechanisms. The drive theory is part of the disease model of addiction [42] and states that addiction is the result of pathological changes in the brain that produces overpowering urges. These changes that result in impairments may involve a structural or functional abnormality in the CNS [42]. Among the goal-focused theories of addiction are positive reward theories, acquired need theories, pre-existing need theories, and identity theories. These theories mainly explain addiction in terms of an individual's behavior that satisfies one's physiological or psychological needs, pleasure, and aspects of self-identity [43–47].

Other theories such as cognitive control theory [48], executive dysfunction theory [49–51], self-regulation theory [52], self-determination theory [53, 54], and implementation intentions theory [55, 56], describe addiction as a failure of individual's strategies, ability or skills to self-control or to counteract impulses and motives underlying the addictive behavior. The biological theories describe that addiction involves specific neural circuitry or mechanisms [57–62] and is primarily a brain disease' characterized by dysfunction of neural pathways such as those that subserve executive function. The Reflective Choice Theories focus on the individual's decisions, preferences, and actions that are made based on reasons and analysis. Therefore, according to these theories, addiction is a rational choice made by individuals in favor of the benefits of the addictive behavior over the costs. The Inhibition dysfunction theories suggest that addiction is an ongoing dysregulation of the ability to inhibit a rewarded behavior due to impairment of impulse controlling mechanisms [63]. In other words, addiction involves impairment of the inhibitory system of the brain regions related to features of response selection, inhibition, and motivation of compulsive behaviors associated with drugs. The hedonic homeostatic dysregulation theory also states that addiction is a cycle of escalating dysregulation of the brain reward systems that gradually increases and facilitates the act of compulsive drug use and a loss of control over drug-taking behavior, which are the basic concepts that underlie the addiction cycle [64].

Drug addiction is a disorder that is chronically relapsing and manifested in terms of compulsive behavior to seek and consume the drug, significant loss of ability to control and limit drug intake, and the emergence of negative and distressful emotional states such as irritability, anxiety, and dysphoria. Drug addiction is conceptualized as a three-stage cyclic disorder that consists of impulsivity and compulsivity and involves neuroplastic changes in the brain reward, stress, and executive functions [64, 65]. Impulsivity often dominates the early stages of the cycle and compulsivity dominates the terminal stages. The three stages are considered to interact with each other, become more intense, and eventually lead to the pathological state known as addiction.

Drug addiction is an excessive drug-taking behavior in which individuals compulsively seek and take drugs and lose their ability to control in limiting their drug intake. One of the multiple motivational mechanisms that drive such behavior is the development of a negative emotional state when access to the drug is prevented or discontinued, which results in dysregulation of hedonic homeostasis [64]. At the neurobiological level, two neuroadaptive models, sensitization and counter-adaptation, have been hypothesized to contribute to the changes in motivation for drug-seeking and compulsive use (hedonic homeostatic dysregulation) and the neurobiological mechanisms, such as the mesolimbic dopamine system, opioid peptidergic systems, and brain and hormonal stress systems [64]. While sensitization has been conceptualized to be a shift in an incentive-salience state since it involves a progressive rise in the effect of a certain drug due to its frequent administration (21), counteradaptation hypotheses (20), on the contrary, were closely related to hedonic tolerance and involve the reduction of dopaminergic and serotonergic neurotransmission in the nucleus accumbens during drug withdrawal (22). Critical neurobiological sites with specific neurotransmitters and hormones have been identified that may regulate the hedonic dysregulation and provide the substrates that convey both vulnerabilities to, and protection against drug addiction. Dysregulation of key neurochemical elements in both reward and stress systems, such as decreases in dopamine and opioid peptide functions in the ventral striatum and recruitment of brain stress systems known as corticotropin-releasing factor (CRF) in the extended amygdala is hypothesized to produce the negative emotional state that initiates a condition of negative reinforcement [66]. An individual who uses a drug impulsively starts using it compulsively when a shift has occurred from positive reinforcement driving the motivated behavior to negative reinforcement driving the motivated behavior. Impulsivity and compulsivity often coexist in the different stages of the addiction cycle. This occurrence reflects the role of dysregulated reward and stress systems in the negative emotional states associated with the withdrawal/negative affect and preoccupation/anticipation stages of the addiction cycle that drive drug-seeking behavior [67].

The addiction cycle becomes more severe and well-established as a person continues substance use and as it produces dramatic changes in the functioning of certain brain areas that reduce the person's ability to control his or her substance abuse. Three neurobiological circuits have been recognized to have empirical value for the study of the neurobiological changes associated with the development and persistence of drug addiction linked to the three-stage cycle (**Figure 1**). The key elements of the ventral tegmental area and ventral striatum are the focal points for the binge/intoxication stage and mediate the acute reinforcing effects of drugs of abuse. Acute withdrawal symptoms such as increased anxiety and dysphoria are associated with the second stage, the withdrawal/ negative affect stage, and are most likely the results of disruption in the function of the extended amygdala reward system and the recruitment of the brain stress neurocircuitry [68]. The preoccupation/ anticipation (craving) stage is a widely distributed network and involves the stress-induced processes at the central brain stress systems in the basolateral amygdala, the orbitofrontal cortex–dorsal striatum, prefrontal cortex, and the hippocampus. The prefrontal cortex is mainly responsible for executive functions like organizing thoughts and activities, prioritizing tasks, managing time, and making important decisions, including limiting substance consumption [65].

This three-stage model of addiction is largely attributed to the extensive works of George Koob [69] and his colleagues and is supported by several animal and human research findings which provide useful means to understand the aspects and symptoms of addiction and design prevention, intervention, and treatment strategies [70]. It is worth noting that the three stages of addiction being discussed do not have absolute temporal distinctions that some components of addiction such as craving, conditioned cued craving, incentive-salience related craving, craving linked to

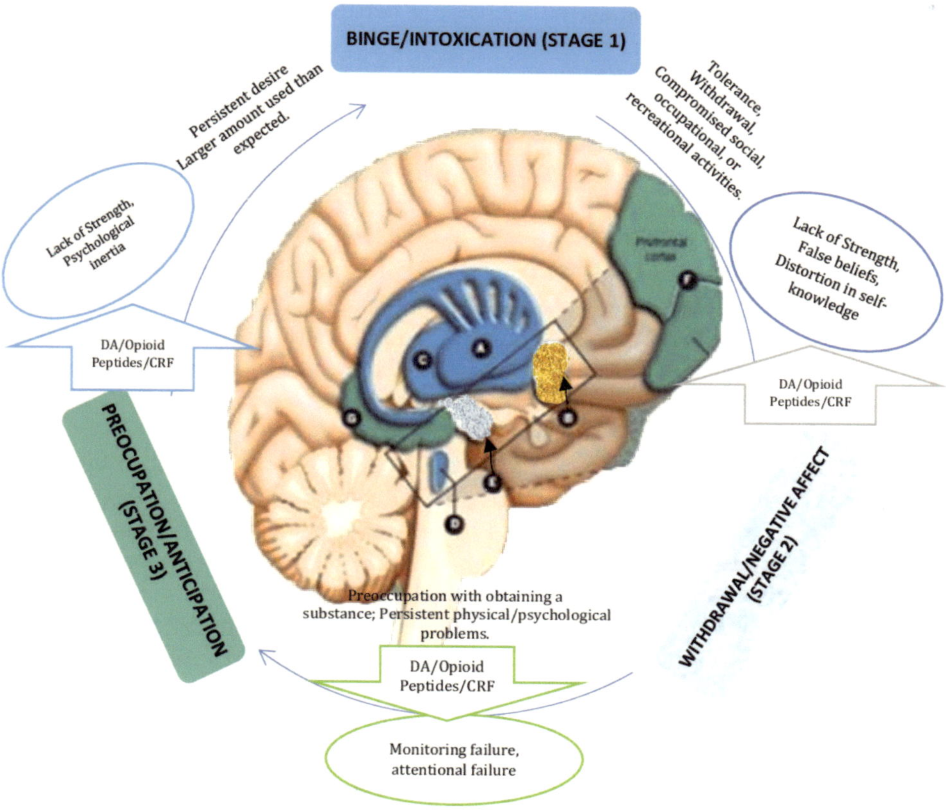

Figure 1.
A diagram depicting the spiralling distress – addiction cycle from social psychological and neurobiological viewpoints. NB. Stage 1: The reward circuit is overstimulated, resulting in a lack of control and bingeing. (A) Basal Ganglia refers to interconnected regions that are linked to learning, reward, and habit formation. (B) Nucleus accumbens (NAs) receives dopamine from Ventral Tegmental area, helps to control desire, satiation, and inhibition. (C) Thalamus is a centre that transmits sensory information and regulates arousal. (D) Ventral tegmental area: Dopamine is generated in this major structure near the top of the brain stem. Stage 2: After long-term exposure to addictive substances, the number of dopamine receptors in the nucleus accumbens decreases (B), requiring more of the addictive substance or action to feel the same. (B) The nucleus accumbens (NAs) is heavily implicated in the first and second stages of the addiction cycle. (E) The amygdala is linked to memory and emotions, particularly anxiety and dread. Stage 3: People who are addicted have a compulsive need to engage in the addictive behaviour again. The frontal cortex is thought to be affected by drug abuse. (F) The frontal cortex is in charge of ideas and actions. The orbitofrontal cortex is hypothesised to be involved in behaviour control. (G). Hippocampus: consolidated of memory. The three-stage addiction cycle incorporates some of the factors of possible self-regulation failure, such as under regulation and mis regulation, as well as the multiple DSM-5 criteria for substance dependence. The arrows depict the possible roles of several neurochemical and endocrine systems in the addiction cycle. Increased functional activity of DA, dopamine, Opioid Peptide, and CRF, corticotropin-releasing factor, is indicated by the arrows. It's worth mentioning that the addiction cycle is depicted as a circular pattern that rises in amplitude with repeated exposure, eventually leading to addiction as a pathological condition.

withdrawal, etc. appear at many places in the addictive process and that the impacts of these aspects of craving and their neural basis remain to be further elucidated.

2.1 Stage 1: binge/intoxication

In most cases, addiction is started by abusing substances that have hedonic properties. Many factors contribute to the transition from drug use to drug addiction, including availability (route of administration), genetics [71], prior drug use history, stress, and life events [72] . Initial; experimentation of drug abuse may be the result of peer pressure due to the rewarding effects of conforming to the peer group. In some cases, the first use of a substance may be related to its therapeutic properties, such as opiate analgesics for the treatment of pain or stimulants such as amphetamine for the treatment of attention-deficit hyperactivity disorder [73].

In humans, the majority of drug users do not develop into drug abusers or drug addicts [74]. Similarly, even with intravenous drug administration in limited-access situations, stable drug intake can be observed in animals without pronounced signs of dependence. The current challenge is to discover the contribution of neurobiological factors to individual differences in drug addiction vulnerability [64]. It is broadly accepted that the key elements of the reinforcing effects of drugs of abuse involve their ability to activate large amounts of extracellular dopamine in limbic regions and the nucleus accumbens. Brain imaging studies in humans revealed that drug-induced increases in dopamine in the ventral striatum, where the nucleus accumbens is located, are significantly linked to subjective correlates of reward such as pleasure, high, and euphoria [27, 75].

The nucleus accumbens (NAs) and the dorsal striatum (DS) are the two sub-regions in the basal ganglia which are particularly important in substance use disorders. While the NAs is involved in motivation and the experience of reward the DS is responsible for forming habits and other routine behaviors [76]. The NAs is located strategically to collect important limbic information from the amygdala, frontal cortex, and hippocampus that could be transformed into motivated behavior (the acute reinforcing effects of drugs) through its connections with the extrapyramidal motor system [70]. It is the primary site mediating reward behavior and thought to directly involve in reinforcing addictive behaviors in response to drug use. It is hypothesized that the initial action of drug reward depends on dopamine release in the nucleus accumbens for cocaine, amphetamine, and nicotine; activation of the opioid peptide receptor in the VTA (dopamine activation) and nucleus accumbens (independent of dopamine activation) for opiates; and activation of the GABAA systems in the nucleus accumbens and amygdala for alcohol [70].

The dopaminergic projection from the VTA to the nucleus accumbens is known as the mesolimbic dopamine system (the mesolimbic pathway) and is strongly associated with the dependence-producing potential of addictive substances [77]. Many drugs of abuse directly or indirectly exert their powerful effects on this pathway and contribute to the development of dependence by signaling to the brain that addictive substances are especially important from a motivational perspective. The direct activation of dopamine, serotonin, opioid peptides, and GABA systems in the basal forebrain facilitates the acute reinforcing effects of drugs of abuse [74]. There are several supporting pieces of evidence for the hypothesis that addictive drugs dramatically activate the mesolimbic dopamine system and the serotonin systems, specifically, those involving 5-hydroxytryptamine-1B (5-HT1B) receptor activation in the nucleus accumbens, during limited-access self-administration [78, 79]. Several studies have shown that most addictive drugs including cocaine, amphetamine, and nicotine [79], either directly or indirectly, activate neurons that release dopamine. They produce their rewarding effects by stimulating the nucleus accumbens through the activation of the brain's dopamine and opioid signaling system. Brain imaging studies in humans who use alcohol, nicotine, and other substance have shown activation of dopamine and opioid neurotransmitters during use [80, 81]. In the same manner, the primary psychoactive component of marijuana, tetrahydrocannabinol (THC), targets the brain's endogenetic cannabinoid system and affects the reward system by influencing the function of dopamine neurons and the release of dopamine in the nucleus accumbens [30, 31].

Another key component of the binge/intoxication stage involves a second sub-region of the basal ganglia, the dorsal striatum. This part of the brain is mainly related to habit formation [82]. With repeated drug use, the release of dopamine, glutamate (an excitatory neurotransmitter), and activation of brain opioid systems trigger changes in the dorsal striatum and strengthens substance-seeking and substance-taking habits. Studies on humans showed that the rise of DA level in the dorsal striatum was significantly correlated with the increase of craving for cocaine, [83, 84]. Likewise, pharmacological blockade of the dorsolateral striatum after forced abstinence resulted in the reduction of drug-seeking behavior in rats [85–87].

As addiction progresses compulsive drug use results and neuroadaptive changes in the structure and function of the brain occur. Neuroadaptations involve changes in the reward circuitry systems that promote compulsive drug use through sensitization and counteradaptation, by increasing a drug's positive and negative reinforcing effects, respectively [82]. Sensitization arises from repeated administration of addictive drugs and is mediated by the mesolimbic dopamine system [84]. It is an increased response to a drug effect which represents a with-in system mechanism of neuroadaptation [82]. Animal studies posit that direct injections of opiates or amphetamine into the ventral tegmental area which alter the function of the dopamine neurons ultimately produce sensitization to later injections of these drugs in the periphery [83]. However, like tolerance, sensitization may develop to a certain drug effect but not to another [82]. The second system that plays an important role in sensitization, representing a between-systems mechanism of neuroadaptation, is the CRF (corticotropin-releasing factor) mediated stress-response system [82]. The CRF is a hormone released by the hypothalamus and the amygdala in response to certain stressors. The CRF, in turn, stimulates the release of additional stress hormones into the bloodstream activating a stress response system called the hypothalamic–pituitary–adrenal (HPA) axis. Exposure to a variety of stressors implicates the CRF mediated stress-response system which promotes sensitization to the drug [82]. The role of sensitization in drug dependence is mainly linked to a motivational state described as "wanting" which progressively increases due to repeated exposure to drugs of abuse [85]. As "wanting" increases across repeated exposures to alcohol and drugs of abuse, the likelihood of relapse following periods of abstinence may increase, eventually leading to compulsive drug use [82].

Drug-associated stimuli raise dopamine levels in the dorsal striatum as addiction grows, leading to drug craving and reinforcing the habit of drug use [82]. In the new DSM-5 classification, drug craving as a motivational state for drug-seeking behavior is finally recognized as one of the main features of substance use disorders [88]. Cue reactivity and cue-elicited craving are both influenced by the process of "Positive Reinforcement," which involves learning to associate salient cues with drug-use rewards [89]. Drug craving is a complex neurocognitive emotional–motivational reaction to a variety of stimuli, ranging from internal to external settings, and from drug-related to stressful or affective experiences.

Substance craving, or "wanting" for a drug, is a common element in clinical definitions of addiction, and it appears to play a role in the maintenance of addictive behaviors [90]. According to Robinson and Berridge, sensitization processes which arise from neuroadaptations in brain reward pathways as a result of prolonged drug misuse are responsible for addicted animals' excessive "wanting" or drug-seeking behavior [91]. They propose that these neuroadaptations result in a rise in the motivational salience of drugs so that exposure to drugs and drug-associated cues causes excessive "wanting" or seeking, increasing the risk of relapse [92, 93]. Furthermore, environmental stimuli previously associated with drug use or internal cues such as stress responses, negative affect, and withdrawal-related states associated with drug abuse can function as conditioned stimuli capable of eliciting craving on their own [94, 95]. External drug-related stimuli, such as persons and places associated with drug use, or drug paraphernalia such as needles, drug pipes, cocaine powder, or beer cans, as well as in vivo drug exposure, can increase drug craving and physiological reactivity [96].

In summary, in the nucleus accumbens of the basal ganglia, the "reward circuitry" along with dopamine and naturally occurring opioids play a vital role in the rewarding effects of alcohol and other substances. Furthermore, as the addiction progresses, stimuli or cues associated with that substance use can cause craving, substance seeking, and use. Chronic alcohol or substance use and frequent activation of the "habit circuitry" or the dorsal striatum of the basal ganglia significantly contributes to the compulsive substance seeking and taking that potentially lead to SUD. The involvement of the reward and habit neurocircuits play key roles in substance craving and compulsive substance seeking when addicted individuals are exposed to alcohol and/or other drug cues in their surroundings.

2.2 Stage 2: withdrawal/negative affect

This stage is related to a neurocircuitry pathway known as the extended amygdala and its connections including the major components of the brain stress systems associated with the negative reinforcement [84]. This pathway is composed of the central amygdala (CeA), the bed nucleus of the stria terminalis (BNST), and the NAc shell. When DA is released, it intensively activates a number of areas that belong to the lateral subdivision of the extended amygdala such as the bed nucleus of stria terminalis, BSTM, and central amygdala) [97]. The extended amygdala also integrates brain arousal–stress systems with hedonic processing systems to produce unpleasant emotional states that promote negative reinforcement mechanisms linked to the development of addiction [98]. For example, hyperactivation of amygdala has been observed in individuals with SUDs, associated with cue-induced drug craving [99].

Two primary sources of reinforcement (positive and negative reinforcement) have been implicated to play significant roles in this allostatic process. Dysregulation of specific neurochemical mechanisms in the brain reward circuits (opioid peptides, γ-aminobutyric acid, glutamate and dopamine) and recruitment of brain stress systems (CRF), which are localized in the extended amygdala, are the reinforcing factors that provide the negative motivational state in the process of addiction [16, 100]. These allostatic changes in the reward and stress systems are assumed to maintain hedonic stability and as such contribute to the vulnerability for development of dependence and relapse in addiction [101].

An important component of this stage is the within-system neuroadaptations to chronic drug exposure which is characterized by a reduction in the function of the neurotransmitter systems in the neurocircuits implicated in the acute reinforcing effects of a drug of abuse [102]. One popular theory is that dopamine systems are negatively affected during key stages of the addiction cycle, such as withdrawal, resulting in decreased motivation for non-drug-related stimuli and increased sensitivity to the abused drug [103, 104]. In animal studies, acute drug withdrawal from all major drugs of abuse results in decreased activity of the mesolimbic dopamine system and decreased serotonergic neurotransmission in the nucleus accumbens [105]. Symptoms of withdrawal may occur with all addictive substances, but with varying intensity and duration depending on both the type of substance and the frequency and severity of use. Brain imaging studies have consistently revealed a long-lasting reduction of a particular type of dopamine receptor (the D2 receptor) in substance-addicted individuals compared to their counterparts. The same dose of stimulant causes a smaller release of dopamine in addicted persons than in non-addicted persons [83]. In addition, decreases in the activity of the dopamine system have also been observed during withdrawal from stimulants such as opioids, nicotine, and alcohol [106].

Acute withdrawal mechanisms are likely to be drug-specific and reflect changes in the biological targets of these drugs. For example, during the first few days of cocaine withdrawal, the brain becomes more sensitive to the effects of GABA-enhancing drugs, which may reflect the down regulation of this neurotransmitter in chronic cocaine users [107]. Brain imaging studies have shown decreased levels of endogenous opioids during cocaine withdrawal, which could explain the irritability, tiredness, and dysphoria experienced during the motivational phase of withdrawal [108]. Similarly, Imaging studies have documented hypofunction in dopamine pathways during protracted withdrawal, as evidenced by decreases in D2 receptor expression and decrease in dopamine release, which may contribute to the anhedonia (i.e., decreased sensitivity to rewarding stimuli) and motivation reported by drug-addicted subjects during protract withdrawal [109].

Typical neurochemical changes in these structures include not only reductions in reward system functioning, a within-system opponent processes, but also recruitment of the brain stress systems intermediated by corticotropin-releasing factor (CRF) and dynorphin- k opioid systems in the ventral striatum, extended amygdala, and frontal cortex known as a between-system opponent processes [80]. A between-system neuroadaptation is the second component of the withdrawal/negative affect stage. This process involves the activation of stress neurotransmitters such as corticotropin-releasing factor (CRF), norepinephrine, and dynorphin in the extended amygdala [85]. Regardless of the presence of the drug, the neurochemical systems involved in stress modulation may be triggered within the neurocircuitry of the brain's stress systems to overcome the persistent effects of the distressing substance and restore normal function [110]. These neurotransmitters play a role in the development of negative feelings associated with withdrawal which leads to stress-triggered substance use. Chronic khat chewers attempting to quit chewing, for example, exhibited withdrawal symptoms that followed similar overall patterns, with notable elevations after the quit day. Most of the khat users relapsed within 11 days and very few maintained abstinences [111]. Negative affects including depression, nervousness, tiredness, restlessness, poor motivation, irritability, as well as craving substantially increased and reached their peak on the first week of khat cessation and remained higher there after indicating the persistence and severity of these symptoms over time [112].

The aforementioned phenomena have been well demonstrated both in animal and human studies [113]. Administration of antagonists for neurotransmitters significantly reduced substance intake in response to withdrawal and stress. Similarly stopping the activation of stress receptors in the brain lowered alcohol consumption in both alcohol-dependent rats and humans with alcohol use disorder [86, 87]. Hence, the desire to remove the negative feelings associated with withdrawal can be a strong driving force to continuous consumption of the substance since the taking of the substance at least momentarily relieves the negative feelings caused by the withdrawal. This process is, however, a vicious cycle as taking substances to reduce withdrawal symptoms during the period of abstinence makes it even more difficult to maintain abstaining the next time a person tries to quit the drug of abuse [56].

In summary, this stage of addiction involves a reduction in the function of the brain reward systems involving dopamine receptors and the activation of brain stress hormones and neuropeptide (CRF, dynorphin, and norepinephrine) in the extended amygdala. The combination of these events significantly contributes to providing a powerful neurochemical basis that produces a negative emotional state associated with drug abstinence or withdrawal. Increases in drug desire and physiological reactivity have also been linked to negative affect, stress, or withdrawal-related suffering [114–117]. The strong desire to relieve these adverse feelings, in turn, drives additional sources of negative reinforcement in compulsive substance taking or drug addiction.

2.3 Stage 3: preoccupation/anticipation

The preoccupation/anticipation (craving) stage mainly involves the Prefrontal Cortex, the region that controls executive functions like organizing thoughts and activities, task prioritization, time management, decision making, and regulation of one's actions, emotions, and impulses. Executive function is necessary for a person to make suitable choices about whether or not to submit to strong urges that may compel individuals to use substances, specifically, when the person encounters triggers and cues such as stimuli associated with that substance or stressful circumstances.

The preoccupation/anticipation stage, which is characterized by an increase in drug craving, is triggered by increased sensitivity to conditioned cues. An individual is driven to seek drugs of abuse again after a period of abstinence. Stress promotes relapse to drug-taking behaviors by activating brain circuits involved in reward processing as well as attentional and memory preferences for drug use cues [17, 118]. Chronic relapse is widely acknowledged as the most challenging obstacle in the fight against drug addiction. Long after encountering acute withdrawal symptoms, users are likely to return to compulsive drug use [119]. Chronic drug misuse is believed to cause a gradual restructuring of reward and memory circuits, which is thought to be critical to the mounting of these reactions. In clinical studies, both dopamine and glutamate have been identified as contributing to the neural alterations associated with conditioned responses [120].

The Incentive-Sensitization Theory of Addiction explains that drug-induced sensitization in the brain's mesocorticolimbic circuits, which assign incentive salience to reward-associated events, is the primary cause of addiction [41]. Incentive salience or "wanting," is generated by neural systems that comprise the mesolimbic dopamine. The role of this neural system is to attribute incentive salience or motivational importance to stimuli resulting their being viewed as highly salient, attractive, and "wanted" [40, 121]. Addictive drug administration, both continuous and occasional, causes incremental neuroadaptations in this neuronal system. Associative control of this sensitized neural system causes significantly increased incentive salience to be ascribed to the act of drug taking and stimuli related to drug-taking. This process is believed to occur due to hyperactivation of the dopamine system resulting in drugs and drug associated cues becoming pathologically more "wanted" by the drug user. Irrespective of other motivating variables such as the expectation of drug pleasure or the unpleasant aspects of withdrawal, sensitization of the neural system responsible for incentive salience can motivate addictive behavior such as compulsive drug seeking and drug-taking. The concomitant targeting of sensitized incentive salience to drug-related cues results in the recurrence of addictive behavior in the face of multiple barriers, including the loss of one's reputation, job, home, and family. This shows that drug addiction is motivated by a strong desire for drugs, often labeled as drug craving [122].

The Incentive-Sensitization Theory of Addiction offers a novel neuropsychological explanation for drug addiction. Due to dopamine system sensitization, drug craving is the subjective sensation that comes with the attribution of excessive amounts of incentive salience to drug-related stimuli or their mental images. This system causes pathological incentive motivation "wanting" for drugs that differ from both the unpleasant symptoms of withdrawal and drug pleasure. Although exposure to drug-related stimuli increased self-reported craving, as well as drug-opposite and drug-like effects, the cumulative effects of positive outcome expectancies, cue-specific dysphoria, and cue-specific drug-positive reactions were able to predict 28 percent of the variance in cue-specific craving in a simple additive model [40, 123].

The changes that are taking place in the brain's reward and emotional circuits are followed by changes in the function of the cortical prefrontal cortex involved in the executive processes. Down-regulation of dopamine signals, which obscures the sensitivity of the reward circuits to pleasure, also occurs in the pre-frontal cortex and linked circuits, seriously affecting executive processes including the self-regulation, decision-making, flexibility in action selection, and initiation or assignment of salience (assignment of relativity) [124]. Neuroplastic changes in glutamatergic signals further disrupt the modulation of the reward and emotional circuits of the prefrontal regions. In people with drug addiction, the impaired signaling of dopamine and glutamate in prefrontal brain regions diminishes their ability to withstand strong urges or take strong decisions to stop taking the drug of abuse. These effects explain why people with addiction can be sincere in their desire and intention to stop using a substance while being impulsive and unable to follow through on their determination. Thus, changed signaling in prefrontal regulatory circuits, along with changes in rewards and emotional response circuits, causes an imbalance which is responsible for both progressive development of compulsive behavior in addictive diseases state and the related failure of individuals with addiction to voluntarily reduce the behavior [125].

Some scientists separate the functions of the prefrontal cortex into two opposing systems to better understand how this brain region is engaged in addiction: a "Go system" and a "Stop system" [80]. The Go system assists people in making decisions on topics that need a lot of thought and planning, as well as engaging in behaviors that are necessary for achieving life goals. When substance-seeking behavior is triggered by substance-related environmental cues (incentive salience), the Go circuits of the prefrontal cortex show significant increases in activity. As a result, the nucleus accumbens is stimulated to release glutamate, the brain's principal excitatory neurotransmitter [126]. In addition, the neurons in the Go circuits of the prefrontal cortex stimulate the habit systems of the dorsal striatum through connections that use glutamate and contribute to the impulsivity associated with substance-seeking behavior of a person [127].

Conversely, the Stop system primarily hinders the activity of the Go system [126]. The nucleus accumbens and habit responses driven by the dorsal striatum, that are areas of the basal ganglia implicated in the binge/intoxication stage of addiction, are controlled by Stop system. This system, according to researchers, helps to reduce incentive salience, or the ability of substance-related stimuli to trigger a relapse. The Stop system also plays an important role in relapse triggered by stressful life events or circumstances by exerting control on the brain's stress and emotional systems [126]. As explained above, the brain's stress and emotional systems involve the activation of stress hormones and neurotransmitters (CRF, dynorphin, and norepinephrine) in the extended amygdala caused by prolonged abstinence during the withdrawal/negative affect stage of addiction [109].

Imaging studies using laboratory animals revealed that lower activity in the Stop system of the prefrontal cortex is associated with increased activity of stress circuitry involving the extended amygdala, which increased substance-taking behavior and relapse [109]. Similar studies in humans with addiction show dysfunction of both the Go and Stop circuits [65, 109]. For example, people with alcohol, cocaine, or opioid use disorders exhibit significant deficiencies in executive functions such as impairments in the maintenance of spatial information, disruption of decision-making and behavioral inhibition. These executive function deficits are equivalent to the changes in the prefrontal cortex which suggest decreased activity in the Stop system and greater reactivity of the Go system in response to substance-related stimuli. Moreover, research findings suggest that humans with post-traumatic stress disorder (PTSD), a syndrome that is usually accompanied by drug and alcohol use problems, have decreased prefrontal cortex control over the extended amygdala [75]. These findings add to the growing body of evidence supporting the importance of the prefrontal cortex-extended amygdala circuit in stress-induced relapse and imply that strengthening prefrontal cortex circuits may be crucial for the intervention and treatment of substance use disorders. The preoccupation/anticipation stage of the addiction cycle is characterized by a disruption of executive function caused by a compromised prefrontal cortex [128]. It is a key element of relapse in humans and the basis for defining addiction as a chronic relapsing disorder. While the over-activation of the Go system in the prefrontal cortex is related to habit-like substance seeking, the under-activation of the Stop system in the prefrontal cortex stimulates impulsive and compulsive substance seeking.

Overall, the study of neurobiological changes has identified three neurobiological circuits with heuristic value concerning the development and persistence of SUD. The three stages which involve different brain regions, neuro-circuits, and neurochemicals are interrelated to bring about specific kinds of changes in the brain. Activities in the nucleus accumbens-amygdala reward system, ventral tegmental dopamine input, and local opioid peptide and GABAergic circuits are among the acute reinforcing of drugs involved in the binge/intoxication stage addiction cycle. In contrast, acute withdrawal symptoms that are critical for addiction, such as dysphoria and heightened anxiety, are thought to be caused by reduced function of the extended amygdala reward system and activation of brain stress neurocircuitry during the withdrawal/negative affect stage [78]. The preoccupation/anticipation (or craving) stage of addiction is characterized by the considerable increase of activities in the Go systems of the prefrontal cortex as incentive salience initiates substance seeking behavior. This results in major afferent projections to the nucleus accumbens and extended amygdala, in particular, the prefrontal cortex (for drug-induced reinstatement) and basolateral amygdala (for cue-induced reinstatement). Increased activities in this circuit further boost incentive salience and produces strong desire to use the substance in the presence of drug-related stimuli. The dorsal striatum's habit-response mechanisms are also activated by the Go system, which contributes to the impulsivity associated with substance seeking [126]. It's considered that the shift from ventral striatal-ventral pallidal-thalamic-cortical loops to dorsal striatal-pallidal-thalamic-cortical loops is implicated in compulsive drug-seeking behaviour [129].

Molecular neuroadaptations start with the stage of binge/intoxication and as substance abuse progresses, transitions through the addiction cycle may bring about changes in long-term transcription which may convey a risk of relapse. A person may go through this cycle for weeks or months or progress through it several times in a day due to several factors including the type, amount, and frequency of substances used. There may also be a difference in how a person progresses through the cycle and the intensity with which he/she experiences each of the stages. In addition to this, it is to be noted that there are not absolute functional nor temporal boundaries that can be drawn between the stages in the process of addiction and therefore as the withdrawal/negative affect aspects of addiction develop those effects from stage 1 persist (though reward may be attenuated) and those in stage 3 begin to emerge. Moreover, deficits in executive function are potential risk factors for developing addiction.

3. DSM-5 substance use disorder

Drug abuse, substance-related problems, and substance use disorders (SUDs) have all been viewed in different ways throughout history and cultures. How drug use and SUDs are conceptualized and how symptoms manifest and are interpreted are all influenced by culture. Sociocultural beliefs can influence how people approach and behave when it comes to substance use and misuse. Individuals' assumptions regarding potential drug-related problems are shaped in large part by their culture [130]. While in some cultures alcohol use was heavily controlled and was allowed only for ceremonial purposes [131], acculturation, on the other hand, has made significant contribution to accelerated abuse of alcohol and use of illegal drugs among certain groups of people [132, 133].

Although the characterization of substance problem syndromes as medical diseases or disorders has a long history, drug abuse and inebriety were historically regarded from a moralistic perspective [134]. Attempts to define and refine diagnostic criteria for SUDs began in the mid-twentieth century and are still ongoing. Research has identified some limitations in the existing diagnostic criteria for SUDs, which can help with the conception of future classification systems [135].

According to modern theories of substance dependence, chronic substance use can cause neuroadaptations in brain systems involved in reward, motivation, emotional regulation, inhibitory control, and tolerance/withdrawal, all of which can lead to compulsive drug use behavior [136]. Illicit drug usage has been documented all over the world with the highest estimates in Europe, North America, and Australasia. Regular use, "problem drug use," and drug addiction are less commonly measured, although they are critical to quantify in order to determine disease burden and risk factors for illicit drug use [137]. To better understand the harms associated with illicit drug dependency, future research should focus on collecting better estimates of mortality and morbidity.

Substance use and SUDs follow standard epidemiological age-related trends, with an onset often in late adolescence or early adulthood, showing peak prevalence in emerging adulthood, and then a decline. Although substance abuse is less common among older persons, often has a greater impact when it does occur, making it a public health concern [137]. A careful review of the population-based empirical literature reveals the importance of considering substance use in the context of development, with specific developmental aspects linked to the origin, course, and resolution of the problem.

SUDs are defined and thought of in a variety of ways. They have a lot in common with other chronic, recurrent diseases like diabetes or high blood pressure from a public health standpoint. Chronic diseases with significant behavioral health components may necessitate a lifelong commitment to manage and control. Many professionals believe that SUDs are inherently progressive. To put it another way, if these diseases are not treated, they tend to worsen over time. This chronic disease viewpoint has sparked significant controversy. For example, there is abundant evidence that many people, especially those suffering from the most severe kinds of addiction, follow a chronic, relapsing, escalating cycle. However, many people with SUDs seem to "recover" without undergoing professional therapy. This pattern, however, does not apply to everyone who has been diagnosed with a SUD. Many persons with milder, earlier-stage SUDs do not relapse and their substance-related problems do not progress [138]. Some experts, on the other hand, contend that, despite their history of chronic substance abuse, these individuals may not have been suffering from a severe SUD. Because of the great degree of individual variability in the course of addiction, it appears imprudent to employ a single treatment approach for all people diagnosed with the illness [138]. Despite age-related norms, significant individual course variability seems to be observed and contemporary statistical approaches have found numerous unique prototypic courses that appear to differ in their factors and outcomes. Research on substance use and misuse from a lifetime perspective has significant implications for the design and implementation of successful, developmentally informed diagnosis, prevention, and intervention programs [136].

The Diagnostic and Statistical Manual of Mental Disorders (DSM) is a classification manual for mental illnesses. It establishes a classification system for clinicians, insurance providers, researchers, and policymakers to utilize during diagnosing, researching, and treating mental illness. The 4th edition (DSM-IV) of the DSM, which had been in use for almost a decade, was replaced in 2013 by the 5th edition (DSM-5) [134, 135]. This version included organizational modifications as well as significant revisions to the diagnostic criteria for nearly every DSM-IV disorder. Some SUDs had just minor wording modifications, while others had significant criterion revisions. Some disorders have been added to and some removed from the list [136].

The transition from DSM-IV to DSM-5 has relevance in a multitude of settings, and it is essential for diagnosing and treating mental illness and SUD, as well as medical billing procedures and mental health research. Furthermore, if the modifications result in significant changes in the estimate of illness burden in the United States, they may be relevant to policymaking [136]. Every year, the National Survey on Drug Use and Health (NSDUH) gathers data on substance abuse and mental health from roughly 70,000 occupants of households and noninstitutional group quarters (e.g., shelters, rooming houses, and dormitories) as well as civilians residing on military bases. The NSDUH data give current, relevant information on the nation's substance use and mental health status to the drug use and mental health prevention, treatment, and research communities. Stakeholders and policymakers can utilize this data to learn more about the disease burden, temporal patterns, and repercussions of substance abuse and mental illness, as well as identify high-risk groups [136]. Professionals in the United States currently rely extensively on the diagnostic method outlined in the DSM-5 for diagnosing substance use disorders [136]. Many nations throughout the world use the 11th edition World Health Organization's (WHO, 2016) International Statistical Categorization of Diseases and Related Health Problems version 10, (ICD-10).

According to the DSM-5, SUDs are a type of a class of disorder (substance-related disorders) that are "associated to the use of a drug of abuse (including alcohol)". Although there are changes at various levels in the shift from DSM-IV to DSM-5 for SUDs, the core criteria stay the same [134, 135, 139]. However, there have been changes at the category/class level (see **Table 1** for the specific disorders considered within the overall group of disorders), substance level (which substances are considered "drugs of abuse"), disorder level (the template of criteria that is applied, with some deviations, across all substances), and individual criteria level (the number and types of symptoms needed to meet criteria for a disorder) [140]. Changes in relation to categorization refer to a disorder's "class," which is used in the DSM to designate groups of related disorders (e.g., personality disorders and anxiety disorders). The DSM-5 includes several revisions to the classification system, one of which is the classification of SUDs. SUDs were classified as substance-related disorders in the DSM-IV, which contained solely substance/drug-based illnesses. Gambling disorder has been added to this classification in DSM-5, and the section has been renamed Substance-Related and Addictive Disorders [136]. Changes from DSM-IV to DSM-5 in the types of substances assessed have been minor, but some reclassification has occurred. Based on empirical evidence since they have similar mechanisms of action (boosting synaptic dopamine), symptom profiles, consequences, and prognoses, cocaine (including crack) and amphetamines have been merged with other stimulants (except caffeine) into a distinct stimulant class [140].

Characteristic	DSM-IV	DSM-5
Disorder Class	Substance-related disorders, included only SUDs	Substance-related and addictive disorders now include SUDs and gambling disorders (formerly pathological gambling)
Disorder Types1	Because of the hierarchical diagnostic guidelines for abuse and dependence, people who met the criteria for dependence were never diagnosed with abuse for the same class of substance.	SUD, substance abuse, and dependence have all been replaced with one diagnosis, SUD.
Substances Assessed	11 classes of substances assessed, plus 2 additional categories	10 classes of substances assessed, plus 2 additional categories
	Alcohol	Alcohol
	Amphetamine and similar sympathomimetics	Stimulant use disorder, which includes amphetamines, cocaine, and other stimulants
	Caffeine (intoxication only)	Caffeine (intoxication and withdrawal)
	Cannabis (no withdrawal syndrome)	Cannabis (with withdrawal syndrome)
	Cocaine	Combined with other stimulants (e.g., amphetamines) under stimulant use disorder
	Hallucinogens Phencyclidine and similar arylcyclohexylamines	Separated into phencyclidine use disorder and other hallucinogen use disorder
	Inhalants (no withdrawal syndrome)	Inhalants (no withdrawal syndrome)
	Nicotine (dependence only)	Tobacco
	Opioids	Opioids
		Merged with hallucinogens
	Sedatives, hypnotics, and anxiolytics	Sedatives, hypnotics, and anxiolytics
	Other drug abuse/dependence	Any other SUD
	Polysubstance dependence	Dropped polysubstance use disorder

Table 1.
Comparison of DSM-IV and DSM-5 Substance Use Disorder Assessment.

The merging of substance abuse disorder and substance dependency disorder into a single SUD is a fundamental alteration in the criteria for substance use disorders from DSM-IV to DSM-5. DSM-5 has combined what had previously been considered as two distinct and hierarchical disorders (substance abuse and substance dependence) into a single construct, SUD, classifying it as mild, moderate, or severe, with the severity of an addiction based on how many of the established criteria are met. Diagnosis of SUD requires two out of eleven criteria to be met in a 12-month period. In addition, the DSM-5 has included a craving criterion to replace the abuse criterion associated with recurring substance-related legal difficulties (e.g., arrests for substance-related disorderly conduct). Due to low endorsement, poor fit with other items, and poor discrimination of this item (nearly everyone endorsing the legal criteria also endorsed other criteria), the legal problems criterion was omitted (see **Table 2**) [136, 141]. The majority of cases that met DSM-IV abuse criteria will not receive a DSM-5 diagnosis since they do not meet the minimum two-criterion threshold for a mild SUD. Most DSM-IV abuse cases will now be classified as mild SUD if they also endorsed two dependence criteria, but those who endorsed multiple (i.e., two or three) abuse criteria and two to three dependence criteria will now be classified as moderate SUD [137]. DSM-IV dependence cases that met three dependence criteria and no more than two abuse criteria will be classified as moderate SUDs in DSM-5, whereas nearly all cases that met four or more dependence criteria will be classified as severe SUDs [140]. The withdrawal dependence criterion is another criterion that has undergone some changes in DSM-5. Unlike other criteria, withdrawal symptoms are unique to the substance's physiological action (see **Table 2**). Withdrawal is manifested by (1) a person experiencing the substance's characteristic withdrawal symptoms, or (2) a person taking the same or a closely comparable substance to avoid the substance's unique withdrawal symptoms in both DSM-IV and DSM-5. Except for cannabis, the DSM-IV and DSM-5 withdrawal criteria remain intact [136].

For that category of substances, the DSM-IV requires the endorsement of one or more symptoms (out of four, at any time) and no history of substance dependency (see **Table 2** for the specific criteria) [136]. In addition, in order to meet the substance dependence criteria, three or more symptoms (out of seven) have to be confirmed in 12-month period. According to DSM-IV diagnostic hierarchy standards, people who met both substance abuse and substance dependence criteria for a particular substance were labeled as having substance dependence alone. The objective of this was to highlight the severity of dependence as compared to the abuse diagnosis [136].

The separate abuse and dependence disorders have been eliminated from DSM-5 for several reasons: (1) the separation has little guidance for treatment; (2) the separation created "diagnostic orphans" (those who endorsed two dependence symptoms but no abuse symptoms and hence did not meet any diagnostic criteria); (3) the hierarchical structure did not follow the expected relationship between abuse and dependence (that abuse was largely a less severe symptom of dependence); and (4) the division caused the abuse diagnosis to suffer from substantial reliability problems [136, 140, 142, 143].

A cluster of symptoms related to cannabis withdrawal has been uncovered in research undertaken following the release of the DSM-IV, and this new information has been included in the DSM-5 [2]. The presence of three or more symptoms occurring within one week of stopping severe and persistent cannabis use is known as cannabis withdrawal syndrome. (1) irritability, anger, or depression; (2) nervousness or anxiety; (3) sleep problems (e.g., insomnia or unpleasant/vivid dreams); (4) decreased appetite or weight loss; (5) restlessness; (6) depressed mood; and (7) at least one physical symptom that causes considerable discomfort such as abdominal pain, shakiness/tremors, sweating, fever, chills, or headache, are all possible symptoms [136].

The severity Criteria were another significant change between the two versions of diagnostic criteria. The DSM-IV did not directly measure the severity of SUDs, though dependence was generally thought to be more severe than abuse, and patients who were diagnosed with dependence did not obtain an abuse diagnosis even if the criteria for abuse were met [136]. A symptom count-based severity indicator has been added to DSM-5, with two to three symptoms classified as mild, four to five symptoms categorized as moderate, and six or more symptoms categorized as severe. A study found that a simple symptom count was as successful at evaluating severity as more advanced algorithms [144], prompting the establishment of a severity index [136].

	DSM-IV	DSM-5
Disorders Assessed	**Substance abuse:**	**SUD: Two out of 11 criteria clustering in a 12-month period**
One or more symptoms	Recurrent substance-related legal problems	Dropped
	The substance is used in larger amounts or for a longer period of time than was intended (1).	Same
	There is a persistent desire or unsuccessful efforts to cut down or control substance use (2).	Same
	A great deal of time is spent in activities necessary to obtain the substance, use the substance, or recover from its effects (3)	Same
	Craving (4): no craving	Added
Three or more symptoms in the same 12-month period (or one symptom if dependence criteria have been met previously in the lifetime	**Substance dependence:**	
	Recurrent substance use resulting in a failure to fulfill major role obligations at work, school, or home (5)	Same
	Continued substance use despite continuous or recurring social or interpersonal issues created or aggravated by the substance's effects (6).	Same
	Important social, occupational, or recreational activities are given up or reduced because of substance use (7)	Same
	Recurrent substance use in situations where it is physically hazardous (8)	Same
	Substance use is continued despite knowledge of having a persistent or recurrent physical or psychological problem that is likely to have been caused or exacerbated by substance use (9)	Same

	DSM-IV	DSM-5
	Tolerance, as defined by either: (1) a need for markedly increased amounts of substance to achieve intoxication or desired effect or (2) a markedly diminished effect with continued use of the same amount of the substance (10)	Same
	Withdrawal, as manifested by either: (1) the characteristic withdrawal syndrome for the substance (excludes Cannabis, Hallucinogens, and Inhalants) (2) the substance (or a similar substance) is taken to relieve or avoid withdrawal symptoms (11).	Withdrawal, as manifested by either: (1) withdrawal syndrome characteristic for the substance (excludes Phencyclidine, Other Hallucinogens, and Inhalants) (2) the substance (or a closely related substance) is taken to relieve or avoid withdrawal symptoms (Except for those taking opioids, sedatives, hypnotics or anxiolytics, or stimulant medications solely under appropriate medical supervision).
Severity	No severity criteria	Severity is determined by the number of symptoms Mild: 2 to 3 symptoms. Moderate: 4 to 5 symptoms. Severe: 6 or more symptoms.
Additional Specifications	With or without physiological dependence, early full remission, early partial remission, sustained full remission, sustained partial remission, on agonist therapy, and in a controlled environment	Early or sustained remission and if the person is in a controlled environment where access to the substance is restricted

Table 2.
Comparison of DSM-IV and DSM-5 Substance Use Disorder Criteria.

3.1 Criteria for diagnosing substance use disorders

Drug addiction is a progressive and chronically relapsing disorder that develops from infrequent, limited, and regulated use of a substance to compulsive usage [145]. When people are unable to obtain the substance to which they are addicted, they suffer from unpleasant emotional states (dysphoria, anxiety, irritability, and other negative feelings) due to low level of reward, excessive stress, and compromised executive function. Eventually, the individual returns to excessive drug-seeking and excessive drug taking behavior. This, in turn, activates CRF in the medial PFC accompanied by executive function deficits that may aid the transition to compulsive like behavior [146].

The addiction process is cyclic and consists of three stages which are interconnected and can lead to a recurrent sequence of addictive behaviors characterized by increasing and persistent levels of psychological and physical problems over time [145]. Each of the components of the cycle involves a distinct psychosocial and behavioral manifestation relevant to the DSM-5 diagnostic criteria (see **Figure 1**).

The changes in various components of reward neurocircuitry may represent the different social psychological and behavioral components involved in the addiction cycle. The social-psychological components of lack of strength and self-regulation with regard to controlling substance use, for example, may reflect increased activity in the stress system and be linked to individuals' failures despite their persistent desire to limit or quit using addictive substances and using them in larger quantities than intended (refer to **Figure 1**). This process signifies the preoccupation/anticipation stage which eventually leads to a cycle of binge use and relapse [68]. In this stage, increased dopaminergic and opioidergic neurotransmission may be involved, resulting in sensitization. On the other hand, monitoring or attentional failures are linked to people's preoccupation with getting drugs, and they may reflect cognitive alterations impacted by broadly distributed brain monoamine systems. In this situation, counteradaptation is caused by compromised dopamine, serotonin, and opioidergic neurotransmission, as well as increased stress neurotransmitters, which may be responsible for the negative emotional state developed due to withdrawal. The combination of a change in the hedonic set-point caused by repeated counter-adaptation and a different mechanism for sensitization would provide a powerful motivational drive for drug addiction to persist [68].

The DSM-5 states that a person must fulfill certain criteria to be diagnosed with a substance use disorder. Currently, there are 11 criteria (see **Table 2**) used to make such a diagnosis which can be divided into four categories [141].

a. **Impaired control:** Impaired control can manifest itself in a variety of ways: (1) Using a substance for longer than the intended time or in higher amounts than intended; (2) Wanting to cut down on usage yet failing to do so; (3) Excessive time spent obtaining, using, and recovering from drug use; (4) Cravings that are so strong that thinking about anything else is difficult.

b. **Social impairment** (5) Substance use negatively affects the ability to fulfill responsibilities at home, workplace, and school. People may continue to use despite recurring and worsening social problems or problems with work, school, or family/social obligations. This might include repeated work absences, poor school performance, neglect of children, or failure to meet household responsibilities. (6) Addiction may also be suggested if a person continues to use substances while having interpersonal problems due to substance use. Interpersonal problems may include arguments with family members concerning substance use, as well as the loss of vital friendships as a result of prolonged substance use. (7) Giving up Important social, work, and recreational activities for the sake of substance use. Substance abuse may cause important and meaningful social and leisure activities to be abandoned or curtailed. A person may spend less time with his or her family or quit outdoor plays with his or her friends.

c. **Risky Use:** The central issue of this criterion is the failure to quit using the substance despite the harm it causes.

(8) Addiction may be indicated when someone takes substances in physically unsafe or dangerous conditions regularly. For instance, using alcohol or other drugs while operating machinery or driving a car. (9) Some people continue to use addictive substances even if they are aware that addictive substances are creating or exacerbating bodily and psychological problems. An individual may continue to smoke cigarettes despite having a respiratory condition such as asthma or chronic obstructive pulmonary disease (COPD), such as chronic bronchitis.

d. **Pharmacological indicators: Tolerance and Withdrawal**

This criterion describes how the body adjusts or attempts to maintain homeostatic equilibrium to the sustained and frequent usage of a substance. For most people, tolerance and withdrawal are hallmark markers of progressing addiction. (10) Tolerance develops when people require a higher dose of a substance to obtain the same effect. To put it another way, it's when someone gets less of a result with the same amount of effort. Either the desire to avoid withdrawal symptoms or to become high could be the "desired effect." Tolerance is experienced differently by different people, i.e., people's sensitivities to different drugs differ. The rate at which tolerance develops and the dose required for tolerance to develop will differ depending on the substance [88]. (11) Withdrawal is the body's reaction to abrupt discontinuation of a drug once the body has built a tolerance to it. Each drug produces a distinct set of (sometimes unpleasant and lethal) symptoms (refer to the previous section for the unique symptoms in each category of substance). Although withdrawal is painful, it usually does not necessitate medical intervention. However, withdrawing from certain drugs, on the other hand, can be so deadly that medical advice may be critical before trying to quit them after a long period of use [88].

While an individual must meet at least two of the above criteria to be diagnosed with a SUD, the severity of the addiction is decided by the number of criteria met. A mild SUD might be the diagnosis, if two or three of these symptoms are present. A moderate SUD would be a more appropriate diagnosis if a person exhibits four or five of these symptoms. Ultimately, a severe SUD occurs when a person exhibits six or more of these symptoms. Substance withdrawal, however, is a distinct diagnosis that may or may not be associated with a substance use disorder diagnosis [88].

4. Conclusion

Addiction is caused by the brain's gradual adaptation of neuronal activity to long-term drug exposure, which results in fundamental neuroplastic changes. The extended amygdala (EAc) is a network made up of the central amygdala and the stria terminalis' bed nucleus. This important location is in charge of controlling drug cravings and seeking behaviors [147]. Drug addiction signifies a three-stage intense dysregulation of motivational circuits due to a combination of excessive incentive salience and habit formation [148], reward deficits and excessive stress, and impaired executive function [64, 80, 126].

Changes in dopamine and opioid peptides in the basal ganglia are involved in the rewarding effects of drugs of abuse, the development of incentive salience, and the development of drug-seeking habits in the binge/intoxication stage. In the withdrawal/negative affect stage, decreases in the function of the dopamine component of the reward system, as well as recruitment of brain stress neurotransmitters like corticotropin-releasing factor and dynorphin in the neurocircuitry of the extended amygdala, lead to an increase in negative emotional states and dysphoric and stress-like responses. The dysregulation of critical afferent projections from the prefrontal cortex and insula, particularly glutamate, to the basal ganglia and extended amygdala, causes craving and executive function deficiencies in the preoccupation/anticipation stage [68].

Almost all addictive substances have the common property of increasing mesolimbic dopamine function. The mesolimbic dopamine (DA) pathway by which the DA cells in the ventral tegmental area (VTA) projecting into the nucleus accumbens (NAc) seems to be crucial for drug rewards. Most psychostimulants such as cocaine [149] amphetamine [150] narcotic analgesics [151], nicotine [152], alcohol [153], and phencyclidine [150] stimulate dopamine transmission in the nucleus accumbens [151], the main area of the ventral striatum. A couple of other dopamine pathways the mesostriatal (DA cells in substantia nigra [154] projecting into dorsal striatum) and the mesocortical (DA cells in VTA projecting into frontal cortex) are recently recognized to have a contribution to drug reward and addiction. Alcohol and other substances of abuse are fundamentally rewarding in that they are consumed by humans or self-administered by laboratory animals. As a result, individuals exposed to drugs, though small in percentage, will become addicted and move from controlled drug use to compulsive and uncontrolled drug consumption despite adverse consequences.

The three stages involving the different neurochemicals and regions of the brain are integrated and feed each other producing strong drives for substance seeking. The addiction cycle tends to intensify over time and progress to greater physical and psychological harms. People with such disorders may have distorted thinking and abnormal behaviors as a result of changes in the brain's structure and functions. Brain imaging studies on people who frequently use psychoactive substances show marked changes in the areas of the brain that are linked to judgment, decision making, learning, memory, and behavioral control, which can last long after the period of intoxication.

Even though there are no specific biological markers of substance abuse disorders currently on use, there are a number of intriguing neurobiological aspects of substance abuse disorders that can help in the diagnosis of substance use, misuse, and SUD. An impaired reward system, overactive brain stress systems, and compromised orbitofrontal/prefrontal cortex function are some of the major neurobiological changes in the brain revealed in both human and animal studies which are quite relevant for the diagnosis of substance use, misuse, and SUD [155]. Although addictive substances have common properties, there are still considerable variabilities among classes of drugs in terms of primary and long-term physical and psychological effects, mechanisms of action, development of tolerance, and withdrawal. Differences in the availability, cost, legality, marketing, and cultural attitudes towards addictive substances and their use also influence which substances are used, and the development of dependence upon them. Thus, the study of substance use disorder and addiction must take these factors into account, while at the same time noting the similarities across drug classes.

Conflict of interest

The authors declare no conflict of interest.

Author details

Samson Duresso
University of Tasmania, Hobart, Australia

*Address all correspondence to: samson.duresso@utas.edu.au

References

[1] Morse, R.M. and D.K. Flavin, *The definition of alcoholism. The Joint Committee of the National Council on Alcoholism and Drug Dependence and the American Society of Addiction Medicine to Study the Definition and Criteria for the Diagnosis of Alcoholism.* JAMA, 1992. **268**(8): p. 1012-4.

[2] Robinson, B.E. and P. Post, *Risk of addiction to work and family functioning.* Psychol Rep, 1997. **81**(1): p. 91-5.

[3] Wang, M.Q., et al., *Social influence on southern adolescents' smoking transition: a retrospective study.* South Med J, 1997. **90**(2): p. 218-22.

[4] Wise, R.A., *Addiction becomes a brain disease.* Neuron, 2000. **26**(1): p. 27-33.

[5] *Addiction and the brain--Part II.* Harv Ment Health Lett, 1998. **15**(1): p. 1-3.

[6] Friedman, D.P., *Drug addiction: a chronically relapsing brain disease.* N C Med J, 2009. **70**(1): p. 35-7.

[7] Wu, P.H. and K.M. Schulz, *Advancing addiction treatment: what can we learn from animal studies?* ILAR J, 2012. **53**(1): p. 4-13.

[8] Kramer, J., et al., *Mechanisms of Alcohol Addiction: Bridging Human and Animal Studies.* Alcohol Alcohol, 2020. **55**(6): p. 603-607.

[9] Cates, H.M., et al., *National Institute on Drug Abuse genomics consortium white paper: Coordinating efforts between human and animal addiction studies.* Genes Brain Behav, 2019. **18**(6): p. e12577.

[10] Markou, A., T.R. Kosten, and G.F. Koob, *Neurobiological similarities in depression and drug dependence: a self-medication hypothesis.* Neuropsychopharmacology, 1998. **18**(3): p. 135-74.

[11] Kreek, M.J., et al., *Genetic influences on impulsivity, risk taking, stress responsivity and vulnerability to drug abuse and addiction.* Nat Neurosci, 2005. **8**(11): p. 1450-7.

[12] Sentir, A.M., et al., *Polysubstance addiction vulnerability in mental illness: Concurrent alcohol and nicotine self-administration in the neurodevelopmental hippocampal lesion rat model of schizophrenia.* Addict Biol, 2020. **25**(1): p. e12704.

[13] Volkow, N.D. and J.S. Fowler, *Addiction, a disease of compulsion and drive: involvement of the orbitofrontal cortex.* Cerebral cortex, 2000. **10**(3): p. 318-325.

[14] Davidson, R.J., et al., *Neural and behavioral substrates of mood and mood regulation.* Biological psychiatry, 2002. **52**(6): p. 478-502.

[15] Nemeroff, C.B., *The corticotropin-releasing factor (CRF) hypothesis of depression: new findings and new directions.* Mol. Psychiatry, 1996. **1**: p. 336-342.

[16] Sinha, R., *How does stress increase risk of drug abuse and relapse?* Psychopharmacology, 2001. **158**(4): p. 343-359.

[17] Sinha, R., *Chronic stress, drug use, and vulnerability to addiction.* Annals of the New York Academy of Sciences, 2008. **1141**: p. 105-130.

[18] Abasi, I. and P. Mohammadkhani, *Family Risk Factors Among Women With Addiction-Related Problems: An Integrative Review.* Int J High Risk Behav Addict, 2016. **5**(2): p. e27071.

[19] Ranjbaran, M., et al., *Risk Factors for Addiction Potential among College Students.* Int J Prev Med, 2018. **9**: p. 17.

[20] Zimic, J.I. and V. Jukic, *Familial risk factors favoring drug addiction onset.* J Psychoactive Drugs, 2012. **44**(2): p. 173-85.

[21] Cancrini, L., et al., *Social and family factors of teenager drug-addiction.* Eur J Toxicol, 1970. **3**(6): p. 397-401.

[22] Gjeruldsen, S., B. Myrvang, and S. Opjordsmoen, *Risk factors for drug addiction and its outcome. A follow-up study over 25 years.* Nord J Psychiatry, 2003. **57**(5): p. 373-6.

[23] Strang, J., et al., *Route of drug use and its implications for drug effect, risk of dependence and health consequences.* Drug Alcohol Rev, 1998. **17**(2): p. 197-211.

[24] Morales, A.M., et al., *Identifying Early Risk Factors for Addiction Later in Life: A Review of Prospective Longitudinal Studies.* Curr Addict Rep, 2020. **7**(1): p. 89-98.

[25] Odgers, C.L., et al., *Is it important to prevent early exposure to drugs and alcohol among adolescents?* Psychol Sci, 2008. **19**(10): p. 1037-44.

[26] Heilig, M., et al., *Developing neuroscience-based treatments for alcohol addiction: A matter of choice?* Transl Psychiatry, 2019. **9**(1): p. 255.

[27] Volkow, N.D., M. Michaelides, and R. Baler, *The Neuroscience of Drug Reward and Addiction.* Physiol Rev, 2019. **99**(4): p. 2115-2140.

[28] Lein, E.S., et al., *Genome-wide atlas of gene expression in the adult mouse brain.* Nature, 2007. **445**(7124): p. 168-176.

[29] Gardon, O., et al., *Expression of mu opioid receptor in dorsal diencephalic conduction system: New insights for the medial habenula.* Neuroscience, 2014. **277**: p. 595-609.

[30] Kang, S., et al., *Ethanol Withdrawal Drives Anxiety-Related Behaviors by Reducing M-type Potassium Channel Activity in the Lateral Habenula.* Neuropsychopharmacology, 2017. **42**(9): p. 1813-1824.

[31] Baldwin, P.R., R. Alanis, and R. Salas, *The Role of the Habenula in Nicotine Addiction.* Journal of addiction research & therapy, 2011. **S1**(2): p. 002.

[32] Mineur, Y.S. and M.R. Picciotto, *Genetics of nicotinic acetylcholine receptors: Relevance to nicotine addiction.* Biochemical pharmacology, 2008. **75**(1): p. 323-333.

[33] Shorey-Kendrick, L.E., et al., *Nicotinic receptors in non-human primates: Analysis of genetic and functional conservation with humans.* Neuropharmacology, 2015. **96**(Pt B): p. 263-273.

[34] Margolis, E.B. and H.L. Fields, *Mu Opioid Receptor Actions in the Lateral Habenula.* PLOS ONE, 2016. **11**(7): p. e0159097.

[35] Nestler, E.J. and C. Luscher, *The Molecular Basis of Drug Addiction: Linking Epigenetic to Synaptic and Circuit Mechanisms.* Neuron, 2019. **102**(1): p. 48-59.

[36] Lepack, A.E., et al., *Dopaminylation of histone H3 in ventral tegmental area regulates cocaine seeking.* Science, 2020. **368**(6487): p. 197-201.

[37] Wong, C.C.Y., J. Mill, and C. Fernandes, *Drugs and addiction: an introduction to epigenetics.* Addiction, 2011. **106**(3): p. 480-489.

[38] Eddy, N.B., et al., *Drug dependence: its significance and characteristics.* Psychopharmacol Bull, 1966. **3**(3): p. 1-12.

[39] Koob, G.F., R. Maldonado, and L. Stinus, *Neural substrates of opiate withdrawal.* Trends Neurosci, 1992. **15**(5): p. 186-91.

[40] Berridge, K.C. and T.E. Robinson, *Liking, wanting, and the incentive-sensitization theory of addiction.* American Psychologist, 2016. **71**(8): p. 670.

[41] Robinson, T.E. and K.C. Berridge, *The incentive sensitization theory of addiction: some current issues.* Philosophical Transactions of the Royal Society B: Biological Sciences, 2008. **363**(1507): p. 3137-3146.

[42] Gelkopf, M., S. Levitt, and A. Bleich, *An integration of three approaches to addiction and methadone maintenance treatment: the self-medication hypothesis, the disease model and social criticism.* Isr J Psychiatry Relat Sci, 2002. **39**(2): p. 140-51.

[43] Koob, G.F., *Hedonic Homeostatic Dysregulation as a Driver of Drug-Seeking Behavior.* Drug Discov Today Dis Models, 2008. **5**(4): p. 207-215.

[44] Solomon, R.L., *The opponent-process theory of acquired motivation: the costs of pleasure and the benefits of pain.* Am Psychol, 1980. **35**(8): p. 691-712.

[45] Solomon, R.L. and J.D. Corbit, *An opponent-process theory of motivation. II. Cigarette addiction.* J Abnorm Psychol, 1973. **81**(2): p. 158-71.

[46] Solomon, R.L. and J.D. Corbit, *An opponent-process theory of motivation. I. Temporal dynamics of affect.* Psychol Rev, 1974. **81**(2): p. 119-45.

[47] George, O., M. Le Moal, and G.F. Koob, *Allostasis and addiction: role of the dopamine and corticotropin-releasing factor systems.* Physiol Behav, 2012. **106**(1): p. 58-64.

[48] Miller, E.K. and J.D. Cohen, *An integrative theory of prefrontal cortex function.* Annu Rev Neurosci, 2001. **24**: p. 167-202.

[49] Fernandez-Serrano, M.J., et al., *Prevalence of executive dysfunction in cocaine, heroin and alcohol users enrolled in therapeutic communities.* Eur J Pharmacol, 2010. **626**(1): p. 104-12.

[50] Hester, R. and H. Garavan, *Executive dysfunction in cocaine addiction: evidence for discordant frontal, cingulate, and cerebellar activity.* J Neurosci, 2004. **24**(49): p. 11017-22.

[51] Madoz-Gurpide, A., et al., *Executive dysfunction in chronic cocaine users: an exploratory study.* Drug Alcohol Depend, 2011. **117**(1): p. 55-8.

[52] Baumeister, R.F., *Self-regulation, ego depletion, and inhibition.* Neuropsychologia, 2014. **65**: p. 313-9.

[53] Patrick, H. and A. Canevello, *Methodological Overview of A Self-Determination Theory-Based Computerized Intervention to Promote Leisure-Time Physical Activity.* Psychol Sport Exerc, 2011. **12**(1): p. 13-19.

[54] Ryan, R.M. and E.L. Deci, *Self-determination theory and the facilitation of intrinsic motivation, social development, and well-being.* Am Psychol, 2000. **55**(1): p. 68-78.

[55] Gollwitzer, P.M. and B. Schaal, *Metacognition in action: the importance of implementation intentions.* Pers Soc Psychol Rev, 1998. **2**(2): p. 124-36.

[56] Sheeran, P., T.L. Webb, and P.M. Gollwitzer, *The interplay between goal intentions and implementation intentions.* Pers Soc Psychol Bull, 2005. **31**(1): p. 87-98.

[57] Brewer, J.A. and M.N. Potenza, *The neurobiology and genetics of impulse control disorders: relationships to drug addictions.* Biochem Pharmacol, 2008. **75**(1): p. 63-75.

[58] Everitt, B.J. and T.W. Robbins, *Neural systems of reinforcement for drug addiction: from actions to habits to compulsion.* Nat Neurosci, 2005. **8**(11): p. 1481-9.

[59] Schultz, W., *Potential vulnerabilities of neuronal reward, risk, and decision mechanisms to addictive drugs.* Neuron, 2011. **69**(4): p. 603-17.

[60] Hariri, A.R., *The neurobiology of individual differences in complex behavioral traits.* Annu Rev Neurosci, 2009. **32**: p. 225-47.

[61] Muller, D.J., O. Likhodi, and A. Heinz, *Neural markers of genetic vulnerability to drug addiction.* Curr Top Behav Neurosci, 2010. **3**: p. 277-99.

[62] Baker, T.E., et al., *Individual differences in substance dependence: at the intersection of brain, behaviour and cognition.* Addict Biol, 2011. **16**(3): p. 458-66.

[63] Lubman, D.I., M. Yucel, and C. Pantelis, *Addiction, a condition of compulsive behaviour? Neuroimaging and neuropsychological evidence of inhibitory dysregulation.* Addiction, 2004. **99**(12): p. 1491-502.

[64] Koob, G.F. and M. Le Moal, *Drug abuse: hedonic homeostatic dysregulation.* Science, 1997. **278**(5335): p. 52-8.

[65] Goldstein, R.Z. and N.D. Volkow, *Drug addiction and its underlying neurobiological basis: neuroimaging evidence for the involvement of the frontal cortex.* Am J Psychiatry, 2002. **159**(10): p. 1642-52.

[66] Koob, G., *Addiction is a Reward Deficit and Stress Surfeit Disorder.* Frontiers in Psychiatry, 2013. **4**(72).

[67] Berlin, G.S. and E. Hollander, *Compulsivity, impulsivity, and the DSM-5 process.* CNS Spectr, 2014. **19**(1): p. 62-8.

[68] Koob, G.F. and N.D. Volkow, *Neurobiology of addiction: a neurocircuitry analysis.* The lancet. Psychiatry, 2016. **3**(8): p. 760-773.

[69] George F. Koob, Ph.D., *Neurobiology of Addiction.* FOCUS, 2011. **9**(1): p. 55-65.

[70] Koob, G.F. and N.D. Volkow, *Neurocircuitry of addiction.* Neuropsychopharmacology, 2010. **35**(1): p. 217-38.

[71] Duncan, J.R., *Current perspectives on the neurobiology of drug addiction: a focus on genetics and factors regulating gene expression.* ISRN Neurol, 2012. **2012**: p. 972607.

[72] Nurco, D.N., et al., *Differential contributions of family and peer factors to the etiology of narcotic addiction.* Drug Alcohol Depend, 1998. **51**(3): p. 229-37.

[73] Harstad, E. and S. Levy, *Attention-Deficit/Hyperactivity Disorder and Substance Abuse.* Pediatrics, 2014. **134**(1): p. e293-e301.

[74] Koob, G.F. and M. Le Moal, *Drug addiction, dysregulation of reward, and allostasis.* Neuropsychopharmacology, 2001. **24**(2): p. 97-129.

[75] Volkow, N.D. and M. Morales, *The Brain on Drugs: From Reward to Addiction.* Cell, 2015. **162**(4): p. 712-25.

[76] United States. Department of Health and Human Services, *Facing addiction in America : the Surgeon General's report on alcohol, drugs and health*. HHS publication. 2016, Washington, D.C.: U.S. Department of Health & Human Services. 1 volume (various pagings).

[77] Wise, R.A., *Drug-activation of brain reward pathways.* Drug Alcohol Depend, 1998. **51**(1-2): p. 13-22.

[78] Koob, G.F., *The neurobiology of addiction: a neuroadaptational view relevant for diagnosis.* Addiction, 2006. **101 Suppl 1**: p. 23-30.

[79] Nestler, E.J., *Is there a common molecular pathway for addiction?* Nat Neurosci, 2005. **8**(11): p. 1445-9.

[80] Koob, G.F., M.A. Arends, and M. Le Moal, *Drugs, addiction, and the brain.*

2014, Amsterdam ; Boston: Elsevier/AP, Academic Press is an imprint of Elsevier. viii, 342 pages.

[81] Clapp, P., S.V. Bhave, and P.L. Hoffman, *How adaptation of the brain to alcohol leads to dependence: a pharmacological perspective.* Alcohol Res Health, 2008. **31**(4): p. 310-39.

[82] Nestler, E.J., B.T. Hope, and K.L. Widnell, *Drug addiction: a model for the molecular basis of neural plasticity.* Neuron, 1993. **11**(6): p. 995-1006.

[83] Self, D.W., *Neural substrates of drug craving and relapse in drug addiction.* Ann Med, 1998. **30**(4): p. 379-89.

[84] Gilpin, N.W., *Brain reward and stress systems in addiction.* Front Psychiatry, 2014. **5**: p. 79.

[85] Koob, G.F. and M. Le Moal, *Plasticity of reward neurocircuitry and the 'dark side' of drug addiction.* Nat Neurosci, 2005. **8**(11): p. 1442-4.

[86] Vendruscolo, L.F., et al., *Glucocorticoid receptor antagonism decreases alcohol seeking in alcohol-dependent individuals.* J Clin Invest, 2015. **125**(8): p. 3193-7.

[87] Dean, S.F., et al., *Addiction neurocircuitry and negative affect: A role for neuroticism in understanding amygdala connectivity and alcohol use disorder.* Neurosci Lett, 2020. **722**: p. 134773.

[88] Regier, D.A., E.A. Kuhl, and D.J. Kupfer, *The DSM-5: Classification and criteria changes.* World psychiatry : official journal of the World Psychiatric Association (WPA), 2013. **12**(2): p. 92-98.

[89] Jasinska, A.J., et al., *Factors modulating neural reactivity to drug cues in addiction: a survey of human neuroimaging studies.* Neurosci Biobehav Rev, 2014. **38**: p. 1-16.

[90] Dackis, C.A. and M.S. Gold, *Pharmacological approaches to cocaine addiction.* Journal of Substance Abuse Treatment, 1985. **2**(3): p. 139-145.

[91] Robinson, T.E. and K.C. Berridge, *The neural basis of drug craving: an incentive-sensitization theory of addiction.* Brain Res Brain Res Rev, 1993. **18**(3): p. 247-91.

[92] Robinson, T.E. and K.C. Berridge, *The psychology and neurobiology of addiction: an incentive-sensitization view.* Addiction, 2000. **95 Suppl 2**: p. S91-117.

[93] Robinson, T.E. and K.C. Berridge, *Review. The incentive sensitization theory of addiction: some current issues.* Philosophical transactions of the Royal Society of London. Series B, Biological sciences, 2008. **363**(1507): p. 3137-3146.

[94] Stewart, J., H. de Wit, and R. Eikelboom, *Role of unconditioned and conditioned drug effects in the self-administration of opiates and stimulants.* Psychological Review, 1984. **91**(2): p. 251-268.

[95] Rohsenow, D.J., et al., *Cue Reactivity in Addictive Behaviors: Theoretical and Treatment Implications.* International Journal of the Addictions, 1991. **25**(sup7): p. 957-993.

[96] Carter, B.L. and S.T. Tiffany, *Meta-analysis of cue-reactivity in addiction research.* Addiction, 1999. **94**(3): p. 327-340.

[97] Di Chiara, G., et al., *Drug addiction as a disorder of associative learning: role of nucleus accumbens shell/extended amygdala dopamine.* Annals of the New York Academy of Sciences, 1999. **877**(1): p. 461-485.

[98] Heimer, L., et al., *Specificity in the projection patterns of accumbal core and shell in the rat.* Neuroscience, 1991. **41**(1): p. 89-125.

[99] Kilts, C.D., et al., *The neural correlates of cue-induced craving in cocaine-dependent women.* American Journal of Psychiatry, 2004. **161**(2): p. 233-241.

[100] Kalivas, P.W. and N.D. Volkow, *The Neural Basis of Addiction: A Pathology of Motivation and Choice The American Journal of Psychiatry.*

[101] Walker, D.L. and M. Davis, *Role of the extended amygdala in short-duration versus sustained fear: a tribute to Dr. Lennart Heimer.* Brain Structure and Function, 2008. **213**(1): p. 29-42.

[102] Melis, M., S. Spiga, and *M. Diana*, *The dopamine hypothesis of drug addiction: hypodopaminergic state.* Int Rev Neurobiol, 2005. **63**: p. 101-54.

[103] LeDoux, J.E., *Emotion circuits in the brain.* Annu Rev Neurosci, 2000. **23**: p. 155-84.

[104] Neugebauer, V., et al., *The amygdala and persistent pain.* Neuroscientist, 2004. **10**(3): p. 221-34.

[105] Weiss, F., et al., *Ethanol Self-Administration Restores Withdrawal-Associated Deficiencies in Accumbal Dopamine and 5-Hydroxytryptamine Release in Dependent Rats.* The Journal of Neuroscience, 1996. **16**(10): p. 3474.

[106] Vengeliene, V., et al., *Neuropharmacology of alcohol addiction.* Br J Pharmacol, 2008. **154**(2): p. 299-315.

[107] Volkow, N.D., et al., *Association Between Decline in Brain Dopamine Activity With Age and Cognitive and Motor Impairment in Healthy Individuals.* American Journal of Psychiatry, 1998. **155**(3): p. 344-349.

[108] Zubieta, J.-K., et al., *Increased mu opioid receptor binding detected by PET in cocaine–dependent men is associated with cocaine craving.* Nature Medicine, 1996. **2**(11): p. 1225-1229.

[109] Volkow, N.D., et al., *Profound decreases in dopamine release in striatum in detoxified alcoholics: possible orbitofrontal involvement.* J Neurosci, 2007. **27**(46): p. 12700-6.

[110] Koob, G.F., *A role for brain stress systems in addiction.* Neuron, 2008. **59**(1): p. 11-34.

[111] Duresso, S.W., et al., *Stopping khat use: Predictors of success in an unaided quit attempt.* Drug Alcohol Rev, 2018. **37 Suppl 1**: p. S235-S239.

[112] Duresso, S.W., et al., *Khat withdrawal symptoms among chronic khat users following a quit attempt: An ecological momentary assessment study.* Psychol Addict Behav, 2018. **32**(3): p. 320-326.

[113] Koob, G. and M.J. Kreek, *Stress, dysregulation of drug reward pathways, and the transition to drug dependence.* Am J Psychiatry, 2007. **164**(8): p. 1149-59.

[114] Childress, A.R., et al., *Limbic Activation During Cue-Induced Cocaine Craving.* American Journal of Psychiatry, 1999. **156**(1): p. 11-18.

[115] Cooney, N.L., et al., *Alcohol cue reactivity, negative-mood reactivity, and relapse in treated alcoholic men.* J Abnorm Psychol, 1997. **106**(2): p. 243-50.

[116] Mantsch, J.R., et al., *Neurobiological mechanisms that contribute to stress-related cocaine use.* Neuropharmacology, 2014. **76 Pt B**(0 0): p. 383-394.

[117] Sinha, R., D. Catapano, and S. O'Malley, *Stress-induced craving and stress response in cocaine dependent individuals.* Psychopharmacology (Berl), 1999. **142**(4): p. 343-51.

[118] Weiss, F., *Neurobiology of craving, conditioned reward and relapse.* Current opinion in pharmacology, 2005. **5**(1): p. 9-19.

[119] Langleben, D.D., et al., *Acute effect of methadone maintenance dose on brain FMRI response to heroin-related cues.* American Journal of Psychiatry, 2008. **165**(3): p. 390-394.

[120] Everitt, B.J. and T.W. Robbins, *Neural systems of reinforcement for drug addiction: from actions to habits to compulsion.* Nature neuroscience, 2005. **8**(11): p. 1481-1489.

[121] Robinson, T.E. and K.C. Berridge, *The neural basis of drug craving: An incentive-sensitization theory of addiction.* Brain Research Reviews, 1993. **18**(3): p. 247-291.

[122] Robinson, T.E. and K.C. Berridge, *Incentive-sensitization and addiction.* Addiction, 2001. **96**(1): p. 103-114.

[123] Robinson, T.E. and K.C. Berridge, *Incentive-sensitization and drug 'wanting'.* Psychopharmacology, 2004. **171**(3): p. 352-353.

[124] Goldstein, R.Z. and N.D. Volkow, *Dysfunction of the prefrontal cortex in addiction: neuroimaging findings and clinical implications.* Nature Reviews Neuroscience, 2011. **12**(11): p. 652-669.

[125] Britt, J.P. and A. Bonci, *Optogenetic interrogations of the neural circuits underlying addiction.* Curr Opin Neurobiol, 2013. **23**(4): p. 539-45.

[126] Goldstein, R.Z. and N.D. Volkow, *Dysfunction of the prefrontal cortex in addiction: neuroimaging findings and clinical implications.* Nat Rev Neurosci, 2011. **12**(11): p. 652-69.

[127] Goodman, A., *Neurobiology of addiction. An integrative review.* Biochem Pharmacol, 2008. **75**(1): p. 266-322.

[128] Kalivas, P.W., *The glutamate homeostasis hypothesis of addiction.* Nat Rev Neurosci, 2009. **10**(8): p. 561-72.

[129] Koob, G.F. and N.D. Volkow, *Neurobiology of addiction: a neurocircuitry analysis.* Lancet Psychiatry, 2016. **3**(8): p. 760-773.

[130] Abbot, P. and D.M. Chase, *Culture and substance abuse: Impact of culture affects approach to treatment.* Psychiatric Times, 2008. **25**(1): p. 43-43.

[131] Paredes, A., *Social control of drinking among the Aztec Indians of Mesoamerica.* Journal of studies on alcohol, 1975. **36**(9): p. 1139-1153.

[132] Caetano, R., et al., *Acculturation, drinking, and alcohol abuse and dependence among Hispanics in the Texas–Mexico border.* Alcoholism: Clinical and Experimental Research, 2008. **32**(2): p. 314-321.

[133] Welte, J.W. and G.M. Barnes, *Alcohol and other drug use among Hispanics in New York State.* Alcoholism: Clinical and Experimental Research, 1995. **19**(4): p. 1061-1066.

[134] Shorter, E., *The history of nosology and the rise of the Diagnostic and Statistical Manual of Mental Disorders.* Dialogues in clinical neuroscience, 2015. **17**(1): p. 59-67.

[135] Robinson, S.M. and B. Adinoff, *The Classification of Substance Use Disorders: Historical, Contextual, and Conceptual Considerations.* Behavioral sciences (Basel, Switzerland), 2016. **6**(3): p. 18.

[136] Hasin, D.S., et al., *DSM-5 Criteria for Substance Use Disorders: Recommendations and Rationale.* American Journal of Psychiatry, 2013. **170**(8): p. 834-851.

[137] Hasin, D.S., et al., *DSM-5 criteria for substance use disorders: recommendations and rationale.* The American journal of psychiatry, 2013. **170**(8): p. 834-851.

[138] Cunningham, J.A. and J. McCambridge, *Is alcohol dependence best viewed as a chronic relapsing disorder?*

Addiction (Abingdon, England), 2012. **107**(1): p. 6-12.

[139] Hasin, D.S. and B.F. Grant, *The co-occurrence of DSM-IV alcohol abuse in DSM-IV alcohol dependence: results of the National Epidemiologic Survey on Alcohol and Related Conditions on heterogeneity that differ by population subgroup.* Arch Gen Psychiatry, 2004. **61**(9): p. 891-6.

[140] Kopak, A.M., S.L. Proctor, and N.G. Hoffmann, *The Elimination of Abuse and Dependence in DSM-5 Substance Use Disorders: What Does This Mean for Treatment?* Current Addiction Reports, 2014. **1**(3): p. 166-171.

[141] Substance, A. and A. Mental Health Services, *CBHSQ Methodology Report*, in *Impact of the DSM-IV to DSM-5 Changes on the National Survey on Drug Use and Health*. 2016, Substance Abuse and Mental Health Services Administration (US): Rockville (MD).

[142] Kahler, C.W. and D.R. Strong, *A Rasch Model Analysis of DSM-IV Alcohol Abuse and Dependence Items in the National Epidemiological Survey on Alcohol and Related Conditions.* Alcoholism: Clinical and Experimental Research, 2006. **30**(7): p. 1165-1175.

[143] Helzer, J.E., K.K. Bucholz, and M. Gossop, *A dimensional option for the diagnosis of substance dependence in DSM-V.* International Journal of Methods in Psychiatric Research, 2007. **16**(S1): p. S24-S33.

[144] Dawson, D.A., T.D. Saha, and B.F. Grant, *A multidimensional assessment of the validity and utility of alcohol use disorder severity as determined by item response theory models.* Drug and alcohol dependence, 2010. **107**(1): p. 31-38.

[145] Koob, G.F. and E.J. Simon, *The Neurobiology of Addiction: Where We Have Been and Where We Are Going.* J Drug Issues, 2009. **39**(1): p. 115-132.

[146] Koob, G.F., M.A. Arends, and M. Le Moal, *Chapter 2 - Introduction to the Neuropsychopharmacology of Drug Addiction*, in *Drugs, Addiction, and the Brain*, G.F. Koob, M.A. Arends, and M. Le Moal, Editors. 2014, Academic Press: San Diego. p. 29-63.

[147] Befort, K., et al., *Mu-opioid receptor activation induces transcriptional plasticity in the central extended amygdala.* European Journal of Neuroscience, 2008. **27**(11): p. 2973-2984.

[148] Robinson, M.J., T.E. Robinson, and K.C. Berridge, *Incentive salience and the transition to addiction.* Biological research on addiction, 2013. **2**: p. 391-399.

[149] Kuczenski, R. and D.S. Segal, *Differential effects of amphetamine and dopamine uptake blockers (cocaine, nomifensine) on caudate and accumbens dialysate dopamine and 3-methoxytyramine.* J Pharmacol Exp Ther, 1992. **262**(3): p. 1085-94.

[150] Carboni, E., et al., *Amphetamine, cocaine, phencyclidine and nomifensine increase extracellular dopamine concentrations preferentially in the nucleus accumbens of freely moving rats.* Neuroscience, 1989. **28**(3): p. 653-61.

[151] Di Chiara, G. and A. Imperato, *Preferential stimulation of dopamine release in the nucleus accumbens by opiates, alcohol, and barbiturates: studies with transcerebral dialysis in freely moving rats.* Ann N Y Acad Sci, 1986. **473**: p. 367-81.

[152] Imperato, A., A. Mulas, and G. Di Chiara, *Nicotine preferentially stimulates dopamine release in the limbic system of freely moving rats.* Eur J Pharmacol, 1986. **132**(2-3): p. 337-8.

[153] Imperato, A. and G. Di Chiara, *Preferential stimulation of dopamine release in the nucleus accumbens of freely*

moving rats by ethanol. J Pharmacol Exp Ther, 1986. **239**(1): p. 219-28.

[154] Hassen, K., et al., *Khat as a risk factor for hypertension: A systematic review.* JBI Libr Syst Rev, 2012. **10**(44): p. 2882-2905.

[155] Volkow, N.D., G. Koob, and R. Baler, *Biomarkers in substance use disorders.* ACS Chem Neurosci, 2015. **6**(4): p. 522-5.

Chapter 2

The *Juramento*: Secondary and Tertiary Preventive Benefits of a Religious-Based Brief Alcohol Intervention in the Mexican Immigrant Community

Victor Garcia, Katherine Fox, Emily Lambert and Alex Heckert

Abstract

Our chapter addresses the prevention benefits of the *juramento*, a grassroots religious-based brief intervention for harmful drinking practiced in Mexico and the Mexican immigrant community in the United States. With origins in Mexican folk Catholicism, it is a sacred pledge made to Our Lady of Guadalupe to abstain from alcohol for a specific time period; in most cases, at least six months. We draw on our data from a subsample of 15 Mexican workers who made *juramentos* and two priests who administered the *juramento* to the workers. The sample is from a larger qualitative study on the use of the *juramento* among Mexican immigrant and migrant workers in southeastern Pennsylvania. Our findings reveal that, in addition to serving as an intervention, the *juramento* results in secondary prevention—by identifying a harmful drinking before the onset of heavy drinking—and tertiary prevention—by slowing or abating the progression of heavy drinking.

Keywords: *juramentos*, alcohol interventions, prevention, Mexican immigrants, harmful drinking

1. Introduction

In Latinx communities across the country, there are several grassroots interventions for harmful drinking, among them, the *juramento*—a religious-based, brief intervention with origins in Mexican folk Catholicism. Basically, it is a ritualized pledge, or vow, made to *Nuestra Señora de Guadalupe*, or Our Lady of Guadalupe, to abstain from alcohol use for a specific time period. Vows are also made to overcome other addictions, such as drug abuse, smoking, and gambling. The *juramento* arose naturally around the religious beliefs of the common people in Mexico, or *el pueblo*, as they say in Spanish, and as such, is not a formal intervention. It is "intrinsically organic and rooted in culture, which makes it familiar to participants and informs their understanding of the disorder and recovery" [1]. With origins outside of biomedicine, the *juramento* does not fall within the scope of public health research, and as a result, it does not receive much attention in the alcohol intervention and treatment fields.

Although the *juramento* is based on religious traditions and practices, its possible contributions to these fields should not be underestimated. The aim of our book chapter is two-fold: (1) to discuss how the *juramento* is a brief intervention for different types of drinking, and (2) to examine how it offers secondary and tertiary prevention. In public health, secondary prevention refers to medical and public health efforts to catch diseases in their earliest stages, perhaps even before the appearance of signs or symptoms. This can include screening and routine checkups, identification of risk factors, and measures to stop the progression of asymptomatic or early-stage conditions [2]. Tertiary prevention aims to slow or stop progression after a diagnosis [3]. Though the disease is established, tertiary prevention seeks to minimize its damage to the suffer and to avoid the most serious of possible outcomes. Drawing on our ongoing research on the *juramento*, we argue that, although it is not a public health intervention and is not delivered by a medical or health care provider, but by a priest, the *juramento* results in these prevention benefits.

2. Background

2.1 The *juramento*

The *juramento* originated in Mexico and is centuries old, although exactly when the practice began remains unknown [4, 5]. It may be as old as the Shrine of Our Lady of Guadalupe itself, which was first constructed in present-day Mexico City nearly five hundred years ago, after the saint appeared several times at that location. Since then, Mexicans have made pilgrimages to the site, especially on her feast day of December 12. There, they make prayers, called *mandas*, for divine intervention for a problem; *mandas* are often made for a personal health ailment or on behalf of a family member or loved one who is suffering one. The *juramento* is based on this tradition but is solely for problems with alcohol and other substance use. Despite its tradition and popularity among certain segments of Mexican society, such as the poor, the *juramento* is not officially recognized by the Catholic Church. It is viewed as folk Catholicism, in which outdated beliefs and practices remain popular among parishioners and are tolerated by the Catholic Church even though they do not fall within current church doctrine. Nonetheless, parish priests familiar with the *juramento* process make *juramentos* upon request.

The particulars of this ritualized pledge vary according to local traditions. In the United States, especially in our research site in Pennsylvania, the *juramento* is a private affair that only involves the *jurado*, the individual making the pledge, and the priest. Close friends and family members may be present to give moral support. In Mexico, according to Cuadrado and Lieberman [5], *juramentos* are also made in group settings at a church and to other saints, such as *El Sagrado Señor de Chalma* (Sacred Lord of Chalma). At the Chapel of the Juramentos located on the grounds of the Shrine of Our Lady of Guadalupe, *juramentos* are made in groups every day of the week over the course of the year. The chapel can hold up to 50 people, and it is common for family members and friends of the *jurados* to attend.

Despite evidence of *juramento* use among impoverished groups in Mexico, especially in rural communities and regions with strong religious traditions, as well as in Mexican immigrant communities in the United States, it is understudied in both countries. Garcia, Lambert, Fox, Heckert, and Pinchi [1], only found four articles on the *juramento* in their literature review. It does not include a recent publication by some members of the same team, Garcia, Heckert, Lambert, and

Pinchi [6]. From the four articles discussed, they found that the *juramento* is practiced in Catholic parishes with large Latino populations in Pennsylvania, Florida, Texas, New Mexico, Arizona, and California. One binational study in the review, by Cuadrado & Lieberman [5], conducted in both the United States and Mexico documents its use among poor people in Mexico for whom formal alcohol treatment is unavailable. Like Mexican immigrants in the United States, they cannot always access biomedical resources, and turn to their faith, particularly the *juramento*, for help with their drinking. The number of *jurados* in the studies are not identified and as a result missing is information on their demographic characteristics and socioeconomic status.

The existing literature does document the many benefits of the *juramento* as an intervention. Researchers generally agree that the process allows individuals to explore the causes behind their drinking, to engage in a period of abstinence that sets up the right frame of mind for recovery, and to reconnect with estranged family and the larger community. Moreover, the *juramento* provides the *jurado* with church and community support essential for sobriety and recovery. Missing from this discussion is how the *juramento* also provides the individual with secondary and tertiary prevention. As will be discussed, secondary and tertiary prevention, respectively, can slow or stop the progression of drinking behaviors into dependence and mitigate the most serious harms of established alcohol use disorders.

2.2 Alcohol and substance use disorder prevention

Prevention literature, especially in relation to alcohol and substance use disorders, can be a challenging body of scholarship to review. While it highlights the range of avenues through which harm reduction can be achieved, there is a lack of consistency in terms and definitions; what one article may describe as prevention may be characterized as treatment by another. Many studies raise the issue of prevention, but fail to explain exactly what is being prevented, or how the intervention can achieve such results. Furthermore, not all articles that discuss prevention classify their efforts into primary, secondary, or tertiary types. The following sections describe the types of efforts within alcohol and substance use research that are associated with a specific tier of prevention, in order to provide an overall sense of the work that occurs within each category.

2.2.1 Primary prevention

The goal of primary prevention is to eliminate these disorders before they start. To that end, some studies seek to prevent substance abuse through research into underlying causes: Ridenour and Stormshak [7] advance an "Ontogenic Prevention" approach, which tailors prevention efforts to individual needs and characteristics; Moulahoum et al. [8] explore immunologically-based treatments and detection to understand sources of addiction; Volkow and Li [9] discuss addiction as a chronic brain disease that is affected by genetic, developmental, and environmental factors, and that such an understanding should inform prevention. Another significant body of literature focuses on psychological and psychosocial interventions. For example, Peterson and Reid [10] support interventions that promote empowerment to abstain from substance use, and Brooks et al. [11] find that hopefulness is an important component of primary prevention efforts. These approaches are especially common in programs aimed for adolescents, which attempt to deter or delay their engagement in substance use by building social, communication, and coping skills [12–14]. Recent literature also explores new delivery methods for prevention strategies. Through their review of motivational interviewing techniques, which have proven to be beneficial in therapeutic settings, Jiang, Wu, and Gao [15] suggest that this prevention could be expanded to other media such as telephone calls and web-based interactions. Similarly, Hopson, Wodarski and Tang [16] discuss the use of video and online prevention modalities to reach adolescents. Additionally, Mutamba et al. [17] find that using lay community health workers (in place of medical providers) can extend the reach of primary prevention programs.

2.2.2 Secondary prevention

According to the World Health Organization [3], secondary prevention for substance use disorders consists of interventions for individuals who are in early stages of substance use, so as to prevent them from developing problematic or harmful patterns. However, the literature on secondary prevention for SUDs demonstrates more varied goals. Nygaard [18] discusses the merits of screening and brief intervention (SBI) at length, and argues that this method should emphasize the motivational aspects of intervention, and should also include social contacts within the field of the intervention, particularly when individuals describe themselves as "social drinkers." As discussed by Trova et al. [19], secondary prevention included counseling and programming for high-risk groups, in order to help them develop alcohol refusal strategies and behavioral and social skills to resist alcohol use. Referrals to substance abuse treatment [20], as well as work with the close relatives of someone with a substance abuse problem [21], were also considered. For young drug users, effective secondary prevention interventions included behavioral therapy, family therapy, general drug treatment, and residential care, particularly when it included culturally sensitive counseling [22].

Secondary prevention can be particularly effective when expanded beyond behavioral health care providers. In their study of trauma patients, Fernandez Mondejar et al. [23] found that hospital emergency units could be important sources of secondary prevention, due to the frequency of serious accidents and injuries that occur to individuals when intoxicated. Another study advocates for secondary prevention in drug courts, as approximately one third of the clients were low risk offenders who did not demonstrate serious substance abuse and could benefit from early intervention [24].

2.2.3 Tertiary prevention

In the literature on tertiary prevention for alcohol and substance use disorders, a few major themes emerge. One is the goal of maximizing normal life functioning for chronic sufferers of dependence; these therapeutic efforts may promote motivation to abstain from alcohol use or support acquisition of new behaviors to modify problem patterns of alcohol consumption. Such efforts may be offered in tandem with mental health treatment or as part of a case management plan [18, 25, 26]. McAnally [27] argues that tertiary prevention must include motivation to avoid substance use as well as reductions of underlying sources of distress in the sufferer's environment; pharmacotherapies for drug dependence are also included here. A few studies also include, as tertiary prevention, attempts to avoid other types of illness that can occur as a result of or in the process of substance use, such as bloodborne viruses among intravenous drug users [28].

Another group of studies describe tertiary prevention as promotion and support for sobriety. Here, the focus is on prevention of an initial relapse, and then on the management of any relapses that do occur [29] - though some question whether complete sobriety, with no relapses, is a realistic goal [30]. There are many different tactics for reducing relapses, including overdose education [27], peer support and therapeutic groups [31], recovery housing [32], cognitive behavioral approaches [33] and mindfulness-based interventions [34–36]. However, not all relapse prevention studies position themselves as tertiary prevention for substance abuse; many treat relapses as a separate health problem.

2.2.4 Prevention in specific cultures and communities

Present across all studies of prevention for alcohol and substance use disorders, whether they are primary, secondary, or tertiary, is a call to tailor interventions to specific populations and their cultural contexts. For example, Greenfield et al. [37] demonstrate that mindfulness-based relapse prevention varies in efficacy among different racial groups; for Whites, it is more effective in preventing heavy drinking relapse than drug use, but the opposite is true for racial and ethnic minorities. Walton, Blow, and Booth [38] found, among their study participants, that African Americans had greater coping skills and self-efficacy than other racial groups, but that their resource needs were greater; this necessitates different relapse prevention strategies. When dealing with diverse populations, intervention and marketing should be offered in multiple languages, and must also include steps to help marginalized communities feel safe from discrimination or criminalization, particularly for their citizenship status or illicit substance use [39]. Several studies address alcohol or substance abuse concerns within indigenous communities, and argue that they are best served by programs that incorporate cultural knowledge and values, and respond to therapeutics that emphasize connection to traditions ([40–42], among others). In summary, it is clear that successful prevention of alcohol and substance abuse requires careful attention to individual and community needs at every point of contact.

These considerations extend to research with Latinx communities, though less has been done to develop rigorous approaches to prevention. While several researchers investigate rates of and contributing factors to alcohol and substance use in Latinx and immigrant populations [43, 44], they do not offer explicit methods or interventions for prevention. Further, existing literature predominantly focuses on drinking and substance use patterns among Latinx adolescents ([45–47], for example). Unsurprisingly, the limited research on prevention also tends to address adolescents, with several that involve Latinx families as a unit [48, 49]. Indeed, those that deal explicitly with prevention in terms of the primary, secondary, and tertiary tiers all target adolescents [50–52]. There is little evidence with which to address these concerns among other Latinx populations, such as adults or migrant workers.

Moreover, though these studies discuss the importance of customizing formal prevention and treatment, none of them consider grassroots interventions. Grassroots interventions such as the *juramento* are culturally and linguistically specific from their inception and need no further adaptations. They are also familiar to the community and do not require any outreach campaigns. As such, they can bring much-needed therapeutic benefits to marginalized and underserved populations.

3. Methods

We draw on our findings from an ongoing qualitative study on the use of the *juramento* among Mexican workers living and working in southeastern Pennsylvania. Scheduled for three years, the study started in 2017, but was interrupted because of COVID-19. This region is home to the country's largest mushroom production site and has experienced Mexican immigration since the mid-1970s. The subsample for this chapter consists of fifteen (15) Mexican immigrants or migrants, all males, who have made *juramentos*, and two priests at a new Catholic church in the region. The Mexican immigrants and migrants are part of a larger sample that includes individuals who have not made a *juramento* but are seeking help at a local Spanish language AA group. The *jurados* ranged in age from 25 to 55 years, with an average age of 34 years. Eight were married; five, single; and two, separated. All except one completed at least nine years of education. Most of the men in the sample are from small *ranchos* or towns in rural regions in the states of Guanajuato and southern states surrounding Mexico City. The Catholic Church has a strong presence spanning centuries in these regions; prominent religious practices in this area include the cargo system, or sponsoring of saint days, recognition of local saint days and Our Lady of Guadalupe on her feast day, and Passover events.

All the participants were selected using purposive sampling and were interviewed using semi-structured interviews. The two priests helped us recruit the fifteen *jurados*. The interviews with the priests centered around the *juramento* process, especially the counseling session; who makes *juramentos* and why; and the perceived benefits of the *juramento* for the individual and family. In keeping with their practice of confidentiality, the priests did not discuss specific *juramento* cases with us. The interviews with the *jurados* solicited basic demographic information, religious background and beliefs, drinking history, including problems associated with drinking, *juramento* history, reasons for making a *juramento* and the perceived benefits from making one, and information of other treatments pursued. Follow-up interviews were conducted if any of the interviews had missing or unclear information. The *jurados* were also administered the Duke Religious Index, or DUREL [53]. It is a five-item measure of religious involvement, developed for use in large cross-sectional and longitudinal observational studies and designed to assess three major dimensions of religiosity: organizational religious activity, non-organizational religious activity, and intrinsic religiosity (or subjective religiosity).

The men's drinking behaviors prior to making their most recent juramento were self-reported, and as such, were not solicited or measured using a diagnostic nosology, such as the Diagnostic and Statistical Manual of Mental Disorders, Fifth Edition (DSM-5). Self-reports have been found to be valid in assessing drinking practices [54, 55]. Based on their self-reports, we categorized their drinking according to one of the following drinking types: binge drinking, heavy drinking, problem drinking, alcohol dependence, and alcohol abuse, as defined by National Institute of Alcohol Abuse and Alcoholism (NIAAA). These are the five drinking types that increase one's risks for harmful consequences, including an alcohol use disorder, or AUD, such as alcohol dependence. In categorizing the men's drinking, we used one or more of the following criteria, as found in the definitions of the five drinking types: frequency of drinking, the amount of alcohol consumed, the intent behind the drinking, and the harm caused by the drinking. According to NIAAA, binge drinking is the consumption of alcohol with the intent to become inebriated. For the men, it was defined as at least five alcoholic drinks in two hours [56]. Heavy drinking is when an individual binge drinks five or more days in the last month [56]. Problem drinking may include binge drinking and heavy drinking and results in accidents, injuries, and other issues resulting from drinking alcohol [57]. Alcohol dependence, or alcoholism, is when an individual loses his or her control over alcohol intake [58]. It is characterized by intense alcohol cravings, high tolerance, and withdrawal symptoms when a person quits using alcohol. Alcohol abuse occurs when a person is not physically dependent upon alcohol, but drinking is resulting in serious health issues and problems at home or work [58]. Alcohol dependence and alcohol abuse are considered alcohol use disorders because they result in chronic relapsing brain disease characterized by compulsive drinking, loss of control over alcohol intake, and a negative emotional state when not using alcohol.

NVivo software was used to code text and to store, sort, and retrieve relevant text generated from questions in the priest and *jurado* semi-structured interviews. The data was coded by two members of the team, at first independently from each other, and later together for consistency. Inductive coding was used to identify themes, especially emerging themes. When coding, we assigned labels to words and phrases that represent important (and recurring) text in each response. A thematic analysis of the coded text was then performed, as is standard in qualitative research. Themes around drinking were developed around the quantity of alcohol consumed, especially prior to making a *juramento*, frequency, and drinking problems that emerged as a consequence. The drinking was then identified and categorized as binge drinking, heavy drinking, problem drinking, alcohol dependence, and alcohol abuse using standard definitions of each type of drinking. The core elements of the *juramento* were also identified and analyzed, as were ad hoc themes related to making a *juramento*, such as religious beliefs and family and community religious practices as shared by the *jurados*, the nature of religious catharsis of the pledge, and examples of the challenges and moral fortitude needed in keeping the promise of abstinence. Recurrent themes were identified in each category as they emerged through repeated review of the textual data. Descriptive reports were prepared around the different themes and subthemes that were used to prepare manuscripts for publication.

4. Findings

Although records are not kept, the priests report that anywhere from 30 to over 50 *juramentos* are made in any given month at our research site. Despite this high number, the *juramento* is not part of the church's structure because, as discussed earlier, it is not recognized by Catholic Church doctrine. Instead, the *juramento* falls under pastoral care—the visiting, counseling, and helping parishioners who are experiencing a difficult hardship. The church where the *juramentos* are made is part of the first national parish for Hispanics of the region's archdiocese. Prior to its construction a decade ago, the Latinx community attended services at local church parishes, and the *juramentos* were made at a nearby Catholic mission for this community, which housed the offices of the priests who looked after the spiritual welfare of the Latinx population and offered social services. This national parish was established to accommodate the rapidly growing Latinx population in the region, which consists primarily of Mexican immigrants and their U.S.-born children, many of whom are now adults with their own children. Puerto Ricans and Guatemalans comprise other significant Latinx groups in the area. The parish serves an estimated 12,000 Latinx parishioners from several local communities.

4.1 The *juramento* process

The *juramento*, as administered at our site, is a highly ritualized brief intervention around a counseling session and the pledge to Our Lady of Guadalupe to abstain from alcohol use. It is a private affair and only includes the priest and the *jurado*, and occasionally a family member who is present to provide support. Unlike a formal brief intervention, such as SAMSHA's Screening, Brief Intervention and Referral to Treatment, or SBIRT [59], it does not include a screening instrument to assess the drinking problem nor a referral to formal treatment [6]. Four general steps are involved in making a *juramento*. It starts with a counseling session with a priest at his office or in private at the church. The purpose of this session is to discuss the individual's drinking and the problems that it creates for him and his family. The severity of drinking is identified through an informal discussion about his behaviors and any resulting problems. Additionally, they discuss the seriousness of making a pledge to Our Lady of Guadalupe, and the importance of seeking additional help. The second step involves determining an abstinence period, usually no more than one year, and preparing an *estampita*, or prayer card. On one side of the card is the image of Our Lady of Guadalupe, and on the other, a *juramento* prayer, which is written as a pledge with the name of the *jurado*, the abstinence period, and the signature of both the *jurado* and the priest. The prayer card is a symbolic contract to enter and keep a sacred pledge. The third step is the reciting of the *juramento* prayer, together with the priest, preferably in front of the image of Our Lady of Guadalupe. The fourth and last step is the *bendición*, the priest's blessing of the *jurado*. There is no follow-up after the intervention. During the abstinence period, the pledge is fortified with prayers to the saint and with regular attendance at mass. The *juramento* is renewable once it is completed and may be repeated as many times as deemed necessary.

The men made *juramentos* not only in southeastern Pennsylvania, but also in Mexico. While living in Mexico, one man traveled to Mexico City to make two *juramentos* at the Chapel of the Juramentos at the Shrine of Our Lady of Guadalupe. Regardless of where they were made, nearly all the *juramentos* were made to this saint. Only two of those made in Mexico were made to a different religious figure—one to El Señior de las Maravillas and the other to El Señor de Chalma. On average, the men each made two *juramentos*, but individually this number ranged from one to five per person. The abstinence periods were from forty days to five years; however, the majority were for a year. Most of the men remained abstinent after completing their *juramento*, some for years, and did not make another until they saw it necessary, either to fend off the temptation to drink or to stop drinking after having resumed. Nearly all completed their *juramentos* - only two *juramentos*, both made in Mexico, were not fulfilled by the *jurados*. In these two cases, the men sought absolution from the priest who performed the *juramento* and made another.

4.2 Drinking behaviors and prevention

The drinking behaviors of the fifteen men in our sample, prior to making a *juramento*, ranged from occasional binge drinking to heavy drinking. In all, three of the men were classified as occasional binge drinkers and three as binge drinkers, eight as heavy drinkers, and one as an alcohol abuser. None suffered from alcohol dependence. We also did not find any problem drinkers, as defined in the literature.

We divided the binge drinkers into two general types—occasional binge drinkers and binge drinkers. Occasional binge drinkers did not binge drink every week. They were social drinkers who engaged in casual drinking with friends and relatives on a weekly basis, usually on the weekends, and who only engaged in binge drinking once or twice a month without doing so again for weeks and months. Unlike the binge drinkers, their intent in drinking was not to get inebriated but to relax and enjoy the moment socially. However, during certain times of the year, such as Christmas or visits to the homeland, occasional binge drinkers would depart from their established drinking pattern and would binge drink in two or more weeks consecutively. Binge drinkers binged every weekend, with a few exceptions. The drinking would start on a Friday night, after work, and continued through Saturday night. The rest of the week they may have a beer or two after work.

DOI: http://dx.doi.org/10.5772/intechopen.95545

4.2.1 Occasional binge drinkers and secondary prevention

The three occasional binge drinkers only made one *juramento*, either for six months or a year. The men fulfilled their *juramentos* and afterwards remained abstinent. Although their binge drinking was infrequent in comparison to the other binge drinkers, occasional binge drinkers sought a *juramento* because they were concerned about their drinking getting out of hand and resulting in problems over time. There was no evidence that they were harming themselves or others with their drinking, but according to them, the potential to do so was there. Notably, the men did not want their drinking to interfere with work and the sending of remittances back home. These monies cover basic needs for their families, such as shelter, food, and medicine. The money transfers are also used to build a house or start a small business, such as a small general store in the neighborhood or a food eatery, and to invest in the education of their children.

Miguel (pseudonym), an immigrant worker in his thirties from the state of Mexico, is one of the occasional binge drinkers. He is married with four children, all of whom live with him locally. Miguel has 10 siblings: half live in Mexico, and half in the United States. Miguel left Mexico in his late twenties because he could not find gainful employment there. Although he lives in Pennsylvania with his immediate family, Miguel continues to send remittances to his parents on a regular basis.

Miguel only made one *juramento* and is currently fulfilling it. It was made in Pennsylvania. He made the *juramento* for a few reasons, not just one. One of them was his concern about his increased drinking over time. Although he did not drink every week, as do some of his co-workers, he felt that his drinking was getting out of hand. Every time he drank socially, his drinking was no longer limited to a beer or two, as it was when he first started drinking. Miguel had two other major concerns: one was his temptation to drink when he was around others who were indulging, and the other was his general health. He was a diabetic, and he knew that alcohol was not good for him.

Prior to making a *juramento*, Miguel tried several times to stop drinking on his own, but after two or three months, he would return to drinking. After making the *juramento*, this was no longer the case. He now is two months shy of completing it. Miguel credits Our Lady of Guadalupe for his abstinence. In his words,

> *I have always believed in the Virgen of Guadalupe, since I was a child. I have faith in others, other saints, but since I can remember, my mother always had her virgincitas, as is customary. You can say that she is my preferred saint. I always entrust myself to the Virgen of Guadalupe.*

Our Lady of Guadalupe provided him with the necessary strength to abstain. She was present during temptation, as he shared. He used his *juramento* prayer card for strength and to ward off peer pressure to drink. As he puts it,

> *Sometimes, I would have to tell them that I am jurado [under the pledge to Our Lady of Guadalupe] ... If they did not believe me, I would show them my card. I always carry the virgincita with me.*

For Miguel and the two other occasional binge drinkers, it is possible that their *juramentos* contributed to prevention, although more research on the causality between making a *juramento* and prevention is needed. We discuss the need for additional research on this subject later in chapter. The men were already exhibiting early symptoms of harmful drinking, but not signs of heavy drinking or worse. No screening instrument is used in the *juramento* process to determine whether their drinking is harmful or not; the two priests in our sample hold the *juramento* counseling sessions and employ a variation of motivational interviewing to get the men to reflect on their drinking and to consider making changes. The men reach their own conclusions about their drinking and choose what type of help they desire. Risk factors for more serious alcohol use were also identified in the session and discussed. The resulting *juramento* gives them strength to remain abstinent for months, if not years, which is a major goal in achieving sobriety and recovery. The abstinence period may serve to stop the progression of the men's drinking from occasional binge drinking to heavy drinking. During their hiatus from drinking, the men learn that there is another way of living. Instead of drinking or spending time fighting the urge to drink, they focus on themselves and their families, return to their religious convictions, and reaffirm their place in the larger community.

4.2.2 Heavy drinkers, alcohol abusers, and tertiary prevention

The heavy drinkers in our sample made more than one *juramento*, and not always consecutively. Some made a *juramento* immediately after completing one, while others would remain abstinent for months or years before making another. *Juramentos* were made as needed. The heavy drinkers, including the one individual who was abusing alcohol, exhibited evidence of tertiary prevention benefits of the *juramento*—mainly slowing the progression of harmful drinking. The drinking of these men was beyond the level of the occasional binge drinkers, and they were no longer showing early signs of harmful drinking. They were already exhibiting a serious drinking problem, and as such they were outside of the realm of secondary prevention benefits.

Juan Manuel (pseudonym), a migrant in his fifties from the State of Hidalgo, near Mexico City, is one of the heavy drinkers in our sample. He is separated from his wife and has five adult children who live in the same community. Like the other *jurados* in our sample, Juan Manuel is from a rural region with a depressed economy, and like many men there, he migrates to the United States to work. He migrates as needed and periodically spends months and years away from Mexico.

Juan Manuel started drinking at a young age. By the age of 18, he was already binge drinking, and by his twenties, he was drinking heavily when he could afford to buy alcohol. Juan Manuel made his first *juramento* in his thirties, after seeking help with Alcoholics Anonymous in his hometown for five months. He wanted to stop drinking because he was having problems at home. The *juramento* was made at the Chapel of Juramentos at the Shrine of Our Lady of Guadalupe, during a pilgrimage on her feast day. He remembers the counseling session with the priest there, especially the questioning about his commitment to fulfilling the pledge. The second *juramento* was also made there after another pilgrimage, four months after he had completed the first. The abstinence period was for five years. This length of abstinence is unusual, but the priest at the chapel allowed him to make a *juramento* for this time period because Juan Manuel had successfully completed his first one. He chose to make a 5-year *juramento* because he was planning to migrate to the United States for work, and he did not want his drinking to interfere with his stay abroad. Juan Manuel completed the *juramento* while in the United States and did not drink again for another year. However, he resumed drinking again when he returned home and discovered that his wife had been cheating on him while he was away. Six months later, he made his third and last *juramento* in his hometown; it was for one year. Since his last *juramento* he has not consumed alcohol and has no desire to do so.

Luis (pseudonym), also a migrant worker in his fifties, and from a state adjacent to Juan Manuel's home state, is the only one in our sample whose drinking was determined to qualify as alcohol abuse. He is married with four children, all of whom live in Mexico. Luis is an experienced migrant worker who has spent many years working elsewhere in Mexico and the United States. Luis provides for his family by sending remittances on a regular basis.

Luis' drinking trajectory was like Juan Manuel's. He, too, started drinking at a young age and was drinking heavily in his 20s before making his first *juramento*. In all, he has made five: three in Mexico and two in Pennsylvania. Luis made his first *juramento* in his twenties, as Juan Manuel did. The pledge was for a year and a half and was made because his drinking was disrupting his home life. Luis would miss work and lose his employment, and consequently, his family was left in dire straits. He made four other *juramentos*—the second for one year, the third for five years, and the fourth for a year, as was his fifth and last. Like Juan Manuel, Luis made the five-year *juramento* because he was planning to migrate to the United States, and he did not want his alcohol consumption to interfere with work and with his ability to save enough money to construct a house for his family in Mexico. He completed this lengthy *juramento* in the United States, and a year later made another after he started drinking again. At the time of the interview for the study, he had just made his fifth *juramento*.

For Juan Manuel and the other heavy drinkers, including Luis, who were already engaged in harmful drinking and at risk for alcohol dependence, the *juramento* may have played a role in preventing it from occurring. It may have kept them from causing further harm to themselves and their families. In Luis's case, he made several *juramentos* to maintain sobriety over time. These men underwent the same counseling session with the priest as did Miguel and the other occasional binge drinkers. The session did not target them as heavy drinkers in danger of suffering from alcohol dependence, but it did focus on the particulars of their drinking. The priests are not familiar with the different types of harmful drinking, as defined by the NIAAA, and so do not apply such classifications. Like all the counseling sessions, the motivational interviewing centered around getting the men to think of the many perils of their drinking and to consider taking action to change their lives. Moreover, as in the case of Miguel and the other occasional binge drinkers, the abstinence made possible by the *juramento* may have kept the men's drinking from progressing during the *juramento,* and in some cases, for months or years of the post-*juramento* period. It provided them with the necessary time to reflect and work on their drinking.

5. Discussion

Our study suggests that the *juramento* may only be beneficial to those who are religious and turn to their beliefs when troubled. The DUREL scores of all the men were high across the three major dimensions of religiosity: organizational religious activity, non-organizational religious activity, and intrinsic religiosity (or subjective religiosity). The DUREL has an overall score range from 5 to 27, and men's score ranged from 26 to 27. All are devout to their faith, and in particular, to Our Lady of Guadalupe. They practice a religion, Catholicism, that teaches that one is never alone in life and that the saints are always present to help. Crucially, sinners are not excluded from this divine assistance, which means that they can always turn to the saints, even if they feel ashamed or embarrassed to seek help from other people. They were taught this at an early age as children and are reminded of it daily in their communities in Mexico and the United States.

The men's religiosity is of no surprise when their religious backgrounds are considered. All were raised in a religious household where Catholicism was an integral part of daily life. Their childhood homes had altars devoted to Our Lady of

Guadalupe and other saints. The altars, as they explained, were sacred spaces for reflection, prayer, and paying homage to saints. Their families regularly attended church and observed the different feast days of the saints and other religious events. As children and adolescents, the *jurados* attended catechism and learned about Catholic doctrine, and completed the Sacraments of Initiation, such as baptism, confirmation, and the Eucharist. The Sacrament of Penance, or confession, was also commonplace. Some were not always devoted to their faith during their adolescence or later in life, especially when drinking, but they never strayed far from their religious beliefs.

Although the *juramento* is not a formal public health intervention, it goes beyond just facilitating abstinence. It may also result in secondary and tertiary prevention, stopping the progression of the men's drinking. In our sample, the *juramento* may have kept occasional binge drinkers from becoming heavy drinkers and heavy drinkers from becoming alcohol dependent. None of the men were in this drinking category before making their *juramento*. Consequently, we did not get an opportunity to see if the *juramento* also served as an intervention with prevention benefits for those suffering from alcohol dependence, i.e., whether it kept men with alcohol dependence from continuing to drink. However, research shows that abstinence is unlikely to be successful for individuals who already meet the criteria for dependence without some type of formal treatment. This kind of drinker may need more attention than what the *juramento* can provide for achieving abstinence and preventing a return to drinking.

To grasp how the *juramento* intrinsically works and how it could result in secondary and tertiary prevention, you must understand the sacred pledge and dyadic relationship entered with Our Lady of Guadalupe. It starts early in the juramento process, during the making of the vow to Our Lady of Guadalupe. As a 34-year-old immigrant makes clear, she is at the center of the *juramento*:

> *"You keep the pledge because you made it to the virgin, and for Mexicans and Catholics the virgin is like your mother. And not keeping a promise to the virgin is like not keeping a promise to your mother. You value and respect your mother". ... "this is the power of the juramento, when you are truly committed to changing and have strength in your faith ...".*

This saint is the symbolic mother of all Mexicans, including those living abroad. Mothers are revered in Mexican culture and society. In fact, the two most important celebrations in the country are December 12, the feast day of Our Lady of Guadalupe, and May 10th, Mother's Day. The importance of Our Lady of Guadalupe in Mexican life is obvious to the faithful and is not reserved for only the *juramento*. It is believed that she intercedes on their behalf and are close enough to God to prompt an intercession with a difficult problem, including granting a miracle when needed.

The vow made to Our Lady of Guadalupe reconnects the *jurados* to their faith and results in a powerful, religious-based catharsis. It sets the right frame of mind for recovery. The *juramento* creates a sense of hope in both the *jurado* and his family that the drinking will stop, as will the problems that come with it. The men shared that it releases them from shame of drinking and the harm committed to others, and in turn, gives them hope for turning their lives around and gaining lost respect in their families and communities. Further, this spiritual awakening allows them to reconcile with their church, religion, and ultimately God, which they were estranged from because of their drinking. Feeling unworthy of God's grace, they had distanced themselves from their religious beliefs. Now, the men have a renewed sense of worthiness in the eyes of God.

The juramento also gives the *jurados* the necessary fortitude to keep their vows and abstain from alcohol use. The men are no longer alone in dealing with their drinking problem. Instead, the *jurado* now has divine support, and with it, the necessary fortitude to abstain from alcohol use and to work on his drinking problem. From this, he draws the strength to change his life and to atone for the harms committed to self and others. Once a juramento is made, there is an additional moral obligation to subordinate one's drinking indulgences to one's commitments to the saint and God. According to the men, not keeping a vow is a sin. A broken vow is an affront to Our Lady of Guadalupe and God. In light of this, the *jurado* tries his best to persevere in his abstinence because he fears committing an ultimate offense in his religion.

Some benefits are more tangible. Once a *juramento* is made, the *jurado's* reputation is at stake, as is his trustworthiness within his family, community, and church. He knows that he must keep the vow, or risk social as well as divine consequences. The *estampita*, or prayer card, contributes to his resolve: for example, during moments of weakness, reciting the *juramento* prayer on the card helps the men resist temptation. Prayer reminds the men that our Lady of Guadalupe is looking after them, and that they are not alone. It gives them strength. The *estampita* also helps to control peer pressure to drink. When friends offer them a drink, the men reply that they are not drinking because they have made a *juramento* and show their prayer card. In these situations, the *estampita* serves as a credential, a form of proof. It proves that the men are telling the truth and obligates others to respect the *jurado*'s promise.

There is a general debate in the substance abuse field regarding whether sobriety alone results in the life changes needed to stop drinking overtime or whether it needs to be combined with treatment to achieve recovery. Sobriety is often defined as the continued state of being sober, i.e., not drinking, while according to SAMHSA [60], recovery is "a process of change through which individuals improve their health and wellness, live self-directed lives and strive to reach their full potential." Some argue that without additional treatment and/or participation in 12-step meetings, such as those in Alcohol Anonymous, you will not be able to start the journey of recovery or develop a healthy mind, sound body, and supportive relationships. Treatment involves identifying and working on the causes of your harmful drinking. You need to know yourself, understand your true persona, and recognize behaviors that may have contributed to your drinking. Knowing who you are and understanding why you drank may also help you to discover personal strengths that can help in your recovery. Not addressing this will just make you a "dry drunk," an expression used in AA to refer to an individual who is not drinking but is not addressing behaviors and the problems of the past that contributed to harmful drinking.

Our study did not address recovery *per se*, but the findings indicate that the men are making changes in their lives, and they are doing this without treatment. This is distinctly significant to a population that has little or no access to formal health resources. None of the men in our study sought treatment or attended AA meetings after making the *juramento*, as the priest suggested during the *juramento*'s counseling session. While this may be the result of multiple contributing factors, one clear reason is that no alcohol treatment programs exist that are affordable, within a reasonable driving distance, and culturally and linguistically appropriate for Mexican and other Latinx immigrants. Formal treatment is simply not available to this population, in this region.

Nonetheless, there is evidence that, with the divine intervention of Our Lady of Guadalupe, the men are not only staying sober, they are also working on their recovery. The power of religion cannot be underestimated: research has found that the lack of a spiritual or religious connection contributes to the escalation of substance misuse [61]. These men demonstrate some of the four indicators of recovery that accompanied the above definition: 1) addressing problems as they happen, without using, and without getting stressed out; 2) having at least one person he can be completely honest with; 3) having personal boundaries; and 4) taking time to restore physical and emotional states when not tired [60]. Their recovery is not based on a personal catharsis reached in treatment, but on a religious catharsis. This special relationship with Our Lady of Guadalupe enhances the men's coping, confers hope for the future, and provides a heightened sense of control, security, and stability. When asked about how the *juramento* has changed their lives, the men are quick to respond that it has improved their social ties and outlook on life; they no longer feel alone in their quest to live alcohol-free. The *jurados* severed unhealthy relationships, especially with those who continue to drink, and reconnected with family. These renewed bonds, in addition to newly established friendships with others in the community, become important sources of support. Healthier thinking and a new way of living prevails. For example, they try not to be consumed by problems that arise at home or at work, especially those that they cannot do anything about. Prayer helps. Some of the men returned to the church and are learning how to trust again and become part of a larger community. Reconnecting to their religion, through the *juramento*, makes a difference.

6. Limitations

Despite its contributions, our chapter has limitations. The primary objective of our qualitative study was to examine the *juramento* as practiced in a single region to understand how it is used to curtail harmful drinking in the Latinx community. We generated data that allowed us to characterize the *juramento*, how it is made, who makes it, why, and how it works. Prevention was not one of the larger aims, but our data also allowed us to address its potential prevention benefits. More research is needed on this subject if we are to understand the *juramento's* contributions to prevention. In particular, we need to focus on some of the findings presented in the chapter. And as such, more attention needs to be paid to how the *juramento* prevents the men's drinking from progressing, by looking closer at the duration of the *juramentos*, the number of *juramentos* made and the reasons for making more than one, and the time period between the *juramentos*. Specifically, attention should be paid to the abstinence periods between *juramentos*, and how abstinence was achieved, including how the different components of the *juramento* contributed to abstinence. We also need to consider if the *juramento* alone is responsible for bringing about this change or if other social factors also contribute, such as the need to meet family responsibilities in the United States and Mexico. Additionally, our sample only included men who had just made a *juramento* or were abstinent after completing one. It did not include individuals who did not complete their juramento or were drinking again after completing one. These individuals must also be included in the research. Prevention benefits, such as stronger marital and family relations and gainful employment, should also be considered. These inquiries will require going beyond an ethnographic and cross-sectional study such as ours and launching a longitudinal study. Cross-sectional studies do not provide definite information about cause-and-effect relationships because such studies focus on a single moment in time; they do not consider what happens before or after that moment.

7. Conclusions

For decades now, public health has called for the development of cultural and linguistically appropriate prevention and treatment programs for alcohol and substance use. It realizes that there is a need for these programs in the country's increasingly diverse population, especially in regions with concentrations of immigrants, migrants, and refugees. For the most part, this same campaign has overlooked grassroots interventions for these health problems. The *juramento* is one of several grassroots interventions for alcohol and substance use in Latinx communities, which include *anexos*, or 24-hour AA groups, *grupos de cuarto y quinto pasos*, or fourth and fifth step AA groups, and *curanderismo*, or traditional medicine [1]. Like the *juramento*, they are organic, arising from within the community, and they consider cultural traditions and beliefs and language as it is practiced daily. Latinx immigrants have introduced these grassroots interventions to the United States not necessarily because they are trying to recreate as much as possible of their homeland culture in new lands, but because there is a need for them in their U.S. communities. Because of their immigrant status in a country whose federal and state governments are increasing limiting services to all immigrants, they have limited government-sponsored health care and nearly no access to formal alcohol and substance use treatments [1, 62]. For Latinx immigrants, grassroots interventions such as the *juramento* are the only source of help for harmful drinking. Attention to such grassroots practices in public health can support the ways that they already provide care to marginalized populations and help connect the interventions with those who need them.

Author details

Victor Garcia[1,3]*, Katherine Fox[2], Emily Lambert[1] and Alex Heckert[1,4]

1 Mid-Atlantic Research and Training Institute for Community and Behavioral Health, Indiana University of Pennsylvania, Indiana, PA, USA

2 Department of Anthropology, Southern Methodist University, Dallas, TX, USA

3 Department of Anthropology, Indiana University of Pennsylvania, Indiana, PA, USA

4 Department of Sociology, Indiana University of Pennsylvania, Indiana, PA, USA

*Address all correspondence to: vgarcia@iup.edu

References

[1] Garcia V, Lambert E, Fox K, Heckert D, Pinchi NH. Grassroots interventions for alcohol use disorders in the Mexican immigrant community: A narrative literature review. J Ethn Subs Abuse. 2020;6:1-20. Available from: https://doi.org/10.1080/15332640.2020.1803781.

[2] Murrary DM, Villani J, Vargas AJ, Lee JA, Myles RL, Wu J, et al. NIH primary and secondary prevention research in humans during 2012-2017. Am J Prev Med. 2018;55(6):915-925.

[3] WHO, UNDCP. *Primary prevention of substance abuse: A workbook for project operators*. World Health Organization. 2000. Available from: https://www.who.int/substance_abuse/activities/global_initiative/en/primary_prevention_17.pdf.

[4] Garcia V, Gonzalez L. Juramentos and mandas: Traditional Catholic practices and substance abuse in Mexican communities of Southeastern Pennsylvania. NAPA Bulletin. 2009;31(1):47-63. Available from: https://doi.org/1111/j.1556-4797.2009.01018.x.

[5] Cuadrado M, Lieberman L. The Virgin of Guadalupe as an ancillary modality for treating Hispanic substance abusers: Juramentos in the United States. Journal of Religion and Health. 2011;50(4):922-930.

[6] Garcia V, Heckert DA, Lambert E, Hidalgo Pinchi N. Using the juramento as a brief AUD intervention for Mexican immigrant farmworkers. *Hispanic Health Care International*. 2020.

[7] Ridenour TA, Stormshak EA. Introduction and rationale for individualized substance abuse prevention from an ontogenetic perspective. Am J Drug Alcohol Abuse. 2009;35(4):206-208.

[8] Moulahoum H, Zihnioglu F, Timur S, Coskunol H. Novel technologies in detection, treatment and prevention of substance use disorders. J Food Drug Anal. 2019;27(1):22-31.

[9] Volkow ND, Li T. Drugs and alcohol: Treating and preventing abuse, addiction and their medical consequences. Pharmacol Ther. 2005;108(1):3-17.

[10] Peterson NA, Reid RJ. Paths to psychological empowerment in urban community: Sense of community and citizen participation in substance abuse prevention activities. Journal of Community Psychology. 2003;31(1).

[11] Brooks MJ, Marshal MP, McCauley HL, Douaihy A, Miller E. The relationship between hope and adolescent likelihood to endorse substance use behaviors in a sample of marginalized youth. Substance Use & Misuse. 2016;51(13):1815-1819.

[12] D'Amico EJ, McCarthy DM. Escalation and initiation of younger adolescents' substance use: The impact of perceived peer use. Journal of Adolescent Health. 2006;39(4):481-487.

[13] Salazar AM, Noell B, Cole JJ, Haggerty KP, Roe S. Incorporating self-determination into substance abuse prevention programming for youth transitioning from foster care to adulthood. Child & Family Social Work. 2018;23(2):281-288.

[14] Low NC, Lee SS, Johnson JG, Williams JB, Harris ES. The association between anxiety and alcohol versus cannabis abuse disorders among adolescents in primary care settings. Family practice. 2008;25(5):321-327.

[15] Jiang S, Wu L, Gao X. Beyond face-to-face individual counseling: A systematic review on alternative

modes of motivational interviewing in substance abuse treatment and prevention. Addict Behav. 2017;73:216-235.

[16] Hopson L, Wodarski J, Tang N. The effectiveness of electronic approaches to substance abuse prevention for adolescents. J Evid Inf Soc Work. 2015;12(3):310-322.

[17] Mutamba BB, van Ginneken N, Smith Paintain L, Wandiembe S, Schellenberg D. Roles and effectiveness of lay community health workers in the prevention of mental, neurological and substance use disorders in low and middle income countries: A systematic review. BMC Health Services Research. 2013;13(412):1-11.

[18] Nygaard P. Focus on secondary prevention: Implications of a study on intervention in social networks. Substance Use & Misuses. 2006;41(13):1719-1733.

[19] Trova AC, Paparrigopoulos T, Ginieri-Coccossis M. Prevention of alcohol dependence. Psychiatriki. 2015;26(2):131-140.

[20] Kagle JD. Secondary prevention of substance abuse. Social Work. 1987;32(5):446-448.

[21] Orford J. Empowering family and friends: A new approach to the secondary prevention of addiction. Drug and Alcohol Review. 1994;13(4):417-429.

[22] Elliott L, Orr L, Watson L, Jackson A. How effective are secondary prevention interventions for young drug users? Family Therapy. 2005;32(1):15-30.

[23] Fernandez Mondejar E, Guerrero Lopez F, Quintana M, Alted E, Minambres E, Salinas Gabina I, et al. Secondary prevention of alcohol and/or drug abuse in trauma patients: Results of a national survey in Spain. Med Intensiva. 2009;33(7):321-326.

[24] DeMatteo DS, Marlowe DB, Festinger DS. Secondary prevention services for clients who are low risk in drug court: A conceptual model. Crime & Delinquency. 2006;52(1):114-134.

[25] DiClemente CC. Prevention and harm reduction for chemical dependency: A process perspective. Clinical Psychology Review. 1999;19(4):473-486.

[26] Carroll JFX, Tanneberger MA, Monti TC. A tertiary prevention strategy for drug-dependent clients completing residential treatment. Alcoholism Treatment Quarterly. 1998;16(3):51-61.

[27] McAnally HB. Addressing host factors: Primary, secondary, and tertiary prevention of opioid dependence. Opioid Dependence. 2018:265-290.

[28] Treloar C, Laybutt B, Carruthers S. Using mindfulness to develop health education strategies for blood borne virus prevention in injecting drug use. *Drugs: Education,* Prevention & Policy. 2010;17(4):431-442.

[29] Marlatt GA, Witkiewitz K. Relapse prevention for alcohol and drug problems. In: Marlatt A, Donovan DM. (eds.). *Relapse prevention: Maintenance strategies in the treatment of addictive behaviors*. New York, New York: The Guilford Press; 2005. p.1-44.

[30] Van Heeringen KC. The prevention of drug abuse – state of the art and directions for future actions. J Toxicol Clin Toxicol. 1995;33(6):575-579.

[31] Levy MS. Listening to our clients: The prevention of relapse. Journal of Psychoactive Drugs. 2008:167-172.

[32] Jason LA, Olson BD, Ferrari JR, Majer JM, Alvarez J, Stout J. An

examination of main and interactive effects of substance abuse recovery housing on multiple indicators of adjustment. Addiction. 2007;102(7):1114-1121.

[33] Schonfeld L, Dupree LW, Dickson-Fuhrmann E, Royer CM, McDermott CH, Rosansky JS, et al. Cognitive-behavioral treatment of older veterans with substance abuse problems. Journal of Geriatric Psychiatry and Neurology. 2000;13(3):124-129.

[34] Bowen S, Chawla N, Collins SE, Witkiewitz K, Hsu S, Grow J, et al. Mindfulness-based relapse prevention for substance use disorders: A pilot efficacy trial. Substance Abuse. 2009;30(4):295-305.

[35] Witkiewitz K, Bowen S. Depression, craving, and substance use following a randomized trial of mindfulness-based relapse prevention. Journal of Consulting and Clinical Psychology. 2010;78(3):362-374.

[36] Amaro H. Implementing mindfulness-based relapse prevention in diverse populations: Challenges and future directions. Substance Use & Misuse. 2014;49(5):612-616.

[37] Greenfield BL, Roos C, Hagler KJ, Stein E, Bowen S, Witkiewitz KA. Race/ethnicity and racial group composition moderate the effectiveness of mindfulness-based relapse prevention for substance use disorder. Addict Behav. 2018;81:96-103.

[38] Walton MA, Blow FC, Booth BM. Diversity in relapse prevention needs: Gender and race comparisons among substance abuse treatment patients. Am J Drug Alcohol Abuse. 2001;27(2):225-240.

[39] Kearney M, Reynolds L, Blitzstein S, Chapin K, Massey P. Primary prevention of prescription drug misuse among culturally and linguistically diverse suburban communities. Journal of Community Health. 2019;44(2):238-248.

[40] Patchell BA, Robbins LK, Lowe JA, Hoke MM. The effect of a culturally tailored substance abuse prevention intervention with Plains Indian adolescents. Journal of Cultural Diversity. 2015;22(2):3-8.

[41] Kelley A, Witzel M, Fatupaito B. A review of tribal best practices in substance abuse prevention. Journal of Ethnicity in Substance Abuse. 2019;18(3):462-475.

[42] Straits KJ, deMaria J, Tafoya N. Place of strength: Indigenous artists and indigenous knowledge is prevention science. Am J Community Psychol. 2019;64(1-2):96-106.

[43] Cox RB, Roblyer MZ, Merten MJ, Shreffler KM, Schwerdtfeger KL. Do parent–child acculturation gaps affect early adolescent Latino alcohol use? A study of the probability and extent of use. Substance Abuse Treatment, Prevention, and Policy. 2013 Dec 1;8(1):4.

[44] Castro FG, Stein JA, Bentler PM. Ethnic pride, traditional family values, and acculturation in early cigarette and alcohol use among Latino adolescents. The Journal of Primary Prevention. 2009 Jul 1;30(3-4):265-292.

[45] Lac A, Unger JB, Basáñez T, Ritt-Olson A, Soto DW, Baezconde-Garbanati L. Marijuana use among Latino adolescents: Gender differences in protective familial factors. Substance Use & Misuse. 2011 Mar 15;46(5):644-55.

[46] Marsiglia FF, Miles BW, Dustman P, Sills S. Ties that protect: An ecological perspective on Latino/a urban pre-adolescent drug use. Journal of Ethnic

and Cultural Diversity in Social Work. 2002 Sep 1;11(3-4):191-220.

[47] Lorenzo-Blanco EI, Schwartz SJ, Unger JB, Zamboanga BL, Des Rosiers SE, Baezconde-Garbanati L, Huang S, Villamar JA, Soto D, Pattarroyo M. Alcohol use among recent immigrant Latino/a youth: acculturation, gender, and the Theory of Reasoned Action. Ethnicity & health. 2016 Nov 1;21(6):609-27.

[48] Cervantes R, Goldbach J, Santos SM. Familia Adelante: A multi-risk prevention intervention for Latino families. The journal of primary prevention. 2011 Aug 1;32(3-4):225.

[49] Szapocznik J, editor. A Hispanic-Latino Family Approach to Substance Abuse Prevention. DIANE Publishing; 1998.

[50] Jurkovic GJ, Kuperminc G, Perilla J, Murphy A, Ibañez G, Casey S. Ecological and ethicalperspectives on filial responsibility: Implications for primary prevention with immigrant Latino adolescents. Journal of Primary Prevention. 2004 Sep 1;25(1):81-104.

[51] Marsiglia FF, Ayers S, Gance-Cleveland B, Mettler K, Booth J. Beyond primary prevention of alcohol use: A culturally specific secondary prevention program for Mexican heritage adolescents. Prevention Science. 2012 Jun 1;13(3):241-251.

[52] Shetgiri R, Kataoka S, Lin H, Flores G. A randomized, controlled trial of a school-based intervention to reduce violence and substance use in predominantly Latino high school students. Journal of the National Medical Association. 2011 Sep 1;103(9-10):932-940.

[53] Koenig, H.G.; Büssing, A. The Duke University Religion Index (DUREL): A Five-Item Measure for Use in Epidemiological Studies. Religions. 2010, *1*, 78-85.

[54] Del Boca, F.K. and Darkes, J. The validity of self-reports of alcohol consumption: state of the science and challenges for research. Addiction. 2003; 98: 1-12. https://doi.org/10.1046/j.1359-6357.2003.00586.x

[55] Solbergsdottir, E., Bjornsson, G., Gudmundsson, L.S., Tyrfingsson, T., & Kristinsson, J. (2004) Validity of Self-Reports and Drug Use Among Young People Seeking Treatment for Substance Abuse or Dependence, Journal of Addictive Diseases, 23:1, 29-38, DOI: 10.1300/J069v23n01_03

[56] National Institute on Alcohol Abuse and Alcoholism. *Drinking levels defined* [Internet]. (no date). Available from: https://www.niaaa.nih.gov/alcohol-health/overview-alcohol-consumption/moderate-binge-drinking

[57] Editorial Staff. *Problem drinking vs. alcoholism* [Internet]. 2020. Available from: https://www.alcohol.org/alcoholism/or-is-it-just-a-problem/

[58] National Institute on Alcohol Abuse and Alcoholism. *Alcohol use disorder: A comparison between DSM-IV and DSM-5* [Internet]. 2020. Available from: https://www.niaaa.nih.gov/publications/brochures-and-fact-sheets/alcohol-use-disorder-comparison-between-dsm

[59] SAMHSA. *Screening, brief intervention, and referral to treatment (SBIRT)* [Internet]. 2017. Available from: https://www.samhsa.gov/sbirt/

[60] SAMHSA. *National and Regional Resources, Region VIII* [Internet]. 2014. Available from: https://www.samhsa.gov/sites/default/files/samhsa-recovery-5-6-14.pdf

[61] National Center on Addiction and Substance Abuse. *So help me god: Substance abuse, religion and spirituality*.

The National Center on Addiction and Substance Abuse (CASA) at Columbia University. 2001.

[62] Pagano A. Barriers to drug abuse treatment for Latino migrants: Treatment providers' perspectives. Journal of Ethnicity in Substance Abuse. 2014;13(3):273-287.

Chapter 3

Sex Differences between Young Adults in the Czech and Slovak Republics in the Relationship between Alcohol-Related Consequences and Depression

Beata Gavurova, Martin Rigelsky and Viera Ivankova

Abstract

In general, the Czech and Slovak Republic are among the countries with increased alcohol consumption. It is clear that increased consumption can predict the occurrence of negative consequences that may subsequently be associated with various mental disorders. One of these mental disorders is depression, which is common in young adults and brings difficulties into their lives that can turn into problems in the future. The study examined the relationship between alcohol-related consequences and depressive symptoms in a sample of university students from the Czech and Slovak Republics in order to map the situation in these regions, where this problem is still ignored (n = 2514; CZE = 47.5%). The research included data from standardized questionnaires, namely the Young Adult Alcohol Consequences Questionnaire (YAACQ), which can predict alcohol use problems, and Health Questionnaire of depression (PHQ-9). The data was collected during the COVID-19 pandemic. Regarding sex differences, a higher YAACQ score was found in males and, conversely, a higher PHQ-9 score was identified in females. The results of correlation and regression analyses revealed significant associations between the scores in the individual YAACQ subscales and the PHQ-9 score, while low to moderate correlations were found in most cases. In all cases, positive trajectories were identified, meaning that the increased risk of depressive disorder can be associated with experience in selected dimensions of alcohol-related consequences. Stronger associations occurred in females than in males. In terms of practical implications, high priority was given to prevention programs and counseling. Professionals' efforts to help young people should be sex-oriented, while females were more vulnerable to depression, males were prone to the consequences of alcohol use.

Keywords: alcohol addiction, patterns of unhealthy behavior, depression, youth, sex, mental health inequalities, Czech and Slovak students

1. Introduction

The importance of mental health is irrefutable in the lives of individuals as well as in society. Evidence supports the fact that there is no health without mental health, as neuropsychiatric disorders such as depression, alcohol and substance use disorders significantly contribute to the global disease burden [1]. Many studies point to a considerable burden of these disorders in all aspects of society, including individuals, their families, workplaces and also the wider economy [2]. On this basis, mental health should not be overlooked, and it is considered important to know its main factors in different population groups. In this sense, depressive disorder and alcohol-related consequences can be considered as two of these risk factors for mental health. Depression is one of the most common mental disorders, and research into alcohol use and its consequences for depressive symptoms can provide useful information to clinicians and professionals. Therefore, the presented research examined the relationship between alcohol-related consequences and perceived depression in the Czech and Slovak young population with sex differentiation.

Alcohol problems at risk of addiction are considered a significant threat and need to be examined in the socio-economic dimension, including education. Sex differences are equally important in examining the community and its inclination to addictive substances. The present time has changed not only the economic but also the legal status of females, thus removing social barriers to their alcohol consumption. As a result, the number of females consuming alcoholic beverages as well as addicted females has significantly increased [3]. There are many reasons to take into account sex differences and specificities in services for addicted females or females at risk of addiction [4], as evidenced by the findings on hospitalizations of males and females in the member states of the European Union (EU) [3]. In any case, it can be considered important to examine this problem, it can also contribute to knowledge in the diagnostic issues of addiction.

There are many international studies examining the variables predicting alcohol use problems in young adults, while depression and sex differentiation have also played an important role in their research [5]. According to their findings, university students often reported depressed mood and alcohol problems. Attention should be paid to any signal that may be related to the problematic drinking and mental disorder of young people. In any case, Slovak and Czech students are no exception to this problem. The knowledge of this issue enables the implementation of active prevention programs that would eliminate the level of addiction in suffering people, or help prevent the emergence of others. The earlier the addiction is treated, the higher the chance of successful abstinence of the individual.

2. Alcohol-related consequences and depressive disorder as risk factors in the lives of young adults

The presented study focused on alcohol-related consequences predicting alcohol use problems, which can lead to a depressed mood in university students. The purpose of the study was to present the alcohol-depression topic in specific geographical regions, to map the situation in these regions and to emphasize the problem at a professional and practical level.

The intensity of alcohol consumption in individual countries is often conditioned by several aspects, while it still remains true that the Slovak Republic is at the forefront of alcohol consumption among OECD countries and alcohol consumption in the Czech Republic is more moderate [6]. Alcohol consumption does not necessarily indicate directly the consequences of drinking, at least in the short term. At this point, it should be noted that the relationship between alcohol use and alcohol-related consequences is not entirely trivial. In this regard, there is evidence of a similar likelihood of reporting negative alcohol-related consequences at both low and higher levels of alcohol consumption [7]. There are many factors that can play an important role in drinking patterns with consequences. As stated by Rehm and Room [8], the cultural aspect is a determinant of alcohol consumption, while it is possible to speak of differences in the perception of acceptable level of alcohol consumption, up to the level of severity of negative alcohol-related behavior. This study focuses on the consequences of alcohol drinking in young adults, as they are a vulnerable group that may have very noticeable consequences. Several authors [9] attribute to this group an inclination to various types of risky behavior (consequences) associated with alcohol use, from reduced academic performance, through unprotected sex to violent and aggressive behavior. Alcohol consumption alone does not capture these important aspects that are part of problem drinking with the risk of addiction. On the other hand, it was supported that the instrument capturing the consequences of drinking (YAACQ) is also able to predict drinking patterns [10] and to assess the level of drinking risk in university students [11]. This is evidenced by the associations between the YAACQ outcomes and drinking outcomes [12]. These facts offer new opportunities for research into alcohol addiction across the population. The consequences of alcohol use can be a concomitant phenomenon of problem drinking and, at the same time, can indicate addictive behavior.

University students are not just young adults, they are a population group that is the expected driving force of the economy in the future, and they represent potential current and future health care, criminal justice, and social burdens as well. Therefore, it is important to pay special attention to them. In the context of drinking patterns, many university students drink a lot of alcohol and tend to drink more and more heavily than their non-university peers, which has countless negative consequences [13]. These habits of young people can be reflected in various aspects of their lives. Tembo et al. [14] revealed that high levels of alcohol consumption among university students are significantly associated with poor mental health outcomes. In addition, other risky behaviors, use of other addictive substances, psychological symptoms (depression, distress), or low interest in academic activities may prevail among university students with problem drinking at risk of addiction [15]. For all these reasons, many authors call for drinking prevention strategies and interventions in the university environment [16]. The importance of active counseling at universities was emphasized and social support represented a very important aspect [17]. The key factors were also participation in university activities, public discussions on the consequences of excessive alcohol consumption, motivation for healthy behaviors through academic and career success [18]. In other words, evidence from other geographical regions clearly supported effective prevention programs, which, however, have been implemented to a small extent in the Czech and Slovak Republics. Thus, it is essential that research efforts focus on this issue and its implications for the university student population.

It is not difficult to expect various negative alcohol-related problems in the lives of young people [19], while drinking motives play an important role in this issue [20]. The alcohol-related consequences include various negative experiences, such as embarrassing situations, problems with friends and family, problems at school or work, indecent (rude) and risky behavior, excessive drinking, physical symptoms, bad feelings, but also unpleasant sexual situations, physical attacks and blackouts [21]. In the university environment, one of the most appropriate measures to capture alcohol-related consequences is the 48-item Young Adult Alcohol Consequences Questionnaire (YAACQ), the great advantage of which is its subscales providing a method of aggregating the consequences of alcohol use that may be clinically useful [10, 21]. Moreover, its subscales show significant associations with other indices of alcohol involvement (such as drinking frequency or binge drinking frequency) [10], which is also considered important in the issue of alcohol addiction.

In terms of sex, Lemley et al. [22] revealed that the negative consequences of alcohol use differed between male students and female students, while males tended to acquire a higher YAACQ score. This is consistent with the results of Geisner et al. [23], who found more alcohol-related consequences for male students. In this regard, Merrill et al. [20] confirmed significant sex differences in the two dimensions of YAACQ, namely risky behaviors (RISK) and academic/occupational consequences (AC-OCC).

Regarding the results revealed in a study examining the consequences of alcohol use (YAACQ) in Spain, Argentina and the United States, it can be concluded that the obtained score may significantly differ from country to country, but also from subscale to subscale [24]. For example, students from Argentina and Spain acquired greater mean number of alcohol-related consequences than students from the United States [24]. Based on the results of another study from the United States, university students obtained the highest percentage to the maximum score in the subscales, such as blackouts, social interpersonal problems, impaired control and risky behaviors [21].

Depressive disorder is also a frequent psychological burden among university students, which may impair their interpersonal, social and work functioning [25]. Moreover, the prevalence of depression in students increases during their university studies [26]. Feelings of hopelessness and despondency are common to this disorder, which can affect their academic performance [27]. In fact, depressive symptoms along with alcohol use are a serious combination, as there is a risk of suicide proneness [28]. Based on these facts, it is necessary to examine these two critical disorders among university students.

Factors such as lack of social support, heavy alcohol consumption and traumatic experiences can be considered significant predictors [29]. Ibrahim et al. [25] conducted a systematic review of university students and it can be noted that the significant effect of alcohol use was not large. The high prevalence rate of depression among university students (ranging from 10% to 85%) contributes to the perception of students as a high-risk population [25], while females are at higher risk compared to male counterparts [30]. Leppink et al. [31] also revealed that females were significantly predominant in severe depression and this is in line with the findings that sex differences are greater in major depression than in minor depression [25].

One of the most commonly used screening instruments for depression is the Patient Health Questionnaire-9 (PHQ-9) [32, 33]. According to Kroenke and Spitzer [34], the PHQ-9 fulfills a dual purpose, namely to diagnose depression and to assess the severity of depression. In the Slovak Republic, the PHQ-9 measure was used by Hajduk et al. [35], who examined prevalence and correlations of depression and anxiety in university students, they revealed mild depression in their research sample. The authors also found a higher prevalence of depression among students compared to anxiety, and their results showed that students with a higher score tended to perceive their mental health as less satisfactory [35]. The Czech version of the PHQ-9 measure was successfully assessed in the general population by Dansova et al. [36].

Comparing the results in the international studies using the PHQ-9 measure, it can be concluded that 37.7% of students from the United States had mild to moderate depression, and 4.4% of students had severe depression [31]. In Croatia, 60.8% students suffered from depressive disorder, while 30.3% of students reported mild depression, 16.1% of students reported moderate depression, 7.2% of students reported severely moderate depression, and severe depression was identified in 0.2% of students [37]. Interesting results were provided by Honney et al. [38], who compared the prevalence of depression in medical and non-medical students from the United Kingdom. Their results revealed that 32.4%, 10.8%, and 5.6% of medical students suffered from mild, moderate and severe depression. Simultaneously, 28.7%, 17.7%, and 12.7% of non-medical students suffered from mild, moderate and severe depression [38]. This fact indicate that medical students were not at higher risk for moderate to severe depressive disorder than non-medical students.

All of these results suggest that depression is frequent in young people's lives and should not be overlooked; on the contrary, efforts should be made to help people overcome these difficulties. One way is to identify possible risk factors and try to eliminate them. It is the problem of alcohol use with consequences that appears to be an important factor in depressed people, who should be given early intervention. Early interventions in problematic drinking behavior could prevent depressive disorders, which can have other consequences. Every indication of problem drinking is crucial for further action to address and overcome these problems in young people's lives.

2.1 The relationship between alcohol-related consequences and depressive disorder

With a focus on the mentioned behavioral and mental disorders in university students, the findings of several studies revealed that psychological symptoms are associated with drinking consequences and alcohol use [23, 39], while depression is no exception [40, 41]. In this regard, Martens [42] confirmed that depressive symptoms in university students were directly related to the negative consequences of alcohol drinking (using the Rutgers Alcohol Problem Index – RAPI), but not to alcohol consumption itself. This builds on the results of Park and Grant [43], in which the consequences of alcohol drinking were significantly associated with psychological risk as well as protective factors. These facts supported the assumption that alcohol-related consequences and mental disorders, such as depression, are closely linked.

The depression-drinking link among university students was examined in several other studies, in which various tools to measure depression and alcohol-related consequences were used. In any case, correlations were clearly found between depressive disorder and drinking consequences [44]. From the perspective of this study, the findings also showed that depressive symptoms were positively and significantly correlated with negative alcohol-related consequences, as measured by the YAACQ score [45]. Similarly, Ruiz et al. [46] confirmed a positive and significant correlation between psychological discomfort and the YAACQ score. Regarding the PHQ-9 measure, several studies can also be found that confirmed a positive association between depression and problem drinking, while Flesch et al. [47] noted that alcohol abuse can be considered a risk factor for a major depressive episode expressed in the PHQ-9 score.

There is also evidence to suggest that depressive symptoms may predict alcohol use and alcohol-related consequences [48, 49], while self-medication plays an important role in this association [50]. On the other hand, problems with alcohol can lead to an increased risk of depression [51, 52]. In this regard, Schutte et al. [53] found that alcohol-related consequences could lead to depression in males, but not in females. This can be explained by the fact that male university students are characterized by higher alcohol consumption and more negative consequences of drinking [23]. As a result, Geisner et al. [23] confirmed a stronger association between psychological symptoms and the negative consequences of alcohol use in males than in females.

On the other hand, Rosenthal et al. [54] used the Brief Young Adult Alcohol Consequences Questionnaire (BYAACQ) in a sample of female university students, and their findings revealed that experiencing negative alcohol-related consequences, regardless of the amount of alcohol consumption, could lead to a higher risk of depression (PHQ-9). With a focus on casual sex, one of the possible alcohol-related consequences, this experience increased depressive symptoms in female students more than in male students [55]. Accordingly, it can be assumed that female students felt guilty or remorse in this situation and felt that they had violated social expectations [56].

Although indirect evidence has created expectations, the relationship between the YAACQ score and the PHQ-9 score has not yet been examined in some regions. The above-mentioned evidence has suggested that depressive disorder and alcohol-related consequences may show interesting results in higher education, where the issue of mental health and unhealthy behavior is of undeniable importance. Insufficient examination of this issue can also be observed in the regions of the Czech and Slovak Republics. In these regions, the effects of alcohol-related consequences on depressive symptoms remain unknown. For this reason, the presented study filled this gap and provided public policy makers as well as experts with an inspiring perspective. At present, every country needs up-to-date information for responsible decision-making, the development of effective strategies and the implementation of interventions. In addition, at the time of the COVID-19 pandemic, it is necessary to monitor the patterns of behavior of vulnerable groups of the population, which are certainly also students. It has been shown that the COVID-19 pandemic can negatively contribute to students' psychological discomfort and unhealthy behavior [57, 58]. The main reasons for students' discomfort were worries about their health and the health of their loved ones, difficulty concentrating, sleep disorders, physical distancing and increased academic concerns [58]. These facts can lead to more serious consequences and a risk of substance abuse. In any case, all necessary measures to prevent an increase in alcohol-related problems should be adopted [59].

The purpose of the presented study was to assess the situation of alcohol-related consequences and depressive disorder in the Czech and Slovak Republics and to provide a valuable platform for the development of strategies and interventions in these regions. When developing and optimizing diagnostic procedures, prevention and treatment, it is desirable to specify potential patients. One way in the specification process is to differentiate according to sex characteristics.

3. Materials and methods

The analyses included data obtained using the YAACQ [21] and PHQ-9 [33] measures. The PHQ-9 measure was successfully validated in several studies aimed at university students [60, 61]. Its reliability and psychometric properties are evidenced by the fact that this measure has been included in many studies on the mental health of university students from various countries, such as Australia [62], the United Kingdom [38], the United States [31] or Croatia [37]. In terms of cross-cultural comparison, the usefulness of PHQ-9 was supported by a study at universities in Germany and China [63] and a study focusing on young adults from Poland and Korea [64]. The PHQ-9 consisted of nine survey items with a four-point scale (0 not at all; 1 several days; 3 more than half the days; 4 nearly every day) aimed at screening for depressive disorder among university students. This brief measure of depression could reach a score ranging from 0 to 27. On this basis, it was possible to know the probability of major or subthreshold depressive disorder at various cut points defining the lower limits of mild, moderate, moderately severe, and severe depression [32, 33]. The score was decisive in the assessment, while the higher the value, the more intense the depressive disorder. In assessing, several studies used score assigned at intervals (0–4 none; 5–9 mild; 10–14 moderate; 15–19 moderately severe; 20–27 severe). For the purposes of this research (i.e. application of regression and correlation analysis), it was more appropriate to use the gross score obtained by the students.

In general, the YAACQ measure covers from mild to more severe alcohol-related consequences and includes the following eight subscales: (1) social interpersonal problems – SOC, (2) impaired control – CONTR, (3) self-perception – SELF-P, (4) self-care – SELF-C, (5) risky behaviors – RISK, (6) academic/occupational consequences – AC-OCC, (7) physiological dependence – PHYS-DEP, and (8) blackout drinking – BLKOUT. Interestingly, two subscales (impaired control, self-care) take into account problem areas that are not fully assessed by other existing measures [10]. It can also be noted that the total YAACQ score correlated with another similar measure (RAPI), which supports the validity of this measure [21]. The advantages of YAACQ have been proven in several studies conducted among students [9, 20, 65] and the use of this eight-factor structure has been supported across countries and cultures [12, 21]. As in the previous case, the gross score was used for the YAACQ measure. A dichotomous scale is commonly used for this instrument (0 no; 1 yes), but in this research, the scale was extended (1 strongly disagree; 2 disagree; 3 undecided; 4 agree; 5 strongly agree). The total score of YAACQ or its individual subscales was formed by the sum of the individual items. The dichotomous scale had a number of benefits that were evident in the diagnostics, as the overall score reflected a number of consequences and it was not difficult to complete. The conversion to a 5-point scale could be more accurate and offer the use of more statistical methods. The use of an extended scale was more appropriate for research and academic purposes. There was some risk when comparing the results with the dichotomous scale, but this risk was minimal.

3.1 Research sample and data collection

The data collection was performed in two parallel levels. First, university representatives as well as teachers were contacted by e-mail with a request to distribute the questionnaire to students. Second, the questionnaire was distributed through student groups on social networks (universities, faculties, dormitories, student communities). The research sample consisted of university students from the Czech and Slovak Republics, who stated that they had consumed alcohol in the last 3 months. Data collection was conducted in 2020, when it is necessary to take into account the coronavirus disease 2019 (COVID-19) pandemic. The questionnaire was distributed electronically. The total sample consisted of 2514 respondents (CZE: n = 1193, 47.5%). The data were cleaned up. First, respondents who answered doubtfully to the control question (in numerical terms, one million has six zeros – the scale of agreement/disagreement) were excluded (n = 179), then erroneous responses caused by the system (blank items, even if it was a mandatory item) were excluded (n = 27) and last, foreign students were excluded (n = 87).

The collection process can be characterized as quota sampling with a focus on the approximate proportionality of the responses in each country. The field of study can be considered as the main quota criterion (there was an effort to collect at least 30 responses per study field in each country). Efforts have also been made to include most universities (with the exception of foreign universities and foreign detached institutions). The quota sampling criteria were met and the research sample included the vast majority of all universities. **Table 1** provides the basic characteristics of the research sample.

The study and its concept were approved by the ethics committee of the General University Hospital in Prague as individual research (Ref. 915/20 S–IV). All

Variable	ALL n (%)	CZE n (%)	SVK n (%)
Residence – school:			
Dormitory	759(30.19)	194(16.26)	565(42.77)
Private accommodation	372(14.8)	256(21.46)	116(8.78)
With family	215(8.55)	164(13.75)	51(3.86)
With a friend	57(2.27)	31(2.6)	26(1.97)
At home	1111(44.19)	548(45.93)	563(42.62)
Field of study:			
Education	283(11.26)	223(18.69)	60(4.54)
Humanities and arts	150(5.97)	87(7.29)	63(4.77)
Social, economic and legal sciences	1089(43.32)	568(47.61)	521(39.44)
Natural Science	95(3.78)	42(3.52)	53(4.01)
Design, technology, production and communications	203(8.07)	74(6.2)	129(9.77)
Agricultural and veterinary sciences	102(4.06)	58(4.86)	44(3.33)
Health service	187(7.44)	44(3.69)	143(10.83)
Services (tourism, sports, security, etc.)	258(10.26)	57(4.78)	201(15.22)
Informatics, mathematics, ICT	147(5.85)	40(3.35)	107(8.1)
Form of study:			
Full-time	2112(84.01)	885(74.18)	1227(92.88)
Part-time	402(15.99)	308(25.82)	94(7.12)
Degree of study:			
1st degree	1441(57.32)	545(45.68)	896(67.83)
2nd degree	659(26.21)	326(27.33)	333(25.21)
Combined 1st and 2nd degree	78(3.1)	43(3.6)	35(2.65)
3rd degree	336(13.37)	279(23.39)	57(4.31)
Sex:			
Males	779(30.99)	297(24.9)	482(36.49)
Females	1735(69.01)	896(75.1)	839(63.51)

Table 1.
Characteristics of respondents.

respondents who participated in the research confirmed their informed consent at the beginning of the questionnaire. All aspects in this research were conducted with respect to the seventh revision of the World Medical Association–Declaration of Helsinki [66] and the second revision of the Farmington Consensus [67].

3.2 Statistical analysis

The statistical processing in this study consisted of two main parts, namely the first part focused on the statistical description of the data and the second part focused on the examined relationship. Descriptive statistics included the basic characteristics (mean (Mean), median (Median), standard deviation (SD), kurtosis (Kurt), skewness (Skew), minimum (Min), maximum (Max)), which were presented generally without classification of respondents as well as in the sex classification of respondents. Subsequently, Pearson's correlation coefficient (r) and Spearman's correlation coefficient (Spearman's ρ) were used to analyze the associations. Prior to this statistical procedure, normality (the Henze-Zirkler test for multivariate normality) and the presence of outliers (a quantile method based on Mahalanobis distance) were verified. The hypothesis of normality was rejected. However, it should be noted that due to the size of the sample, the normality tests may have been skewed and may have tended to reject the normality hypothesis. This was followed by regression analysis using a simple OLS model, before which the assumptions for use were verified (the Bonferroni outlier test, the Breusch-Pagan test). A simple quantile regression analysis (τ = 0.25, 0.50, 0.75) was applied to assess the effects, and the standard error was estimated by Powell's kernel version for the covariance matrix estimate on the commonly used Hall-Sheather bandwidth rule. IBM SPSS Statistic software (IBM Corp., Armonk, NY, USA) and R v 4.0.2 (RStudio, Inc., Boston, MA, USA) were used for statistical processing.

4. Results

Figure 1 shows the intensity of the total YAACQ and PHQ 9 scores. This visualization consists of the mean values of the percentage expression to the maximum value in terms of selected indicators. The presented figure provides some information, the most important of which is the low probability that the values of outputs in the Slovak Republic and the Czech Republic have acquired significant differences. This was evidenced by the result of the Wilcoxon nonparametric test, which in both indicators showed a p-value higher than 0.05 for the countries (p-value: YAACQ = 0.156; PHQ-9 = 0.137). On the other hand, it is possible to observe certain differences between regions in both indicators. Thus, a significant difference between the individual regions was found using the Kruskal Wallis test (YAACQ: χ^2 = 36.404, p-value = 0.020; PHQ-9: χ^2 = 33.311, p-value = 0.043). Sex characteristics were also taken into account in terms of differences, and the Wilcoxon test confirmed significant differences between males and females in both indicators at a level lower than 0.001 (mean YAACQ % to max: females = 32.7%, males = 36.8%; mean PHQ-9% to max: females = 23.1%, males = 20.2%). On this basis, the inclusion of sex characteristics in subsequent calculations were warranted. More intense color

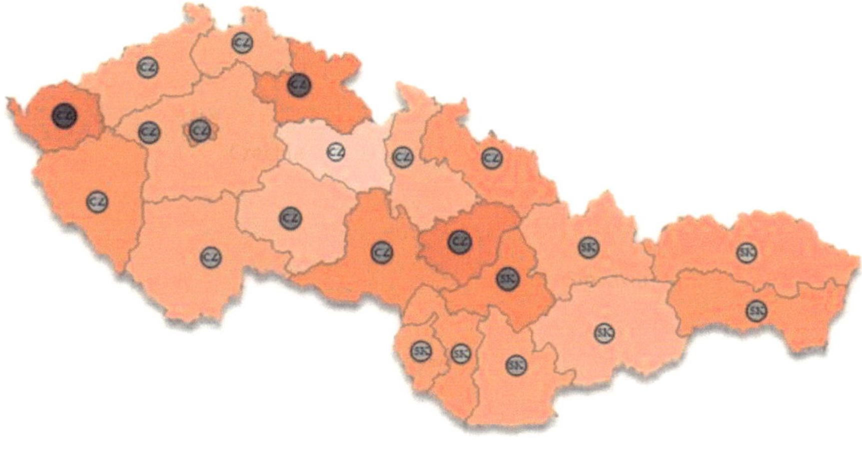

Figure 1.
Relationship between the YAACQ score and the PHQ-9 score (% to max - mean) in the Czech Republic and the Slovak Republic. Note: Color shading of choropleth map – YAACQ (% to max - mean); circles in regions – PHQ-9 (% to max - mean); CZ – Czech Republic; SK – Slovak Republic.

shading represents a higher value (in the case of the PHQ-9 indicator, the higher value is represented not only by color shading, but also by the size of the circle). In this context, a certain relationship could be observed between the YAACQ and PHQ-9 indicators, as in several regions with a higher intensity of the YAACQ indicator, a higher intensity of the PHQ-9 indicator can also be found. This fact was also supported by Spearman's correlation coefficient (ρ – 0.262; p-value <0.001). This secondarily declared the appropriateness of choosing a quantile regression model.

The first row of **Table 2** (TheoryM) shows the theoretical interval of the analyzed indicators, i.e. the lowest and highest value that the respondent could obtain. In this table, it is also possible to observe descriptive characteristics for all respondents (without classification), as well as separately for males and females. The significance of differences in all indicators was assessed using the Wilcoxon test. As the scales can take on different intervals of values (TheoryM), the results can be seen through the share of the maximum of the theoretical interval. Based on this, the highest score was found in the SOC subscale (mean = 12.376; 41.25% of the TheoryM maximum) and the BLKOUT subscale (mean = 14.585; 41.67% of the TheoryM maximum). On the other hand, the assessment of standard deviations (SD) has the highest added value in terms of comparing the values obtained for males and females. Apart from the PHQ-9 score, all of the cases showed lower values for females, meaning that the responses of females were more constant. As can be seen, the indicators associated with the negative consequences of alcohol use (YAACQ) were more common in males. On the other hand, the indicator of depressive disorder was more common in females.

In general, the PHQ-9 score indicates the level of intensity of perceived depression in five intervals. The results showed that exactly 50% of the students were identified in the "none" interval, a slightly increased depression in the "mild" interval was found in 29.8% of the students, the share of the "moderate" interval showed 11.6%, the share of the students with "moderately severe" depression was 5.5% and the group with the highest level of perception of depressive symptoms in the "severe" interval included 3.1% of the students.

The following part is devoted to the assessment of the associations between the selected indicators of alcohol-related consequences and depression in general, as well as in the sex classification. In the first step, the Henze-Zirkler test for multivariate normality was used, which showed significant deviations from the normal distribution in all of the analyzed cases. Also, the presence of outliers was assessed using a quantile method based on Mahalanobis distance, and a significant proportion of outliers were found. At this point, it should be noted that the research included a relatively large set of data, in which tests tend to reject the hypothesis of normality. For this reason, the results are provided in both parametric (Pearson's r) and nonparametric (Spearman's ρ) alternatives.

As mentioned above, **Table 3** shows both parametric and non-parametric alternatives to the bivariate analysis of associations. The double use of the correlation test minimized the statistical error resulting from the computational processes. In most cases, the parametric alternative of the test (Pearson's r) acquired slightly higher values than the nonparametric alternative (Spearman's ρ). Each analyzed association was significant at the level of $\alpha < 0.001$. Focusing on the results in the given table, the strength of the association up to 0.30 can be interpreted as low to medium, up to 0.50 as medium to substantial and up to 0.70 as substantial to very strong. Accordingly, most of the associations between the selected YAACQ subscales could be considered as substantial to very strong. The associations between the score in the individual YAACQ subscales and the PHQ-9 score were shown to be low to medium. In general, SELF-P and SELF-C could be considered the most

Statistic	SOC	CONTR	SELF-P	SELF-C	RISK	AC-OCC	PHYS-DEP	BLKOUT	PHQ-9
TheoryM	6–30	5–25	4–20	8–40	9–45	5–25	4–20	7–35	0–27
Mean	12.376	8.727	6.682	13.231	13.833	7.138	4.965	14.585	6.002
Median	11	7	5	11	12	5	4	13	4.5
SD	5.317	4.299	3.759	6.332	6.075	3.473	1.798	6.645	5.328
Kurt	0.486	1.693	2.110	1.590	3.435	5.329	7.186	0.140	1.675
Skew	0.963	1.444	1.643	1.425	1.760	2.187	2.416	0.869	1.358
Min	6	5	4	8	9	5	4	7	0
Max	30	25	20	40	45	25	18	35	27
Males									
Mean	13.126	9.367	6.902	14.281	15.250	7.942	5.371	16.108	5.465
Median	12	8	5	12	13	6	4	15	4
SD	5.689	4.541	3.828	6.778	7.093	4.106	2.056	7.142	5.107
Kurt	0.382	0.835	1.511	0.859	2.104	3.442	3.096	−0.380	2.063
Skew	0.918	1.204	1.474	1.194	1.502	1.832	1.738	0.623	1.454
Min	6	5	4	8	9	5	4	7	0
Max	30	25	20	40	44	25	16	35	27
Females									
Mean	12.040	8.439	6.583	12.759	13.197	6.777	4.783	13.901	6.244
Median	11	7	5	10	11	5	4	13	5
SD	5.107	4.155	3.724	6.064	5.441	3.081	1.638	6.292	5.409
Kurt	0.428	2.246	2.437	2.042	3.806	6.059	11.126	0.468	1.532
Skew	0.958	1.573	1.728	1.545	1.810	2.319	2.898	0.976	1.319
Min	6	5	4	8	9	5	4	7	0
Max	30	25	20	40	45	25	18	35	27
Wilcoxon rank sum test (Sex)									
W	749127	768035	712307	776281	795381	794436	790832	798066	612152
p-value	<0.001	<0.001	0.023	<0.001	<0.001	<0.001	<0.001	<0.001	<0.001

Table 2.
Descriptive statistics.

predictive subscales in terms of the PHQ-9 score. However, the differences in the correlation of individual scales were often very small. Due to the fact that the increased rate of associations between individual subscales was also confirmed, a simple regression model was applied in the following part focused on regression analysis.

The application of regression analysis (OLS) itself was determined by several tests of assumptions. The Bonferroni outlier test did not show any outliers at the level of $\alpha < 0.01$, but the Breusch-Pagan test identified all the models as heteroskedastic, at the mentioned level of significance. Therefore, a white estimator of HC3 was used to assess the effect.

The results in **Table 4** show that all the associations were significant at the level of significance $\alpha < 0.001$. Simultaneously, the coefficients were positive, which

ρ \ r	SOC	CONTR	SELF-P	SELF-C	RISK	AC-OCC	PHYS-DEP	BLKOUT	PHQ-9
SOC		0.622	0.579	0.552	0.678	0.515	0.388	0.626	0.225
CONTR	0.613		0.678	0.656	0.562	0.582	0.497	0.586	0.218
SELF-P	0.549	0.606		0.636	0.503	0.461	0.394	0.495	0.262
SELF-C	0.529	0.635	0.607		0.554	0.627	0.487	0.531	0.243
RISK	0.698	0.590	0.516	0.567		0.581	0.426	0.648	0.201
AC-OCC	0.479	0.562	0.433	0.590	0.55		0.484	0.554	0.208
PHYS-DEP	0.342	0.448	0.345	0.446	0.394	0.417		0.399	0.203
BLKOUT	0.636	0.610	0.489	0.536	0.656	0.553	0.390		0.187
PHQ-9	0.208	0.195	0.257	0.231	0.208	0.177	0.163	0.196	
MALES									
SOC		0.633	0.550	0.58	0.694	0.542	0.402	0.643	0.185
CONTR	0.611		0.690	0.652	0.547	0.583	0.509	0.549	0.199
SELF-P	0.515	0.615		0.622	0.491	0.460	0.392	0.481	0.286
SELF-C	0.528	0.620	0.587		0.544	0.650	0.512	0.546	0.238
RISK	0.720	0.582	0.484	0.550		0.558	0.417	0.630	0.167
AC-OCC	0.515	0.586	0.462	0.608	0.577		0.497	0.562	0.220
PHYS-DEP	0.339	0.437	0.349	0.463	0.383	0.445		0.411	0.200
BLKOUT	0.640	0.572	0.467	0.532	0.630	0.586	0.381		0.128
PHQ-9	0.162	0.210	0.279	0.222	0.148	0.170	0.149	0.135	
FEMALES									
SOC		0.61	0.593	0.530	0.665	0.490	0.366	0.609	0.257
CONTR	0.610		0.673	0.652	0.566	0.576	0.480	0.598	0.239
SELF-P	0.563	0.603		0.644	0.515	0.467	0.397	0.504	0.257
SELF-C	0.524	0.635	0.617		0.551	0.605	0.458	0.511	0.260
RISK	0.685	0.583	0.532	0.566		0.581	0.408	0.649	0.245
AC-OCC	0.452	0.540	0.416	0.574	0.521		0.453	0.534	0.227
PHYS-DEP	0.335	0.444	0.342	0.425	0.380	0.386		0.368	0.227
BLKOUT	0.631	0.616	0.498	0.528	0.653	0.520	0.377		0.237
PHQ-9	0.242	0.207	0.255	0.255	0.258	0.203	0.197	0.249	

Note: Above the diagonal is a parametric alternative (Pearson's r) and below the diagonal is a nonparametric alternative (Spearman's ρ). The p-values are not shown, as all of the analyzed relationships were significant at the level of $\alpha < 0.001$.

Table 3.
Correlation analyses.

means that an increased risk of depressive disorder can be associated with experience in selected dimensions of alcohol-related consequences. The multiple R2 showed relatively low values, which can be considered a certain limitation.

The most important output of the presented study is shown in **Table 5**, which is devoted to the assessment of the effects of the score in the individual YAACQ

PHQ-9	SOC	CONTR	SELF-P	SELF-C	RISK	AC-OCC	PHYS-DEP	BLKOUT
α (SE)	3.21† (0.28)	3.65† (0.26)	3.30† (0.26)	3.56† (0.28)	3.56† (0.28)	3.73† (0.27)	3.02† (0.37)	3.81† (0.26)
β (SE)	0.23† (0.02)	0.27† (0.03)	0.20† (0.02)	0.18† (0.02)	0.18† (0.02)	0.32† (0.04)	0.60† (0.08)	0.15† (0.02)
R2	0.05	0.05	0.07	0.06	0.04	0.04	0.04	0.04

Note: SE – standard error;
† p-value <0.001.

Table 4.
Assessment of the effects of YAACQ on PHQ-9 (OLS model).

PHQ-9	τ	ALL		MALES		FEMALES	
		α(SE)	β(SE)	α(SE)	β(SE)	α(SE)	β(SE)
SOC	0.25	1.00†(0.22)	0.10†(0.02)	**0.50(0.43)**	0.10***(0.03)	0.61**(0.28)	0.15†(0.02)
	0.5	2.20†(0.30)	0.20†(0.03)	2.59†(0.56)	0.12***(0.04)	2.00†(0.36)	0.23†(0.03)
	0.75	4.33†(0.48)	0.33†(0.04)	3.60†(0.74)	0.30†(0.06)	3.38†(0.66)	0.46†(0.06)
CONTR	0.25	1.00†(0.21)	0.14†(0.02)	**<0.01(0.38)**	0.20†(<0.01)	1.23†(0.27)	0.15†(0.03)
	0.5	2.50†(0.29)	0.25†(0.03)	1.75†(0.48)	0.25†(0.05)	2.61†(0.38)	0.28†(0.05)
	0.75	5.08†(0.45)	0.38†(0.05)	4.33†(0.73)	0.33†(0.08)	4.50†(0.52)	0.50†(0.06)
SELF-P	0.25	1.27†(0.18)	0.18†(0.03)	**<0.01(0.36)**	0.25†(0.05)	1.14†(0.23)	0.21†(0.04)
	0.5	2.67†(0.26)	0.33†(0.04)	1.40***(0.45)	0.40†(0.07)	2.67†(0.31)	0.33†(0.05)
	0.75	4.87†(0.41)	0.53†(0.06)	3.60†(0.61)	0.60†(0.09)	4.67†(0.51)	0.58†(0.08)
SELF-C	0.25	0.89†(0.21)	0.11†(0.02)	**−0.14(0.41)**	0.14†(0.03)	1.00†(0.27)	0.13†(0.02)
	0.5	2.20†(0.28)	0.20†(0.02)	1.40***(0.49)	0.20†(0.04)	1.75†(0.35)	0.25†(0.03)
	0.75	4.73†(0.42)	0.27†(0.03)	3.56†(0.66)	0.28†(0.05)	4.47†(0.54)	0.32†(0.04)
RISK	0.25	1.23†(0.24)	0.08†(0.02)	2.00†(<0.01)	**<0.01(0.03)**	0.82***(0.30)	0.13†(0.02)
	0.5	2.13†(0.32)	0.19†(0.02)	2.56†(0.60)	0.12***(0.04)	1.86†(0.41)	0.24†(0.03)
	0.75	4.43†(0.51)	0.29†(0.04)	3.88†(0.60)	0.23†(0.05)	3.40†(0.67)	0.40†(0.05)
AC-OCC	0.25	1.17†(0.17)	0.16†(0.04)	1.20***(0.42)	**0.01*(0.05)**	0.75**(0.31)	0.25†(0.05)
	0.5	2.50†(0.30)	0.30†(0.04)	1.94†(0.52)	0.29†(0.07)	2.00†(0.43)	0.40†(0.07)
	0.75	4.50†(0.53)	0.50†(0.06)	4.00†(0.54)	0.40†(0.07)	5.50†(0.58)	0.50†(0.08)
PHYS-DEP	0.25	0.67†(0.31)	0.33†(0.06)	2.00†(0.59)	**<0.01(0.11)**	**0.29(0.39)**	0.43†(0.08)
	0.5	2.00†(0.39)	0.50†(0.08)	2.67†(0.69)	0.33**(0.13)	**1.00(0.64)**	0.75†(0.14)
	0.75	4.50†(0.71)	0.88†(0.15)	5.00†(0.84)	0.50***(0.15)	3.00***(0.95)	1.25†(0.20)
BLKOUT	0.25	1.00†(0.21)	0.08†(0.01)	2.00†(0.41)	**<0.01(0.03)**	0.83***(0.27)	0.12†(0.02)
	0.5	2.57†(0.28)	0.14†(0.02)	3.13†(0.52)	0.07**(0.03)	2.00†(0.34)	0.20†(0.03)
	0.75	4.75†(0.44)	0.25†(0.03)	5.62†(0.77)	0.13***(0.05)	4.00†(0.49)	0.33†(0.04)

Note: SE – standard error;
**p-value <0.1;*
***p-value <0.05;*
****p-value <0.01;*
† p-value <0.00;
non-significant associations are highlighted in bold.

Table 5.
Assessment of the effects of YAACQ on PHQ-9 (quantile regression).

subscales on the PHQ-9 score. When assessing the results, it is most appropriate to focus on the β coefficients (independent variable). The standard error should also be taken into account when interpreting, while the lower the value, the more stable the model. This has the highest added value when comparing the β coefficients in males and females, while the results revealed lower values predominantly in the female models. Based on the results, the significant effects of alcohol-related consequences on depressive disorder can be clearly confirmed in the vast majority of analyzed cases. The associations that cannot be considered significant at the level of $\alpha < 0.05$ were found only in ten cases (highlighted in bold). In all cases that supported to be significant, positive regression coefficients were found, which can be understood in the sense that alcohol-related consequences may be a risk factor for depressive disorder. In other words, an increased PHQ-9 score may be associated with an increased score in the YAACQ subscales. By focusing on the differences between females and males, the results suggested that females had a higher intensity of effects based on regression coefficients.

5. Discussion

In order to develop successful addiction diagnosis programs and strategies, it is necessary to know the variables that predict the development of substance use problems. This study contributed to this knowledge, as diagnostic information on university students with alcohol problems in the Czech and Slovak Republics could be useful for the development of effective prevention strategies in addiction issue. Although many countries have effective strategies and can be an inspiration, the countries examined in this study implement active interventions and prevention aimed at students to a very small extent. This issue is little discussed at professional, political and social level, and therefore, the need to address it is overlooked. There is a lack of support for university counseling centres for students and, in addition, information on the current situation is insufficient.

The successful development of addiction prevention policy requires the availability of multidimensional analyses and the creation of specific databases that would make it possible to assess the effectiveness of policy in individual geographically defined areas [68]. Many national researches were initiated within international institutions [69]. These facts were the motivation for conducting research in national conditions. The main aim of the presented study was to assess the relationship between alcohol-related consequences and depressive disorder. This aim was met in a sample of university students from the Czech and Slovak Republics.

Based on the results of the descriptive analysis, it can be concluded that males acquired a higher score in all subscales of alcohol-related consequences. Similarly, Geisner et al. [23] revealed more alcohol-related consequences for male students and Merrill et al. [20] found significant sex differences in risky behaviors (RISK) and academic/occupational consequences (AC-OCC). This is consistent with the findings of Lemley et al. [22], who revealed that sex was a significant predictor for negative alcohol-related consequences, while male students tended to obtain a higher YAACQ score. This may be explained by the fact that male students are more prone to excessive alcohol consumption than female students [23], while their heavier drinking can be associated with alcohol-related consequences [70]. Males also perceived alcohol-related consequences less negatively than females [71]. In this regard, females were less likely to be exposed to risk factors and alcohol-related consequences. In contrast, protective factors against alcohol-related consequences predominated in females, as they perceived greater social sanctions for drinking and they were less likely to have characteristics associated with excessive drinking, such as aggressiveness, uncontrollable behavior, sensation-seeking, and others [72]. On the other hand, there is also interesting evidence that although female students consumed less alcohol, they were more likely to experience negative consequences when drinking [73]. This can be explained by the fact that females have less alcohol dehydrogenase than males, they are less efficient at metabolizing alcohol and thus more vulnerable to its effects.

In the Czech and Slovak regions, students acquired the highest percentage to the maximum score in blackouts (41.67%), while different values could be found in other countries, such as the United States (56.71%) [21], Argentina (26%) and Spain (29,43%) [24]. In terms of impaired control, Czech and Slovak students obtained a comparable percentage to its maximum score (34.91%) as students from the mentioned countries (the United States = 35.33% [21]; Argentina = 35.8%; Spain = 28.8% [24]). Similar results with students from the United States (32%) [21] could be observed in risky behaviors (the Czech and Slovak Republics = 34.58%).

Regarding depression, female students acquired a higher PHQ-9 score than their male counterparts. This fact follows the evidence that depressive disorder (PHQ-9) is more common in females [74]. There are several other findings confirming that depression is a more frequent mental problem for females [30], while sex predispositions to mental disorders remain unclear. Albert [75] tried to explain this on the basis of biological factors that may contribute to a higher prevalence of depression in females as well as to their mental vulnerability. There are also insights into this issue that addressed sex differences in depression during adolescence, and their results showed that the causes of depression were more common in females, who were also more likely to develop risk factors for depressive disorder than males [76]. In the context of the main idea of this study, it should be noted that the main risk factors for depression among female students include low economic status, chronic illness, and unhealthy patterns of behavior [77].

In general, the results in this study also showed that 29.8%, 11.6%, 5.5% and 3.1% of students suffered from mild, moderate, moderately severe and severe depression. This can be compared with the findings of Hajduk et al. [35], who identified depression in 35.5% of Slovak students. For comparison, similar results were found in university students from the United Kingdom [38]. Croatian students also reported depressive disorder with a similar prevalence (mild = 30.3%, moderate = 16.1%, moderately severe = 7.2%, severe = 0.2%) [37]. Students from the United States had mild to moderate depression in a prevalence of 37.7%, and 4.4% of students suffered from severe depression [31]. This suggests that depression in Slovak and Czech students reached a comparable level with other countries even during the COVID-19 pandemic. By comparing depression, the measured scores did not differ much from the scores before the COVID-19 pandemic [35]. Due to the lack of information on the YAACQ score obtained by Czech and Slovak students, it was not possible to compare the values before the COVID-19 pandemic. At the same time, there is a need to compare the reported depression and the consequences of alcohol use after the COVID-19 pandemic.

The results also indicated the existence of significant and positive associations between all the examined indicators (individual alcohol-related consequences, depression), while the associations between the consequences of alcohol use and depressive disorder were identified in low to medium intensity. The findings in this study agree with the findings of other international studies that have revealed that depression is associated with alcohol-related consequences [42, 45]. This was also confirmed between psychological discomfort, such as distress, and the YAACQ score [46]. In this study, a stronger association was found in female students. Also, similar results were revealed in regression models, and the significant effects of alcohol-related consequences on depressive disorder were confirmed in the vast majority of the analyzed cases. Correlation analysis as well as regression analysis provided an output with positive coefficients, meaning that the increased risk of depressive disorder can be associated with experience in selected dimensions of alcohol-related consequences. Specifically, the findings of Geisner et al. [23] showed a stronger association between psychological symptoms and alcohol-related consequences in males, who were also characterized by higher alcohol consumption and more negative alcohol-related consequences. The results presented in this study partially agree with the findings of Schutte et al. [53], who revealed that alcohol-related consequences could cause depression in males, but not in females. On the contrary, the results of this study support the findings of Rosenthal et al. [54], who revealed that experiencing negative alcohol-related consequences (BYAACQ) may lead to a higher risk of depression (PHQ-9) among female students. The study conducted by Miller et al. [78] should also be emphasized, while their findings showed that blackouts were associated with other consequences of alcohol use (BYAACQ), which in turn were associated with depressive disorder (PHQ-8). In other words, blackouts showed direct and indirect effects on depression in young adults [78]. Focusing on other alcohol-related consequences, the experience of casual sex also increased depressive symptoms in females more than in males [55], while guilt, remorse, feelings that violated societal expectations played an important role in this situation [56]. Last but not least, the findings of this study are close to the knowledge that alcohol use disorder may increase the risk of subsequent depressive disorder [40, 41].

These findings could be useful to support the development of diagnostic variables for alcohol addiction in Czech and Slovak university students. Effective diagnostic measures and prevention programs exist in many other regions, which can be an inspiration. The examined regions should implement them in the university environment. It seems that strategies should also include monitoring the consequences of alcohol use and subsequent depressive symptoms, while experts should distinguish between the individual dimensions of the consequences. The idea is whether chronic alcohol use causes brain changes associated with depression [79], or whether there are genetic or other variables that could explain the relationship revealed in this study. The findings provide great potential for clinical and diagnostic research, that can build on this study.

6. Conclusion and implications

The results of this study represent valuable outputs for national policy makers, as well as for national and international research communities, whose ambition is to examine psychological and behavioral predictors and sex differences in addictive behaviors. All of the above-mentioned findings suggested that the consequences of alcohol use should be an integral part of policy and professional discussions on young people's mental health, as these consequences can be an important factor in the increased risk of depressive disorder. Also, students represent a group of the population of society that is to become an active productive part of it, and they represent potential current and future health care, criminal justice, and social burdens as well. Therefore, it is necessary to point out these aspects and to support the development of prevention addiction programs for this population group as well.

For this reason, public health policies should be strengthened in order to raise people's awareness of the threats of alcohol use and other consequences that may affect the mental health of individuals. Policy makers should strive to integrate mental health into all aspects of social and health policies, strategies and interventions. This research supports the idea that alcohol use with a risk of addiction and consequences contributes negatively to the symptoms of depression in young people. Specifically, the dimensions of self-perception and self-care appear to be the most important among Slovak and Czech young adults. This fact requires a special attention in the development of diagnostic procedures and the implementation of interventions in the field of addiction in these geographical regions. As the YAACQ is able to predict drinking patterns [10] and the level of drinking risk [11], it is welcome if the dimensions of alcohol-related consequences are also taken into account in alcohol addiction policies. In fact, prevention and education should also play a key role in universities and counseling centres. It would be beneficial if prevention programs for female students focused on coping and overcoming depressive symptoms. On the other hand, there is a need to focus on helping male students with alcohol use disorders and the subsequent consequences of drinking. In general, there is a lack of university counseling centres to help students overcome difficult situations in their lives. Professionals providing adequate help should also focus on the individual alcohol-related consequences as an accompanying aspect of diagnosing alcohol addiction, which would also lead to the prevention of mental disorders such as depression. Promoting an active lifestyle will continue to play an important role in this issue.

In the regions of the Czech and Slovak Republics, alcohol use disorders, together with the consequences of drinking, do not have the necessary attention and are overlooked not only at universities, but also in society as a whole. It is important to be aware of the importance of this issue at both professional and political level. Interventions are urgently needed to prevent young people from becoming addicted.

Health literacy is also considered as an important part of prevention programs at various stages of addiction [80–82]. In the Slovak and Czech Republics, there is no health literacy system that would include specific programs for different population groups [83]. Therefore, it is very difficult to estimate the extent to which the emergence and development of addiction among university students is determined by an insufficient level of health literacy (or its complete absence) and the extent to which it is determined by socio-economic factors. The family and the quality of the previous educational process also play an important role in problem drinking.

In any case, regional differences in addiction need to be examined, while it is also important to examine the consequences of alcohol use, the level of addiction, the mental health of the population and the economic parameters of the region, which may provide greater opportunities for addiction [84]. The ambition in this differentiating perspective was to point out the sex-differentiated effects of problem drinking with consequences, specifically in terms of the higher prevalence of depression in females than in males. Taking these differences into account can also significantly support the development of sex-differentiated services and programs [4, 85, 86]. From an international perspective, the European Monitoring Centre for Drugs and Drug Addiction (EMCDDA) [87] also pointed to the limited nature of services specialized for females. Although there is at least one such facility in almost every EU country, the demand is much higher and it is therefore necessary to ensure greater availability of specialized health care.

One of the strengths of this study is the fact that the research was conducted in a relatively large geographically area. The sample size is not negligible, as the sample in this study covered the vast majority of Czech and Slovak universities. The study also has several weaknesses that need to be taken into account when interpreting the results. The limitations of the presented research may include the fact that the sample was not random, and thus certain questions may arise regarding the representativeness of the research sample. Given the size of the sample and the fact that quota sampling was used, it was not expected that the findings would be significantly distorted due to the non-random sampling. Also, the questionnaire was distributed electronically and there is no guarantee that students have read all the attached information, which can be considered a limitation. There was also a possible limitation when comparing the results with the results of other authors, as a multilevel scale was used in this research, which is perceived as more accurate. It is not known how the COVID pandemic influenced access to alcohol, and this may be a weakness of the study.

As already emphasized, there is a need for scientific interest in the issue of addictive behavior and mental disorders. Future research will focus on uncovering other hidden differences in terms of health, mental disorders and alcohol use. In more detail, it is planned to compare these indicators between different fields of study. The ambition is to extend the research sample and to make a comparison between all countries belonging to the Visegrad Group. The time frame of data collection in this research also provides space for comparing the results aimed at evaluating changes in the addictive behavior of university students during the COVID-19 pandemic with the period after this pandemic situation. The international dimension of the research will provide an insight into the strength of the impact of the socio-economic changes caused by the COVID-19 pandemic on the emergence and development of the young generation's addiction.

Acknowledgements

This research was supported by the Internal Grant Agency of FaME Tomas Bata University in Zlin: RVO/2020: "Economic quantification of marketing processes that focus on value increase for a patient in a process of system creation to measure and control efficiency in health facilities in the Czech Republic".

Conflict of interest

The authors have no conflict of interest, financial or otherwise. The funders had no role in preparing the study; in data processing; in writing the manuscript or deciding on the publication of the results.

Notes/thanks/other declarations

We thank the students for their participation in the research. We also thank the university representatives, scientific, pedagogical and administrative workers for their willingness to distribute the questionnaire.

Author details

Beata Gavurova[1*], Martin Rigelsky[2] and Viera Ivankova[2]

1 Center for Applied Economic Research, Faculty of Management and Economics, Tomas Bata University in Zlin, Zlin, Czech Republic

2 Faculty of Management, University of Presov in Presov, Presov, Slovakia

*Address all correspondence to: gavurova@utb.cz

References

[1] Prince M, Patel V, Saxena S, Maj M, Maselko J, Phillips MR, Rahman A. No health without mental health. The Lancet. 2007;370(9590):859–877. DOI: 10.1016/s0140-6736(07)61238-0

[2] Doran CM, Kinchin I. A review of the economic impact of mental illness. Australian Health Review. 2019;43(1): 42–48. DOI: 10.1071/ah16115

[3] Schnitzerova E, Antonicova L. Gender aspects in the context of cosial work and services for drug users. Alkoholizmus a drogové závislosti - Protialkoholický obzor. 2011;46(4):241–251. Available from: https://www.adzpo.sk/images/articles/adzpo-2011-46-4-241-251.pdf [Accessed: 2020-12-29]

[4] Kalina K. Ženy a muži jako specifické cílové skupiny. In: Kalina K, et al. editors. Základy klinické adiktológie. 1st ed. Praha: Grada; 2008. p. 265–274. ISBN 978–80–247-1411-0

[5] Kim SS, Lee HO, Kiang P, Kalman D, Ziedonis DM. Factors associated with alcohol problems among Asian American college students: gender, ethnicity, smoking and depressed mood. Journal of Substance Use. 2013;19(1–2):12–17. DOI: 10.3109/14659891.2012.709912

[6] OECD. Health at a Glance 2019: OECD Indicators [Internet]. 2019. Paris: OECD Publishing. Available from: https://doi.org/10.1787/4dd50c09-en [Accessed: 2020-12-29]

[7] Skogen JC, Bøe T, Thørrisen MM, Riper H, Aas RW. Sociodemographic characteristics associated with alcohol consumption and alcohol-related consequences, a latent class analysis of The Norwegian WIRUS screening study. BMC Public Health. 2019;19(1). DOI:10.1186/s12889-019-7648-6

[8] Rehm J, Room R. The cultural aspect: How to measure and interpret epidemiological data on alcohol-use disorders across cultures. Nordisk Alkohol- & Narkotikatidskrift. 2017;34 (4):330–341. DOI: 10.1177/1455072517704795

[9] Pilatti A, Read JP, Caneto F. Validation of the Spanish version of the Young Adult Alcohol Consequences Questionnaire (S-YAACQ). Psychological Assessment. 2016;28(5): e49–e61. DOI: 10.1037/pas0000140

[10] Read JP, Merrill JE, Kahler CW, Strong DR. Predicting functional outcomes among college drinkers: Reliability and predictive validity of the Young Adult Alcohol Consequences Questionnaire. Addictive Behaviors. 2007;32(11):2597–2610. DOI: 10.1016/j.addbeh.2007.06.021

[11] Read JP, Haas AL, Radomski S, Wickham RE, Borish SE. Identification of hazardous drinking with the Young Adult Alcohol Consequences Questionnaire: Relative operating characteristics as a function of gender. Psychological Assessment. 2016;28(10): 1276–1289. DOI: 10.1037/pas0000251

[12] Keough MT, O'Connor RM, Read JP. Replication and validation of the Young Adult Alcohol Consequences Questionnaire in a large sample of Canadian undergraduates. Alcoholism-Clinical and Experimental Research. 2016; 40(5):1093–1099. DOI: 10.1111/acer.13039

[13] Merrill JE, Carey KB. Drinking over the lifespan: Focus on college ages. Alcohol Research-Current Reviews. 2016;38(1):103–114.

[14] Tembo C, Burns S, Kalembo F. The association between levels of alcohol consumption and mental health problems and academic performance among young university students. Plos One. 2017;12(6):e0178142. DOI: 10.1371/journal.pone.0178142

[15] dos Reis TG, de Oliveira LCM. Alcohol consumption among students of a Brazilian public university and consequences associated with this consumption. Bioscience Journal. 2017; 33(5):1371–1380.

[16] Larimer ME, Cronce JM. Identification, prevention, and treatment revisited: Individual-focused college drinking prevention strategies 1999–2006. Addictive Behaviors. 2007; 32(11):2439–2468. DOI: 10.1016/j.addbeh.2007.05.006

[17] Lamis DA, Ballard ED, May AM, Dvorak RD. Depressive symptoms and suicidal ideation in college students: The mediating and moderating roles of hopelessness, alcohol problems, and social support. Journal of Clinical Psychology. 2016;72(9):919–932. DOI: 10.1002/jclp.22295

[18] Murphy JG, Barnett NP, Goldstein AL, Colby SM. Gender moderates the relationship between substance-free activity enjoyment and alcohol use. Psychology of Addictive Behaviors. 2007; 21(2):261–265. DOI: 10.1037/0893-164x.21.2.261

[19] Bravo AJ, Pearson MR, Pilatti A, Read JP, Mezquita L, Ibanez MI, Ortet G. Impulsivity-related traits, college alcohol beliefs, and alcohol outcomes: Examination of a prospective multiple mediation model among college students in Spain, Argentina, and USA. Addictive Behaviors. 2018;81: 125–133. DOI: 10.1016/j.addbeh.2018.02.009

[20] Merrill JE, Wardell JD, Read JP. Drinking motives in the prospective prediction of unique alcohol-related consequences in college students. Journal of Studies on Alcohol and Drugs. 2014;75(1):93–102. DOI: 10.15288/jsad.2014.75.93

[21] Read JP, Kahler CW, Strong DR, Colder CR. Development and preliminary validation of the Young Adult Alcohol Consequences Questionnaire. Journal of Studies on Alcohol. 2006;67(1):169–177. DOI: 10.15288/jsa.2006.67.169

[22] Lemley SM, Kaplan BA, Reed DD, Darden AC, Jarmolowicz DP. Reinforcer pathologies: Predicting alcohol related problems in college drinking men and women. Drug and Alcohol Dependence. 2016;167:57–66. DOI: 10.1016/j.drugalcdep.2016.07.025

[23] Geisner IM, Larimer ME, Neighbors C. The relationship among alcohol use, related problems, and symptoms of psychological distress: Gender as a moderator in a college sample. Addictive Behaviors. 2004;29 (5):843–848. DOI: 10.1016/j.addbeh.2004.02.024

[24] Bravo AJ, Pilatti A, Pearson MR, Read JP, Mezquita L, Ibanez MI, Ortet G. Cross-cultural examination of negative alcohol-related consequences: Measurement invariance of the Young Adult Alcohol Consequences Questionnaire in Spain, Argentina, and USA. Psychological Assessment. 2019;31 (5):631–642. DOI: 10.1037/pas0000689

[25] Ibrahim AK, Kelly SJ, Adams CE, Glazebrook C. A systematic review of studies of depression prevalence in university students. Journal of Psychiatric Research. 2013;47(3):391–400. DOI: 10.1016/j.jpsychires.2012.11.015

[26] Ludwig AB, Burton W, Weingarten J, Milan F, Myers DC, Kligler B. Depression and stress amongst undergraduate medical students. BMC Medical Education. 2015;15(1):141. DOI: 10.1186/s12909-015-0425-z

[27] Awadalla S, Davies EB, Glazebrook C. A longitudinal cohort study to explore the relationship between depression, anxiety and academic performance among Emirati

university students. BMC Psychiatry. 2020;20(1):448. DOI: 10.1186/s12888-020-02854-z

[28] Dvorak RD, Lamis DA, Malone PS. Alcohol use, depressive symptoms, and impulsivity as risk factors for suicide proneness among college students. Journal of Affective Disorders. 2013;149(1–3):326–334. DOI: 10.1016/j.jad.2013.01.046

[29] Asante KO, Andoh-Arthur J. Prevalence and determinants of depressive symptoms among university students in Ghana. Journal of Affective Disorders. 2015;171:161–166. DOI: 10.1016/j.jad.2014.09.025

[30] Angst J, Gamma A, Gastpar M, Lepine JP, Mendlewicz J, Tylee A. Gender differences in depression: Epidemiological findings from the European DEPRES I and II studies. European Archives of Psychiatry and Clinical Neuroscience. 2002;252(5):201–209. DOI: 10.1007/s00406-002-0381-6

[31] Leppink EW, Lust K, Grant JE. Depression in university students: Associations with impulse control disorders. International Journal of Psychiatry in Clinical Practice. 2016;20(3):146–150. DOI: 10.1080/13651501.2016.1197272

[32] Kroenke K, Spitzer RL, Williams JBW. The PHQ-9: Validity of a brief depression severity measure. Journal of General Internal Medicine. 2001;16(9):606–613. DOI: 10.1046/j.1525-1497.2001.016009606.x

[33] Kroenke K, Spitzer RL, Williams JBW, Lowe B. The Patient Health Questionnaire somatic, anxiety, and depressive symptom scales: A systematic review. General Hospital Psychiatry. 2010;32(4):345–359. DOI: 10.1016/j.genhosppsych.2010.03.006

[34] Kroenke K, Spitzer RL. The PHQ-9: A new depression diagnostic and severity measure. Psychiatric Annals. 2002;32(9):509–515. DOI: 10.3928/0048-5713-20020901-06

[35] Hajduk M, Heretik A, Vaseckova B, Forgacova L, Pecenak J. Prevalence and correlations of depression and anxiety among Slovak college students. Bratislava Medical Journal. 2019;120(9):695–698. DOI: 10.4149/BLL_2019_117

[36] Dansova P, Masopustova Z, Hanackova V, Kickova K, Korabova I. The Patient Health Questionnaire-9: the Czech version. 2016;60(3):468–481.

[37] Milic J, Skrlec I, Vranjes IM, Podgornjak M, Heffer M. High levels of depression and anxiety among Croatian medical and nursing students and the correlation between subjective happiness and personality traits. International Review of Psychiatry. 2019;31(7–8):653–660. DOI: 10.1080/09540261.2019.1594647

[38] Honney K, Buszewicz M, Coppola W, Griffin M. Comparison of levels of depression in medical and non-medical students. The Clinical Teacher. 2010;7(3):180–184. DOI: 10.1111/j.1743-498x.2010.00384.x

[39] Weitzman ER. Poor mental health, depression, and associations with alcohol consumption, harm, and abuse in a national sample of young adults in college. The Journal of Nervous and Mental Disease. 2004;192(4):269–277. DOI: 10.1097/01.nmd.0000120885.17362.94

[40] Boden JM, Fergusson DM. Alcohol and depression. Addiction. 2011;106(5):906–914. DOI: 10.1111/j.1360-0443.2010.03351.x

[41] Li J, Wang H, Li M, Shen Q, Li X, Zhang Y, Peng J, Rong X, Peng Y. Effect of alcohol use disorders and alcohol intake on the risk of subsequent depressive symptoms: a systematic review and meta-analysis of cohort

studies. Addiction. 2020;115(7):1224–1243. DOI: 10.1111/add.14935

[42] Martens MP, Martin JL, Hatchett ES, Fowler RM, Fleming KM, Karakashian MA, Cimini MD. Protective behavioral strategies and the relationship between depressive symptoms and alcohol-related negative consequences among college students. Journal of Counseling Psychology. 2008; 55(4):535–541. DOI: 10.1037/a0013588

[43] Park CL, Grant C. Determinants of positive and negative consequences of alcohol consumption in college students: alcohol use, gender, and psychological characteristics. Addictive Behaviors. 2005;30(4):755–765. DOI: 10.1016/j.addbeh.2004.08.021

[44] Kenney SR, Lac A, LaBrie JW, Hummer JF, Pham A. Mental Health, Sleep Quality, Drinking Motives, and Alcohol-Related Consequences: A Path-Analytic Model. Journal of Studies on Alcohol and Drugs. 2013;74 (6):841–851. DOI: 10.15288/jsad.2013.74.841

[45] Preonas PD, Lau-Barraco C. Affective factors explaining the association between depressive functioning and alcohol outcomes among college students. Journal of American College Health. 2019. DOI: 10.1080/07448481.2019.1683565

[46] Ruiz P, Pilatti A, Pautassi RM. Consequences of alcohol use, and its association with psychological distress, sensitivity to emotional contagion and age of onset of alcohol use, in Uruguayan youth with or without college degree. Alcohol. 2020;82:91–101. DOI: 10.1016/j.alcohol.2019.09.001

[47] Flesch BD, Houvessou GM, Munhoz TN, Fassa AG. Major depressive episode among university students in Southern Brazil. Revista de Saude Publica. 2020;54:11. DOI: 10.11606/s1518-8787.2020054001540

[48] Dennhardt AA, Murphy JG. Associations between depression, distress tolerance, delay discounting, and alcohol-related problems in European American and African American college students. Psychology of Addictive Behaviors. 2011;25(4):595–604. DOI: 10.1037/a0025807

[49] Wang J, Patten SB. A prospective study of sex-specific effects of major depression on alcohol consumption. The Canadian Journal of Psychiatry. 2001;46 (5):422–425. DOI: 10.1177/070674370104600507

[50] Kuo PH, Gardner CO, Kendler KS, Prescott CA. The temporal relationship of the onsets of alcohol dependence and major depression: using a genetically informative study design. Psychological Medicine. 2006;36(8):1153. DOI: 10.1017/s0033291706007860

[51] Fergusson DM, Boden JM, Horwood LJ. Tests of causal links between alcohol abuse or dependence and major depression. Archives of General Psychiatry. 2009;66(3):260. DOI: 10.1001/archgenpsychiatry.2008.543

[52] Hasin DS, Grant BF. Major depression in 6050 former drinkers: Association with past alcohol dependence. Archives of General Psychiatry. 2002;59(9):794. DOI: 10.1001/archpsyc.59.9.794

[53] Schutte KK, Hearst J, Moos RH. Gender differences in the relations between depressive symptoms and drinking behavior among problem drinkers: A three-wave study. Journal of Consulting and Clinical Psychology. 1997;65(3):392–404. DOI: 10.1037/0022-006x.65.3.392

[54] Rosenthal SR, Clark MA, Marshall BDL, Buka SL, Carey KB, Shepardson RL, Carey MP. Alcohol consequences, not quantity, predict major depression onset among first-year female college students. Addictive

Behaviors. 2018;85:70–76. DOI: 10.1016/j.addbeh.2018.05.021

[55] Grello CM, Welsh DP, Harper MS. No strings attached: The nature of casual sex in college students. Journal of Sex Research. 2006;43(3),255–267. DOI: 10.1080/00224490609552324

[56] Foster C, Caravelis C, Kopak A. National College Health Assessment Measuring Negative Alcohol-Related Consequences among College Students. American Journal of Public Health Research. 2014;2(1):1–5. DOI: 10.12691/ajphr-2-1-1

[57] Panno A, Carbone GA, Massullo C, Farina B, Imperatori C. COVID-19 related distress is associated with alcohol problems, social media and food addiction symptoms: Insights from the italian experience during the lockdown. Frontiers in Psychiatry. 2020;11:577135. DOI: 10.3389/fpsyt.2020.577135

[58] Son C, Hegde S, Smith A, Wang X, Sasangohao F. Effects of COVID-19 on college students' mental health in the United States: interview survey study. Journal of Medical Internet Research. 2020;22(9):e21279. DOI: 10.2196/21279

[59] Ramalho R. Alcohol consumption and alcohol-related problems during the COVID-19 pandemic: a narrative review. Australasian Psychiatry. 2020;28(5):524–526. DOI: 10.1177/1039856220943024

[60] Adewuya AO, Ola BA, Afolabi OO. Validity of the patient health questionnaire (PHQ-9) as a screening tool for depression amongst Nigerian university students. Journal of Affective Disorders. 2006;96(1–2):89–93. DOI: 10.1016/j.jad.2006.05.021

[61] Du N, Yu K, Ye Y, Chen S. Validity study of Patient Health Questionnaire-9 items for Internet screening in depression among Chinese university students. Asia-Pacific Psychiatry. 2016;9 (3):e12266. DOI: 10.1111/appy.12266

[62] Farrer LM, Gulliver A, Bennett K, Fassnacht DB, Griffiths KM. Demographic and psychosocial predictors of major depression and generalised anxiety disorder in Australian university students. BMC Psychiatry. 2016;16(1). DOI: 10.1186/s12888-016-0961-z

[63] Zhou Y, Xu J, Rief W. Are comparisons of mental disorders between Chinese and German students possible? An examination of measurement invariance for the PHQ-15, PHQ-9 and GAD-7. BMC Psychiatry. 2020;20:480. DOI: 10.1186/s12888-020-02859-8

[64] Zajenkowska A, Jasielska D, Melonowska J. Stress and sensitivity to frustration predicting depression among young adults in Poland and Korea - Psychological and philosophical explanations. Current Psychology. 2019; 38:769–774. DOI: 10.1007/s12144-017-9654-0

[65] Corbin WR, Waddell JT, Ladensack A, Scott C. I drink alone: Mechanisms of risk for alcohol problems in solitary drinkers. Addictive Behaviors. 2020;102:106147. DOI: 10.1016/j.addbeh.2019.106147

[66] World Medical Association. Declaration of Helsinki—Ethical principles for medical research involving human subjects [Internet]. 2013. Available from: https://www.wma.net/policies-post/wma-declaration-of-helsinki-ethical-principles-for-medical-research-involving-human-subjects/ [Accessed: 2020-12-24]

[67] International Society of Addiction Journal Editors. The Farmington Consensus [Internet]. 2017. Available from: http://www.isaje.net/farmington-consensus.html [Accessed: 2020-12-24]

[68] Sopko J, Kocisova K. Key indicators and determinants in the context of the financial aspects of health systems in selected countries. Adiktologie. 2019;19

(4):189–202. DOI: 10.35198/01-2019-004-0003

[69] Megyesiova S, Gavurova B. Multivariate analysis of alcohol consumption and death rates resulting from alcohol consumption in EU and OECD member states. Adiktologie. 2019;19(4):179–187. DOI: 10.35198/01-2019-004-0002

[70] Foster DW, Young CM, Bryan J, Steers MLN, Yeung NCY, Prokhorov AV. Interactions among drinking identity, gender and decisional balance in predicting alcohol use and problems among college students. Drug and Alcohol Dependence. 2014;143:198–205. DOI: 10.1016/j.drugalcdep.2014.07.024

[71] Gaher RM, Simons JS. Evaluations and expectancies of alcohol and marijuana problems among college students. Psychology of Addictive Behaviors. 2007;21(4):545–554. DOI: 10.1037/0893-164x.21.4.545

[72] Nolen-Hoeksema S. Gender differences in risk factors and consequences for alcohol use and problems. Clinical Psychology Review. 2004;24(8):981–1010. DOI: 10.1016/j.cpr.2004.08.003

[73] Rose PA, Schuckman HE, Oh SS, Park EC. Associations between gender, alcohol use and negative consequences among Korean college students: A national study. International Journal of Environmental Research and Public Health. 2020;17(14):5192. DOI: 10.3390/ijerph17145192

[74] Ngasa SN, Sama CB, Dzekem BS, Nforchu KN, Tindong M, Aroke D, Dimala CA. Prevalence and factors associated with depression among medical students in Cameroon: A cross-sectional study. BMC Psychiatry. 2017;17(1):216. DOI: 10.1186/s12888-017-1382-3

[75] Albert P. Why is depression more prevalent in women? Journal of Psychiatry & Neuroscience. 2015;40(4): 219–221. DOI: 10.1503/jpn.150205

[76] Nolen-Hoeksema S, Girgus JS. The emergence of gender differences in depression during adolescence. Psychological Bulletin. 1994;115(3): 424–443. DOI: 10.1037/0033-2909.115.3.424

[77] Acikgoz A, Dayi A, Binbay T. Prevalence of depression among female university students and associated factors. Cukurova Medical Journal. 2018;43(1):131–140. DOI: 10.17826/cumj.340629

[78] Miller MB, DiBello AM, Merrill JE, Neighbors C, Carey KB. The role of alcohol-induced blackouts in symptoms of depression among young adults. Drug and Alcohol Dependence. 2020;211: 108027. DOI: 10.1016/j.drugalcdep.2020.108027

[79] Shor C, Zuo W, Eloy JD, Ye J-H. The Emerging Role of LHb CaMKII in the Comorbidity of Depressive and Alcohol Use Disorders. International Journal of Molecular Sciences. 2020;21(21):8123. DOI: 10.3390/ijms21218123

[80] Degan TJ, Kelly PJ, Robinson LD, et al. Health literacy in substance use disorder treatment: A latent profile analysis. Journal of Substance Abuse Treatment. 2019;96:46–52. DOI: 10.1016/j.jsat.2018.10.009

[81] Aaby A, Friis K, Bo C, Rowlands G, Maindal HT. Health literacy is associated with health behaviour and self-reported health: A large population-based study in individuals with cardiovascular disease. European Journal of Preventive Cardiology. 2017; 24(17):1880–1888. DOI: 10.1177/2047487317729538

[82] Bostock S, Steptoe A. Association between low functional health literacy and mortality in older adults: Longitudinal cohort study. BMJ-British

Medical Journal. 2012;344:e1602. DOI: 10.1136/bmj.e1602

[83] Rolova G, Gavurova B, Petruzelka B. Exploring health literacy in individuals with alcohol addiction: A mixed methods clinical study. International Journal of Environmental Research and Public Health. 2020;17 (18):6728. DOI: 10.3390/ijerph17186728

[84] Gavurova B, Kovac V, Kulhanek A, Bartak M. Territorial distribution of alcohol and drug addictions mortality concerning regional disparities in the Slovak Republic from year 1996 to year 2015. Adiktologie. 2019;19(3):125–134. DOI: 10.35198/01-2019-003-0005

[85] Kuruc A, Smitkova H. Rod/gender ako sociálna kategória v psychoterapii a poradenstve. Československá Psychologie. 2007;51(3):269–278.

[86] Miovsky M. Evaluace adiktologických programu a služeb. In: Kalina K, et al. editors. Základy klinické adiktológie. Praha: Grada; 2008. p. 307–315. ISBN 978–80–247-1411-0

[87] EMCDDA. 2005. Differences in patterns of drug use between men and women. Technical datasheet [Internet]. 2005. Lisbon: European Monitoring Centre for Drugs and Drug Addiction. Available from: https://www.emcdda.europa.eu/system/files/publications/387/TDS_gender_64783.pdf [Accessed: 2020-12-29]

Chapter 4

Leveraging Advanced Analytics to Understand the Impact of the COVID-19 Pandemic on Trends in Substance Use Disorders

Ewa J. Kleczyk, Jill Bana and Rishabh Arora

Abstract

Coronavirus disease (COVID-19) caused an overwhelming healthcare, economic, social, and psychological impact on the world during 2020 and first part of 2021. Certain populations, especially those with Substance Use Disorders (SUD), were particularly vulnerable to contract the virus and also likely to suffer from a greater psychosocial and psychological burden. COVID-19 and addiction are two conditions on the verge of a collision, potentially causing a major public health threat. There is surge of addictive behaviors (both new and relapse), including use of alcohol, nicotine, and recreational drugs. This book chapter analyzed the bi-directional relationship between COVID-19 and SUD by leveraging descriptive summaries, advanced analytics, and machine learning approaches. The data sources included healthcare claims dataset as well as state level alcohol consumption to help in investigating the bi-directional relationship between the two conditions. Results suggest that alcohol and nicotine use increased during the pandemic and that the profile of SUD patients included diagnoses and symptoms of COVID-19, depression and anxiety, as well as hypertensive conditions.

Keywords: COVID-19, pandemic, addiction, smoking, alcohol, opioid addiction, public health, advanced analytics, linear regression, machine learning model

1. Introduction

The coronavirus disease (COVID-19) has caused a large healthcare, economic, and psychosocial impact on communities in the United States and around the world in 2020 and first part of 2021. Many communities, especially those with low income and Substance Use Disorders (SUD), were particularly vulnerable to contract the infection and likely to suffered from a greater economic and psychosocial burden [1].

Addiction, characterized by a range of mental, physical, and behavioral symptoms, claims the lives of millions of people every year around the world [2]. In their National Survey on Drug Use and Health, Substance Abuse and Mental Health Services Administration estimated that 22.6 million Americans, 12 years of age or older (9.2% of the population), have SUD, including alcohol and tobacco use [3]. Furthermore, the long-term treatment has challenges to due frequent relapse [4]. Alcohol consumption and drug addiction cost around 1.5% of the global burden of disease, and it can be as high as 5% in some countries, according to recent data [2].

There are two basic settings to treat SUD: inpatient and outpatient. The primary goal is for patients affected by addiction to be in the most effective, yet least restrictive environment that allows them to move along a continuum of care, depending on their personal and medical needs. There are four phases of SUD care: outpatient treatment, intensive outpatient treatment, residential treatment, and inpatient hospitalization [5].

Furthermore, SUD treatment programs are often designed based on three basic models:

- Psychological model that includes behavioral therapy and treats emotional challenges as the primary cause of SUD.

- Medical model that requires treatment of SUD symptoms by a healthcare provider. It focuses on the physiological, biological, and genetic causes of the disease.

- Sociocultural model that aims to modify the physical and social environment of a person with SUD [5].

Many patients, receiving SUD treatments, may have also problems in other areas of their life, including but not limited to: physical and mental health issues, relationship problems, inadequate social and work skills, as well as legal or financial challenges. As a result, the treatment options should aim to address the entire spectrum of issues, and not only treat the addiction component [5].

Even with the variety of treatment options for SUD, more than 6,000 people a month died from overdosing before the pandemic started in the US [6]. In addition to the continued loss of lives due to addiction, the pandemic also added other challenges for those suffering from SUD, resulting in additional 2,000 individuals a month dying from SUD between March and August 2020 [6]. The government COVID-19 based restrictions, like home confinement, caused enormous economic burden to communities in the US as well as around the world. Individuals and their families faced various unwelcome emotional, psychological, and behavioral challenges, including excessive substance abuse and depression [4], which further increased the risk for addiction. The COVID-19 related restrictions caused individuals to turn to smoking, alcohol, drugs, including opioids and synthetic drugs like Fentanyl, as well as gaming activities to deal with the COVID-19 pandemic [6–8].

On the other hand, individuals suffering from addiction were often also part of low income communities that already faced many significant challenges related to access to healthcare, quality education, and unemployment. They also were also more prone to contract infection during the COVID-19 pandemic due to their underlying comorbid conditions and immune system deficiencies [8, 9].

In this book chapter, the bi-directional correlation between the COVID-19 diagnoses and SUD was investigated, and insights were provided to better understand the impact of the pandemic on addiction occurrence. The research leveraged multiple analytics methods from descriptive statistics, through a simple linear regression, and selected machine learning models to analyze this relationship. The data sources utilized for the analysis included healthcare claims dataset and the state level alcohol consumption.

2. Literature review

The COVID-19 pandemic caused limited social interactions for individuals around the world due to the strict national, state, and local governmental restrictions [10, 11]. As a result of the restrictions, many individuals started using tobacco, alcohol, and other substances to help with stress related symptoms. On the other hand, the increased restrictions and home confinement reduced the substance exposure, but also resulted in more pronounced cravings and withdrawal effects in current users. Selected articles have cited a substantially increased number of drug – and alcohol – withdrawal cases and hospitalizations, which were potentially putting burden on the already strained health care systems [12, 13].

Opioid addiction and its management was often discussed SUD type in the COVID-19 era. Opioid addicts particularly faced a challenge due to difficulty in accessing healthcare services, imposed restrictions on prescription and over-the-counter drugs, closures of rehabilitation centers, and an increased risk of life-threatening withdrawals [14]. While loosening of restrictions were recommended for home-based self-injections and long-acting formulations of methadone and buprenorphine to mitigate these problems, there was also fear of overdosing and fatalities [15, 16].

Due to the financial burden and an uncertain future as a result of the pandemic, gambling activities also increased to unprecedented levels [17, 18]. Eating disorders and compulsive buying were progressively being reported [19, 20]. COVID-19 pandemic created a vicious cycle of stress, depression, social isolation, anxiety, excess leisure time that led to surge of behavioral addictions, resulting in mood alterations, irritability, anxiety, and stress [19, 20].

3. Data and methodology overview

There were multiple types of data utilized for this research. The first source of the data is represented by the healthcare claims database with the study time period from January 31, 2019 to December 31, 2020. Patient cohorts: study target and control were established, using SUD and COVID-19 ICD 10 diagnosis codes. The diagnoses codes are listed in the appendix. The healthcare claims dataset included diagnosis codes, medical and surgical codes, therapeutics and treatments prescribed at the transactional level. In addition, socioeconomic variables, including age, gender, race, education and incomes levels were leveraged to provide additional insights into the characteristics of patients with SUD during COVID-19 pandemic [21].

The second dataset employed for the study represented the State Level Alcohol Consumption trends for 2019 and 2020. The 2020 data was available, however, only through end of September. For this analysis, alcohol consumption data on per capita, alcohol sales from 19 states (Alaska, Arkansas, Colorado, Connecticut, Delaware, Florida, Illinois, Kansas, Kentucky, Louisiana, Massachusetts, Missouri, North Dakota, Oregon, Tennessee, Texas, Utah, Virginia, and Wisconsin) by type of alcoholic beverage was leveraged. Only information from the states noted above was used due to limited availability of data from other states [22].

A number of analytical methods was employed for the analysis from the rules-based patient qualification criteria, descriptive statistics, linear regression analysis to machine learning algorithms in order to understand the bi-directional relationship between SUD trends and the COVID-19 surge.

3.1 Healthcare claims patient level database

The healthcare claims database is an anonymous longitudinal patient data set that can help researchers, healthcare providers, and pharmaceutical companies in the design of research studies in order to aid comparisons of diagnosis and treatment outcomes that represent individual patient-based experiences and interactions with the US healthcare system [21].

The healthcare claims database leveraged for this study consisted of medical, hospital, and prescription claims across all insurance payment types. As shown in **Figure 1**, the database covers more than 317 million patients in the US, spans over more than 17 years of medical health history, and includes more than 1.9 million healthcare providers [21]. The data elements used for the study included diagnoses codes for SUD and other comorbid conditions, procedures and treatments, payment types: commercial, Medicaid, Medicare and cash, along with patient sociodemographic characteristics like age, gender, race, education and income levels, as well as geography [21].

3.2 Methodology overview: Linear regression introduction

One of the methods utilized to analyze the relationship between addiction and the COVID-19 pandemic was a linear regression approach. In statistics, linear regression is a linear method to modeling the relationship between a scalar response (dependent variable – y) and one or more explanatory variables (independent variables – x):

$$y = f(x) \tag{1}$$

When there is only one explanatory variable, the regression is called a simple linear regression. When there are more than one independent variables, the process is called a multiple linear regression [23].

In a linear regression, the relationships are modeled using linear predictor functions, whose model parameters are estimated from the data [24]. Linear regression focuses on the conditional probability distribution of the response given the values of the predictors, which is the domain of multivariate analysis [24].

There are several metrics often leveraged to evaluate the model performance: R-squared and F-statistic. R-squared also called the coefficient of determination is the proportion of the variance in the dependent variable that can be explained by the variation in the independent variable(s). The value of the metric ranges between 0 and 1, and the higher value represents a better performance of the model [24]. An F-test represents a statistical test often used when comparing statistical models employed on the studied datasets to identify the model that best fits the population from which the data sample was drawn [24].

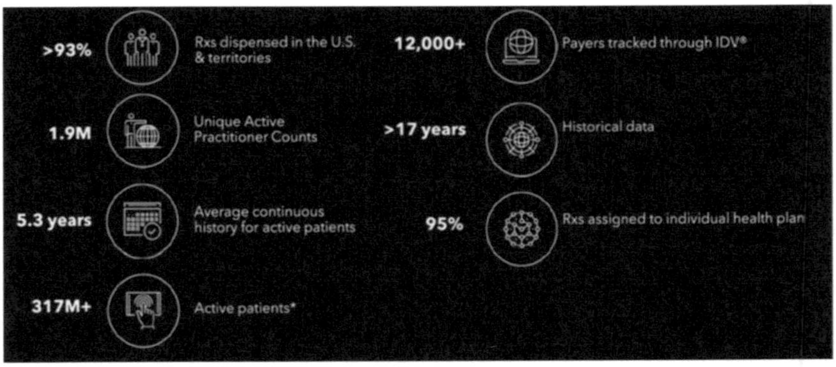

Figure 1.
Healthcare claims patient level database description.

3.3 Machine learning introduction

Machine learning is a subfield of the artificial intelligence area, which includes statistics, mathematics, computer algorithms, etc. focused on building applications that learn and improve their predictive capabilities automatically over time without being specifically programmed to do so. Machine learning models are built upon a statistical framework, since they involve data elements often described, using statistical distributions and assumptions. These algorithms gained in popularity in the recent years due the increased amounts of data availability and significant advancements in the computing power [25].

In this book chapter, selected algorithms were leveraged to analyze the relationship between SUD and COVID-19 diagnoses. The analysis identified factors beyond the pandemic, such as patient characteristics: age, race, education and income levels, comorbid conditions (example: diabetes, hypertension, mental health), concomitant treatments that increased the addiction diagnoses, including patients most likely to struggle with SUD, regions of greater prevalence, and comorbid conditions presented along with SUD and COVID-19 diagnoses.

3.3.1 Supervised learning algorithms

Supervised learning is the process of training or building machine learning algorithms, in which algorithms learn to map from input space (X) to output space (Y) [26].

$$Y = f(X) \tag{2}$$

The major objective is to approximate the mapping function (f) in order to predict (y) outcome when a new data point (x) is added [26]. Supervised learning algorithms are mainly used for classification and prediction problems [27]. The following are examples of supervised algorithms: logistic regression, decision trees (DTs), random forest (RF), extreme gradient boosting (XGBoost), support vector machines (SVMs), naïve bayes, adaptive boosting (AdaBoost), and artificial neural network (ANN) [28].

3.3.2 Unsupervised learning algorithms

Unsupervised learning algorithms, on the other hand, learn the hidden patterns within the input dataset (X) [29]. These models are called unsupervised, because there is no supervision to guide them, and the algorithms learn, discover, and display the patterns in the input data (X) [30]. These algorithms are often employed to uncover the natural clusters, dimension reduction, anomaly detection, etc. Examples of unsupervised algorithms include: k-means clustering, principal component analysis (PCA), factor analysis (FA), singular value decomposition (SVD), apriori algorithm (association rule) [28].

Depending on the study objectives and the available data type, algorithms are tested for performance, data type fit, and are selected accordingly. A random forest and an extreme gradient boosting models were selected to explain the bi-directional relationships of the SUD trends and COVID-19 pandemic surge.

3.3.3 xExtreme gradient boosting

Gradient boosting algorithm is an ensemble of weak prediction models, mostly decision trees [31]. XGBoost starts by creating a first simple tree [32, 33], which than adds other trees, and builds upon the weaker learners. The model learns with each iteration and revises the previous tree until an optimal point is reached [34].

Feature importance is the value mostly generated by tree-based models like decision trees, random forest, XGBoost, etc. [31] and signifies the importance of features in the model in predicting the outcome. It represents how good the feature is at reducing node impurity. It is widely known as 'gini importance' or 'mean decrease impurity,' and is defined as the total decrease in node impurity averaged over all trees of the ensemble [32]. Importance is mostly calculated as: weight, gain and cover, where 'weight' is the number of times a feature is present in a tree, 'gain' is the average gain of splits, while 'cover' is the average coverage of splits, with 'coverage' being defined as the number of samples affected by the split [33].

3.3.4 Random forest

Random forest or random decision forest is an ensemble learning method for classification and regression analysis that constructs an array of decision trees during the training timeframe. The output of the random forest for the classification task is the class selected by the majority of trees, while for the regression task, the output represents the mean or average prediction across individual trees [35, 36].

3.3.5 Chi-square test and p-value

The Chi-square test is one of the most widely used non-parametric tests [37], often utilized to test the independence between observed and expected frequencies of one or more attributes in a contingency table, known as 'goodness of fit test' [38].

The p-value, also used in this study, evaluates the statistical significance of the predictor variables. The significance level was set at the 5% and 10% to aid the feature importance evaluation and statistical results' interpretation [24, 38].

3.3.6 Classification metrics

The following classification metrics were leveraged to validate the machine learning models' performance. A confusion matrix is often generated from the predicted probability values with 0.5 as the classification threshold. Patients with probability value greater than or equal to 0.5 are noted as 1 and below 0.5 are noted as 0 [38].

Confusion matrix:

- True Positive (TP) – Target patient correctly identified by the model as target patient

- False Positive (FP) – Control patient misclassified by the model as target patient

- True Negative (TN) – Control patient correctly classified by the model as control patient

- False Negative (FN) – Target patient misclassified by the model as control patient

Model performance metrics:

- Accuracy: % of total patients correctly identified among total patients

- Positive Predictive Value (PPV, Precision): % of true target patients among total predicted target patients
- True Positive Rate (TPR, Sensitivity, Recall, Hit Rate): % of true target patients who were correctly identified among total target patients
- False Positive Rate (FPR): % of true control patients incorrectly identified among total control patients
- Specificity: % of those control who will have a negative target result
- F1 Score: is the harmonic mean of precision and recall
- AUC: Area Under the Receiver Operating Characteristic (ROC) Curve. To validate the trade-off between true positive rate and false positive rate [38].

4. Analysis results and discussion

4.1 Substance usage disease trends overview

This section provides an overview of SUD trends for 2019 and 2020 when leveraging the healthcare claims dataset that was discussed in the earlier section of the chapter. The summary includes information on the overall trends, patient demographics, and insights into the COVID-19 diagnosis rates. The first part of the analysis was to review and understand the SUD diagnoses trends as well as COVID-19 infection rates within the SUD population. The focus of the analysis was on the SUD population only to understand changes in trends during the pandemic.

The monthly trends of patients with SUD diagnoses presented that the addiction trends stayed consistent over 2019 and 2020, with the exception of April–May 2020 timeframe. The list of SUD diagnoses is presented in the appendix refers to **Tables 6–9**. At the beginning of the pandemic (April–May 2020), there was a decrease in the number of patients with addiction diagnoses. A two sample t-test that compared the SUD diagnosis counts between April–May 2019 and April–May 2020 revealed that the difference in counts was not significant at either the 5% or 10% significance level. However, the directional decline might have been a result of the state enacted restrictions, including home confinement as well as the inability to hold in-person HCP office visits and elective procedures (**Figure 2**).

The SUD diagnoses trend data also involved analyzing trends by splitting the patient cohort into newly diagnosed patients in the last 12 months as well as previously diagnosed patients within the same timeframe. The analysis presented that the share of newly diagnosed patients vs. previously diagnosed declined slightly between 2019 and 2020, but the difference was not statistically significant. In 2020, newly diagnosed patients accounted for 62% of all patients vs. 66% in 2019. In addition, patients diagnosed with addiction as well as COVID-19 represented 3% of the newly diagnosed patients and 4% of those with already a diagnosis.

Furthermore, several different types of SUD experienced a decline in the number of patients diagnosed at the start of the pandemic. Opioid dependence was the leading addiction type with alcohol dependence following as next most frequently diagnosed SUD (**Figure 3**). The counts of opioid dependence diagnosis were statistically different from the counts for other types of SUD. Statistically significant difference in trends at 5% significance level was also observed between opioid dependence and alcohol dependence, opioid dependence vs. cannabis dependence,

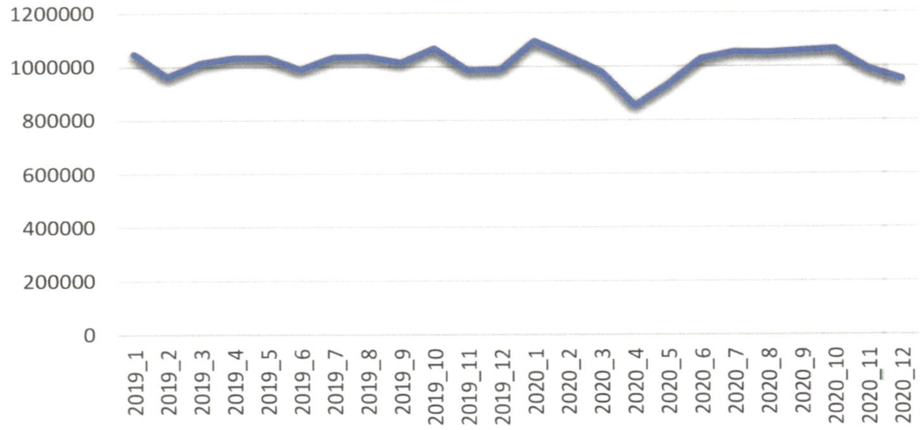

Figure 2.
Addiction monthly patient count trends, 2019–2020.

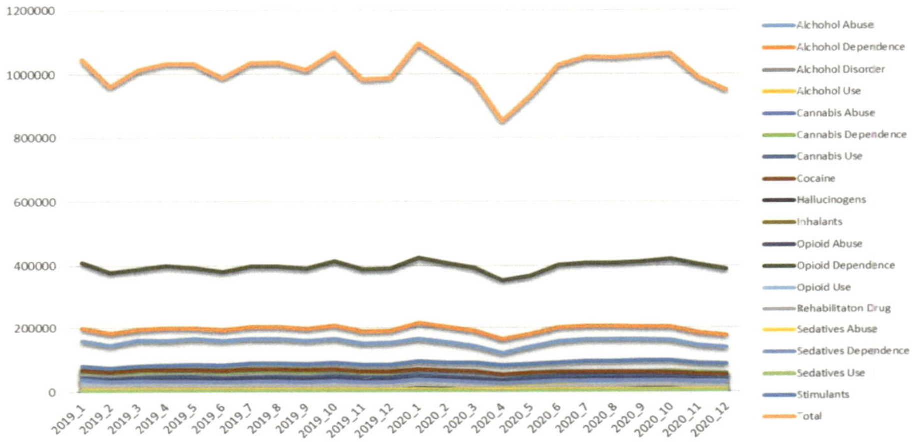

Figure 3.
Addiction monthly patient count trends, 2019–2020.

sedatives dependance vs. cannabis dependance, and sedatives dependence vs. alcohol use. The addiction diagnosis codes are noted in the appendix. Patients with psychoactive type of addiction represented a higher share within the COVID-19 diagnosed population (19%) as compared to the overall share (3%). Psychoactive SUD is referred to as addiction type with hallucinatory symptoms. The COVID-19 patient distribution for other addictions was very similar to the overall addiction population.

An additional analysis of demographic and geographic attributes as presented in **Table 1** revealed that males presented a higher percentage of the SUD population compared to SUD and COVID-19 population, but the percentage was not statistically significantly different from the percentage of women SUD patients. On the other hand, patients using cannabis appeared younger compared to the rest of the SUD population. This finding was statistically significant based on a two sample t-test (p-value = 0.00, statistically significant at 5%).

Most of both SUD and COVID-19 patients had commercially provided insurance coverage (~70%), while ~30% of patients had a government provided healthcare insurance (p-value = 0.00, statistically significant at 5%). Inhalants and rehabilitation drug addiction represented the highest share of patients with commercial insurance with more than 75%.

Diagnosis Group	2020 - Average Age			2020 - % Male for COVID 19 Diagnosed Population		
	Total Addiction Population	COVID 19 Population	Rest of the Addiction Population	Total Addiction Population	COVID 19 Population	Rest of the Addiction Population
Alcohol Abuse	49	56	48	66%	69%	66%
Alcohol Dependence	47	53	46	67%	70%	67%
Alcohol Disorder	55	55	55	68%	70%	68%
Alcohol Use	50	57	48	65%	68%	65%
Cannabis Abuse	35	41	34	57%	58%	57%
Cannabis Dependence	33	38	33	62%	61%	62%
Cannabis Use	37	43	36	54%	55%	54%
Cocaine	44	50	43	62%	65%	62%
Hallucinogens	35	41	34	68%	69%	68%
Inhalants	42	53	39	61%	61%	61%
Opioid Abuse	41	48	40	57%	59%	57%
Opioid Dependence	42	49	41	52%	49%	52%
Opioid Use	48	53	48	48%	50%	48%
Psychoactive	42	49	41	58%	59%	58%
Rehabilitation Drug	41	46	41	52%	49%	52%
Sedatives Abuse	39	49	39	53%	55%	53%
Sedatives Dependence	45	53	44	43%	42%	43%
Sedatives Use	44	49	44	46%	47%	46%
Stimulants	37	42	37	57%	60%	57%

Table 1.
Patient demographic summary (age and gender).

Furthermore, the North East and Midwest regions represented two main geographic areas of the United States with the highest level of patients diagnosed with SUD and covered more than 50% of the total addiction diagnosed patients. The share of patients in these two regions was statistically significantly higher compared to the rest of the US regions (p-value = 0.00, statistically significant at 5%). The West regions on the other hand covered approximately 20% of the addiction diagnosed population.

The SUD treatment pattern analysis revealed that the procedural services, including psychotherapy, recommended to treat SUD patients declined in April and May 2020 and then returned to similar levels before the pandemic and on par with

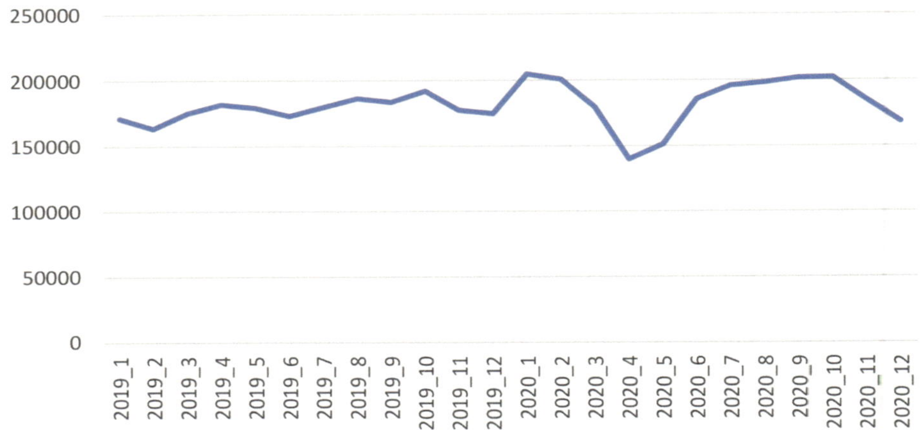

Figure 4.
Procedural treatment trends, 2019–2020.

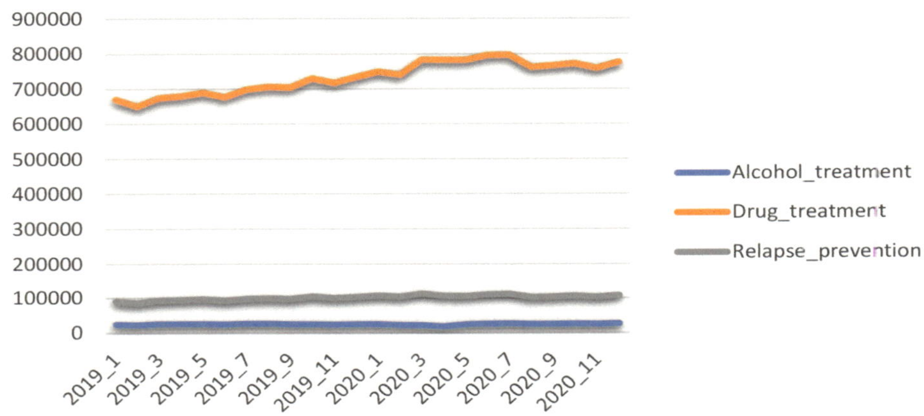

Figure 5.
Addiction Rx treatment monthly patient count trends, 2019–2020, by addiction type.

the 2019 trends (**Figure 4**). The decline was statistically significant at the 10% significance level with a p-value = 0.07. The decline might have been related to the imposed country-wide lockdown during the two months on 2020.

On the other hand, the number of patients treated with prescription medications statistically significantly increased between 2019 and 2020 (p-value = 0.00, statistically significant at 5%), even during the pandemic, the trend continued to increase, implying that patients continuously were receiving patient care (**Figure 5**). The drugs names are presented in the appendix. Prescription treatments for drug related addiction had the highest share of the treatments, followed by addiction relapse treatments. The share of drug prescription treatments was statistically different from the other types of therapy, including relapse and alcohol treatments.

4.2 Alcohol consumption overview

This section of the book chapter provides an overview of alcohol consumption trends for 2019 and 2020. For this analysis, alcohol consumption data on per capita, alcohol sales from 19 states (Alaska, Arkansas, Colorado, Connecticut, Delaware, Florida, Illinois, Kansas, Kentucky, Louisiana, Massachusetts, Missouri, North

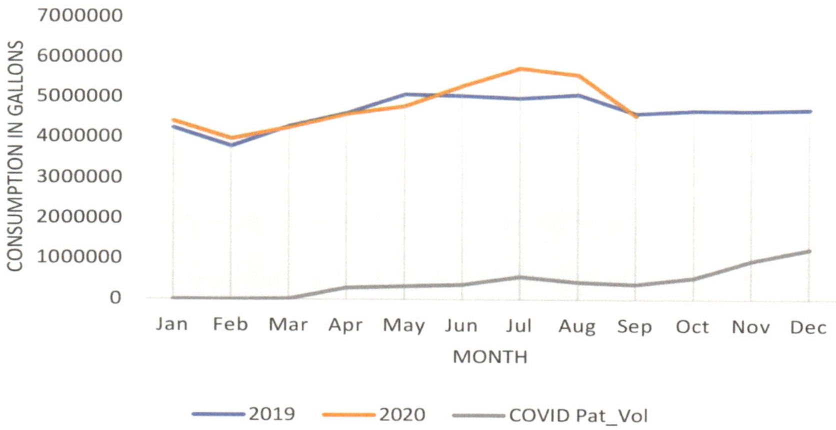

Figure 6.
Monthly avg. of pure alcohol (gallons of ethanol) across United States.

Dakota, Oregon, Tennessee, Texas, Utah, Virginia, and Wisconsin) by type of alcoholic beverage was leveraged. The limited alcohol consumption information by state was due to the limited data availability at source [22].

The monthly trends of pure alcohol (gallons of ethanol) from 2019 and 2020 in **Figure 6** showed that the trend stayed nearly the same, with a only a directional increase in 2020 [22]. A two sample t-test did not present statistically significant differences between the yearly trends. On the other hand, it was observed that with the increase in COVID-19 cases in the middle of pandemic (June–August 2020), there was an associated increase in the consumption of pure alcohol, as evident from the high Pearson correlation coefficient of 0.87 between the alcohol consumption and COVID-19 diagnosed number of patients. The increase in the alcohol use might have been associated with individuals experiencing hardship due to the prolonged lock-downs, loss of job, and the overall changes in lifestyle as a result of pandemic, and alcohol being perceived as a way for coping with the changing environment.

The trends describing gallons of alcohol per capita for age 14 and older (**Figure** 7) showed a statistically significance increase (p-value = 0.04, statistically significant at 5%) in gallons per capita from mid-May 2020, which might be a result of the COVID-19 pandemic spread. This was also apparent from a strong a Pearson correlation coefficient of 0.91 between the pandemic outbreak as denoted by a volume of patients diagnosed with COVID-19 and gallons of alcohol per capita [22].

In order to understand the alcohol consumption over time, the percentage change in gallons of alcohol per capita from 2017 to 2019 (a 3-year average) to 2020

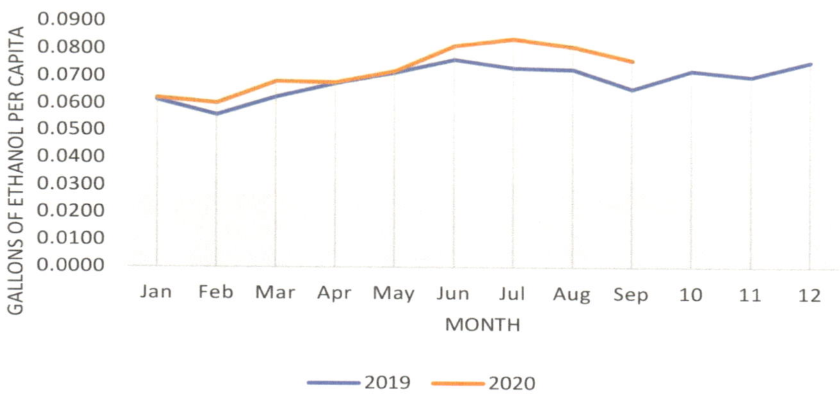

Figure 7.
Gallons of ethanol per capita age 14 and older (2019 and 2020).

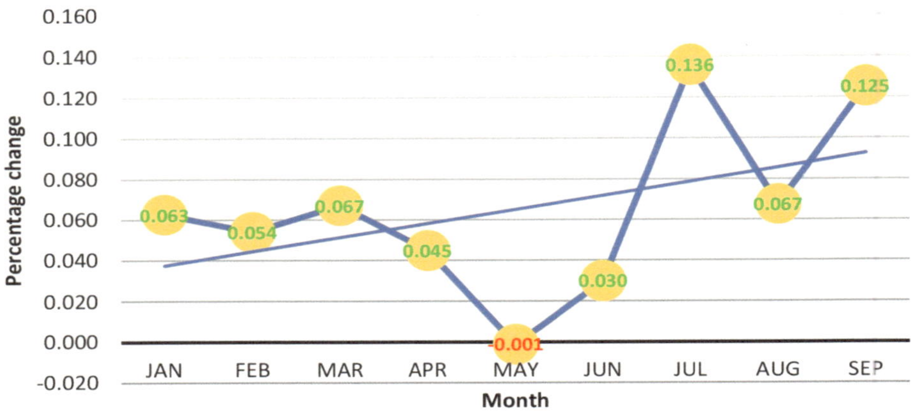

Figure 8.
Percentage change in gallons of ethanol per capita age 14 and older from 2017 to 2019 (3-year average) to 2020. Note: Limited states shown due to unavailability of the data from the source.

was analyzed (**Figure 8**). Overall, a visible increase in the trend was noticed; however, in May 2020, a statistically significant decline in the percentage in alcohol consumption (p-value = 0.06, statistically significant at 10%) was observed due to the COVID-19 imposed lockdowns and closures of liquor stores. From the month of June onwards, a statistically significant increase in the percentage change (p-value = 0.06, statistically significant at 10%) was noted, which might have been associated with the lockdown restrictions being partially lifted, leading to re-opening of liquor stores and increased purchasing levels [22].

Figure 9 depicts a comparison of selected states' gallons of alcohol consumption per capita between 2019 and 2020. As noted earlier, only a few selected states were considered for the analysis due to the limited availability of the data at the source. For most of the states, an increase in alcohol (in gallons) per capita is noticeable in 2020. Delaware's excise tax on liquor of $3.75 per gallon, lower than 72% of the other 50 states, led to the highest increase in per capita alcohol in 2020. Most of the states experienced an increase in per capita alcohol during the COVID-19 pandemic [22].

The alcohol consumption data was also analyzed for each alcohol type. **Figure 10** presents a yearly consumption comparison between 2019 and 2020 for beer, wine and spirits. It was observed that beer consumption was higher in January and February in 2020 compared to January and February in 2019, but after the COVID-19 pandemic started, the consumption decreased from March onwards until May 2020

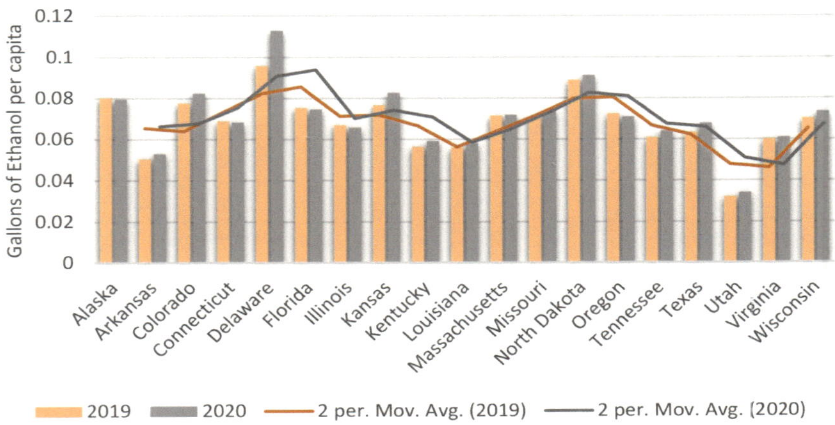

Figure 9.
State wise three-year average gallons of ethanol per capita age 14 and older, 2017–2019 and 2020.

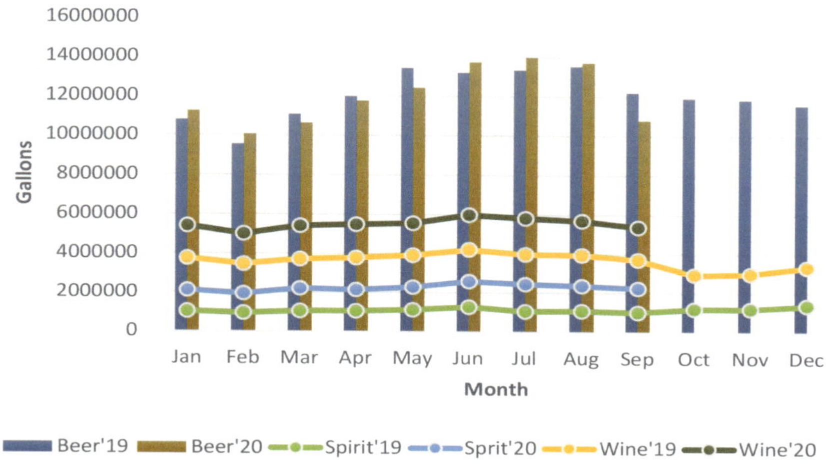

Figure 10.
Average beverage consumption breakout by wine, beer and spirit from 2019 and 2020. Note: 2020 data is available only until Sep due to limited availability from the source.

due to lockdowns and limited liquor facilities opened in each state. For wine and spirits, the trend of consumption showed an increase, starting from January 2020 onwards [21]. It was also evident that the increase in volume of beer, spirit, and wine consumption from 2019 to 2020 was statistically significant based on the two sample t-test, which resulted in a p-value < 0.02 for each alcohol type [22].

4.3 Effects of alcohol and substance use during COVID-19

In this section of the book chapter, the effects of alcohol and SUD during the COVID-19 pandemic were analyzed. An ordinary least square linear regression model was used to investigate the correlation between these events. The dataset employed was a combination of the healthcare claims data and the alcohol consumption data, both aggregated at a state and monthly levels for comparison [21, 22].

The results of the ordinary least square regression are presented in **Table 2**. The analysis results showed that sedatives use, alcohol abuse, and beer consumption were the highly significant variables and positively correlated with the COVID-19 pandemic spread. Sedatives like benzodiazepines are often prescribed for anxiety and insomnia, confirming the finding [39]. Furthermore, an increased consumption of alcohol might have led to seeking treatments to manage the signs of frustration, sadness, mental health conditions, and stress [40], caused by the prolonged isolation during the pandemic.

Other parameters like opioid use, cannabis use/abuse were significant as well, but they were negatively correlated with the pandemic spread. These results were consistent with previous research articles, presenting that drug use declined during the pandemic while at the same time patients suffered from withdraws and other symptoms related to fewer substances available for consumption [12–14, 41, 42]. On the other hand, while beer consumption was positively correlated with COVID-19 pandemic trends, the consumption of spirits presented the reversed correlation, which was contrary to the findings of overall alcohol trend increases. The difference in correlation might have been related to the differences in states regulations of the different types of alcohol, which in turn might impact the alcohol type availability for consumption at the state level [43].

The model significance was evident from the F-statistic value of 14.7 with an adjusted R square value of ~74%, which informed that a relatively high proportion of the variations in the data could be explained by the predictor variables.

OLS Regression Results	
Prob (F-statistic): 3.48e-23	R-squared: 0.790
No. Observations: 124	Adj. R-squared: 0.736
Df Residuals: 98	F-statistic: 14.74
Df Model: 25	Log-Likelihood: -1266.9
Covariance Type: nonrobust	AIC: 2586. BIC: 2659.

Variable	Coef	std err	t	P>|t|
Const	106.4333	2383.339	0.045	0.964
Stimulants_DX	10.739	9.72	1.105	0.272
Psychoactive_DX	8.5724	9.749	0.879	0.381
Alcohol_Disorder_DX	-15.3404	10.442	-1.469	0.145
Opioid_Abuse_Disorder_DX	-12.6339	16.859	-0.749	0.455
Hallucinogens_DX	88.8541	57	1.559	0.122
Cannabis_dependence_DX	-44.6289	21.517	-2.074	0.041
Cocaine_DX	11.2889	17.254	0.654	0.514
Alcohol_Abuse_DX	28.4386	15.069	1.887	0.062
Opioid_Use_DX	-27.898	11.827	-2.359	0.020
Cannabis_Abuse_DX	20.9762	22.25	0.943	0.348
Alcohol_Use_DX	-17.2129	24.825	-0.693	0.490
Opioid_Dependence_DX	1.7466	1.463	1.194	0.235
Sedatives_Abuse_DX	-136.0078	63.427	-2.144	0.034
Alcohol_Dependence_DX	-5.7262	8.12	-0.705	0.482
Rehabitilation_Drug_DX	-2.6533	2.707	-0.98	0.329
Cannbis_Use_DX	-50.8229	22.303	-2.279	0.025
Sedatives_Use_DX	806.6812	169.107	4.77	0.0001
Sedatives_Depedence_DX	0.8243	3.516	0.234	0.815
Drug_Treatment_RX	0.0002	0.003	0.089	0.929
Alcohol_Treatment_RX	0.6266	1.038	0.604	0.547
Relapse_Prevention_RX	-0.4599	0.282	-1.629	0.107
Rehabilitation_PX	-0.5844	0.452	-1.292	0.199
Spirit_Avg_Gallon	-0.0073	0.004	-2.045	0.044
Wine_Avg_Gallon	-0.0005	0.002	-0.222	0.825
Beer_Avg_Gallon	0.0011	0	2.786	0.006

Note: Per capita alcohol sales from 19 states (Alaska, Arkansas, Colorado, Connecticut, Delaware, Florida, Illinois, Kansas, Kentucky, Louisiana, Massachusetts, Missouri, North Dakota, Oregon, Tennessee, Texas, Utah, Virginia, and Wisconsin) by type of alcoholic beverage.

Table 2.
Ordinary least square regression analysis results.

4.4 Machine learning: important features leading to addiction

To understand the parameters associated with SUD and identify if the COVID-19 pandemic impacted the addiction diagnosis rate, supervised classification machine learning algorithms, including random forest and XGBoost were performed.

4.4.1 Dataset overview

As a part of the analysis, two distinct patient cohorts: study target and control groups were developed to allow for analysis of the SUD and COVID-19 trends. The distinction between these two groups permitted the machine learning models to learn the variations in the data and identify the important variables that best distinguished between both groups. The target group was defined by the patients in the data from October 2020 to December 2020, who had at least 2 addiction diagnoses, followed by a treatment after initial diagnosis, and the control group was defined by the patients from October 2019 to December 2019, having two addiction diagnoses, followed by a treatment after initial diagnosis. A sample of ~20,000 records were randomly selected for the modeling exercise based on similar age and gender distribution as in the target group. Two months of historical claims data related to diagnosis, procedures, and pharmacological treatment were pulled from initial diagnosis event along with other demographic data elements like age, gender, income, education, etc. The healthcare claims level data was converted to patient level records, using data preprocessing steps, and a final data structure with ~ 20,000 records and ~15,000 features was created for machine learning modeling [21].

4.4.2 Feature selection

The data elements used for the study included diagnosis, procedures, and pharmacological treatments along with other demographic features like age, gender, income, education, etc. Since the number of features was ~15,000, the data element dimension needed to be reduced to a more manageable number.

In order to reduce the variables' space and select the top features, the LightGBM and Boruta algorithms were leveraged for the purposes of dimension reduction. LightGBM is a gradient boosting framework, which uses tree-based learning, whereas Boruta is a feature selection algorithm, a wrapper built around RF Classification algorithm. The top features from both the algorithms were selected for the machine learning algorithms development [44].

Table 3 below represents a list of selected features important in the preliminary run of the models. Data elements related to the COVID-19 diagnoses and associated symptoms along with alcohol and nicotine use as well as major depressive disorder were noted as important variables, separating the 2020 and 2019 SUD patient cohorts.

4.4.3 Machine learning models overview

In order to understand the underlying factors for the SUD 2020 and 2019 patient cohorts and investigate if there was an association with the COVID-19 pandemic, the following machine learning models were applied: random forest and XGBoost. Hyper tunning process was also performed to optimize the models. Below a brief methodology overview is presented.

Random forest is a classification algorithm, consisting of many decision trees that use bootstrap aggregation, bagging and feature randomness when building each individual tree. It creates an uncorrelated forest of trees whose prediction is more accurate than that of any individual tree. The model outcome provides estimates of variables important in the classification [45].

XGBoost is a decision-tree-based ensemble machine learning algorithm that uses a gradient boosting framework. XGBoost approaches the process of sequential tree building, using parallelized implementation. Each model run learns from the error of previous models and weak learners. It incorporates the error of weak learners in the ensemble model and re-runs the process. It uses bootstrap aggregating technique, also called as bagging, which implies diving the data into sub samples for each iteration of model training. For prediction purposes, the model chooses majority of the vote from all the learners [46].

Hyper parameter tuning is the optimization process of finding the model parameters to improve the model performance. The objective is to minimize the

Features	Description
DX_Z20.828_ICD_10	CONTACT W AND EXPOSURE TO OTH VIRAL COMMUNICABLE DISEASES
PX_U0003	INFECTIOUS AGENT DETECTION BY NUCLEIC ACID (DNA
PX_87635	IADNA SARS-COV-2 COVID-19 AMPLIFIED PROBE TQ
DX_R51.9_ICD_10	HEADACHE, UNSPECIFIED
DX_U07.1_ICD_10	COVID-19
DX_R74.01_ICD_10	ELEVATION OF LEVELS OF LIVER TRANSAMINASE LEVELS
PX_87426	IAAD IA SEVERE AQTRESPIRSYND CORONAVIRUS
DX_Z11.59_ICD_10	ENCOUNTER FOR SCREENING FOR OTHER VIRAL DISEASES
DX_R51_ICD_10	HEADACHE
PX_U0002	2019-NCOV CORONAVIRUS, SARS-COV-2/2019-NCOV (COV
DX_N18.3_ICD_10	CHRONIC KIDNEY DISEASE, STAGE 3 (MODERATE)
DX_N18.30_ICD_10	CHRONIC KIDNEY DISEASE, STAGE 3 UNSPECIFIED
PX_U0004	2019-NCOV CORONAVIRUS, SARS-COV-2/2019-NCOV (COV
PX_H0020	ALCOHOL AND/OR DRUG SERVICES; METHADONE ADMINIST
PX_80307	DRUG TST PRSMV INSTRMNT CHEM ANALYZERS PR DATE
DX_F17.210_ICD_10	NICOTINE DEPENDENCE, CIGARETTES, UNCOMPLICATED
RX_78340	DISULFIRAM
DX_R45.851_ICD_10	SUICIDAL IDEATIONS
DOC_IM	Internal Medicine
DOC_FM	Family Medicine
DX_F32.9_ICD_10	MAJOR DEPRESSIVE DISORDER, SINGLE EPISODE, UNSPECIFIED
DX_I10_ICD_10	ESSENTIAL (PRIMARY) HYPERTENSION
DX_J06.9_ICD_10	ACUTE UPPER RESPIRATORY INFECTION, UNSPECIFIED
DX_R05_ICD_10	COUGH
RX_78312	NARCAN
RX_09110	NAPROXEN
PX_G0480	DRUG TEST(S), DEFINITIVE, UTILIZING (1) DRUG IDE
PX_G2023	SPECIMEN COLLECTION FOR SEVERE ACUTE RESPIRATORY

Table 3.
Preliminary important data features.

cost function, hence reduce the error caused by the model. It uses gradient descent algorithm, which initially randomly assigns the model parameter to calculate the cost function and later improves it at each step, so that the cost function assumes a minimum value. Mathematically, it takes the derivative of the sum of squared residuals and equates it to 0 to find a point where the function is changing [47].

4.4.4 Machine learning analysis details

The machine learning algorithms were evaluated for the different performance metrics as noted in the earlier section of the book chapter. Initially, the models were overfitting, as they seemed to capture most of the variations from the training data, as well as at the same time captured the noise from the data. This resulted in many negative records misclassified as positive, which might have led to a considerably lower precision value.

As noted in **Table 4**, the baseline models, random forest resulted in AUC of 73% and XGBoost resulted in AUC of 74% with recall of 74.08% and 82.80% respectively. While working with healthcare claims data, a higher ratio of false negative records is perceived as a large problem. For example, predicting a sick patient as

	Random Forest		XGBoost	
	Baseline	**Hypertuned**	**Baseline**	**Hypertuned**
AUC ROC	73%	75%	74%	75%
Accuracy	63.63%	58.22%	63.51%	62.55%
Precision	61.29%	54.76%	59.78%	58.59%
Recall/Sensitivity/ True Positive Rate	74.08%	**94.73%**	82.68%	**85.62%**
F1 Score	67.08%	**69.40%**	69.39%	**69.57%**

Table 4.
Machine learning model metrics.

healthy, because ideally the patient should have received the treatment on time, may lead to health complications and even potentially death. Thus, it is advised to minimize the number of false negative observations, which will result in a higher recall, depicting an inverse relationship between the two, also called true positive rate or sensitivity. However, the initial baseline models resulted in a comparatively lower recall. To improve the model accuracy, the hyper parameter tuning was executed to find the best model parameters.

In addition, F1 score was defined as follows:

$$2 * (\text{Precision} * \text{Recall})/(\text{Precision} + \text{Recall}) \qquad (3)$$

which is a function of precision and recall and should be maximized such that both precision and recall both are optimal [45–47]. Hyper parameter tuned models not only improved the recall, but also slightly improved the F1 scores for random forest and XGBoost to 69.4% and 69.57% respectively, implying a robust model sensitive to false negative observations.

The machine learning models were retrained, using a few model parameters, including mex=depth, min-samples_split and max_features. In order to obtain the optimal values of model parameters, k fold cross validation with 5 iterations were used in the hyper parameter tuning process [47].

Using the optimal values of the model parameters obtained from hyper parameter tuning, the models showed an improvement in the model performance, which was evident from the model metrics. As shown in **Table 4**, the recall significantly increased for both of the models and also, the F1 scores slightly improved compared to the baseline models. This resulted in a decrease in the false negatives count, which led to an increase in recall.

Figure 11 depicts the final ROC AUC plot, which shows the relationship between the true positive rate and the false positive rate at different probability thresholds. A true positive rate also known as the sensitivity metric, which informs the proportion of positive records that were correctly classified over the total number of positive records. A false positive rate is the proportion of negative records misclassified over total number of negative records [38]. Both random forest and XGBoost resulted in AUC of 75% with recall of 94.7% and 85.6% respectively, which improved from the baseline models.

4.4.5 Machine learning model interpretation

The random forest and XGBoost models identify features, which were a combination of SUD as well as COVID-19 data elements. **Table 5** presents the top

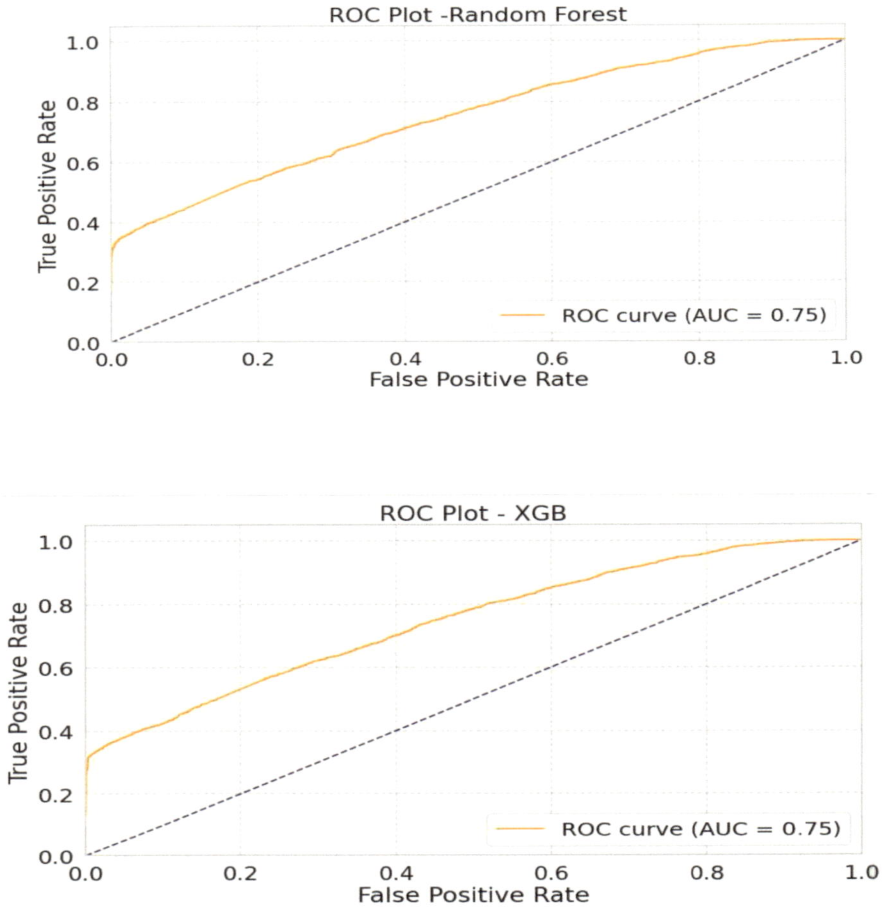

Figure 11.
ROC AUC curve of random forest and XGBoost.

important features. The importance of the features was measured using the 'gini' importance metric, which calculated the impurity in the node. The metric measured how each feature decreased the impurity of the split, while making the decision tree in the algorithm and averaging it over all the trees in the forest, resulting in the measure of feature importance [32, 33].

Features like nicotine dependence, alcohol abuse, long term drug therapy, disulfiram [48], methadone [49] were presented as important in explaining the differences in SUD patient cohorts between 2019 and 2020. For example, the value 0.003 of nicotine dependence importance denoted that the impurity reduced in the node by adding the variable, which thus contributed to the model robustness and a higher accuracy level. The effects of pandemic on individual's lives were not only restricted to patients' physical health, but also affected their mental health, as noted by the major depressive, anxiety diagnoses, and suicidal tendencies as presented in the top most important healthcare data elements. The unexpected and unwanted change enforced on daily lives, drastically increased the stress levels. Difficulties in management of the changing environment and following preventive measures, such as undergoing lockdowns, fueled the stress levels even more. The economic downturn, leading to unemployment, and low consumer confidence played an imperative role in increasing the stress levels as well. As a result of the prolonged stress and anxiety due to the lockdowns, the consumption of alcohol, smoking, and other nicotine-based products increased [12, 13, 41, 42].

Variable	Description	Importance
DX_Z20.828_ICD_10	CONTACT W AND EXPOSURE TO OTH VIRAL COMMUNICABLE DISEASES	0.356
PX_U0003	INFECTIOUS AGENT DETECTION BY NUCLEIC ACID (DNA	0.075
PX_87635	IADNA SARS-COV-2 COVID-19 AMPLIFIED PROBE TQ	0.074
DX_R51.9_ICD_10	HEADACHE, UNSPECIFIED	0.049
DX_U07.1_ICD_10	COVID-19	0.042
DX_R74.01_ICD_10	ELEVATION OF LEVELS OF LIVER TRANSAMINASE LEVELS	0.035
DX_Z11.59_ICD_10	ENCOUNTER FOR SCREENING FOR OTHER VIRAL DISEASES	0.029
PX_87426	IAAD IA SEVERE AQTRESPIRSYND CORONAVIRUS	0.025
DX_R51_ICD_10	HEADACHE	0.024
DX_N18.3_ICD_10	CHRONIC KIDNEY DISEASE, STAGE 3 (MODERATE)	0.021
DX_Z03.818_ICD_10	ENCNTR FOR OBS FOR SUSP EXPSR TO OTH BIOLG AGENTS RULED OUT	0.019
PX_U0002	2019-NCOV CORONAVIRUS, SARS-COV-2/2019-NCOV (COV	0.018
DX_N18.30_ICD_10	CHRONIC KIDNEY DISEASE, STAGE 3 UNSPECIFIED	0.016
PX_99285	EMERGENCY DEPT VISIT HIGH SEVERITY&THREAT FUNCJ	0.015
DX_R74.0_ICD_10	NONSPEC ELEV OF LEVELS OF TRANSAMNS & LACTIC ACID DEHYDRGNSE	0.014
PX_H0020	ALCOHOL AND/OR DRUG SERVICES; METHADONE ADMINIST	0.013
PX_71046	RADIOLOGIC EXAM CHEST 2 VIEWS	0.011
PX_U0004	2019-NCOV CORONAVIRUS, SARS-COV-2/2019-NCOV (COV	0.010
PX_C9803	HOSPITAL OUTPATIENT CLINIC VISIT SPECIMEN COLLEC	0.010
PX_99443	PHYS/QHP TELEPHONE EVALUATION	0.009
PX_99072	ADDL SUPL MATRL&STAF TM DRG PHE RES-TR NFCT DS	0.008
PX_85025	BLOOD COUNT COMPLETE AUTO&AUTO DIFRNTL WBC	0.007
PX_80307	DRUG TST PRSMV INSTRMNT CHEM ANALYZERS PR DATE	0.006
PX_80053	COMPREHENSIVE METABOLIC PANEL	0.005
PX_G2067	MEDICATION ASSISTED TREATMENT, METHADONE; WEEKLY	0.005
PX_G0378	HOSPITAL OBSERVATION SERVICE, PER HOUR	0.005
PX_93010	ECG ROUTINE ECG W/LEAST 12 LDS I&R ONLY	0.005

DX_F17.210_ICD_10	NICOTINE DEPENDENCE, CIGARETTES, UNCOMPLICATED	0.003
PX_80048	BASIC METABOLIC PANEL CALCIUM TOTAL	0.003
DX_K21.00_ICD_10	GASTRO-ESOPHAGEAL REFLUX DIS WITH ESOPHAGITIS, WITHOUT BLEED	0.003
RX_78340	DISULFIRAM	0.003
PX_93005	ECG ROUTINE ECG W/LEAST 12 LDS TRCG ONLY W/O I&R	0.002
DX_R45.851_ICD_10	SUICIDAL IDEATIONS	0.002
PX_85027	BLOOD COUNT COMPLETE AUTOMATED	0.002
PX_84484	ASSAY OF TROPONIN QUANTITATIVE	0.002
PX_G1004	CLINICAL DECISION SUPPORT MECHANISM NATIONAL DEC	0.002
DX_I10_ICD_10	ESSENTIAL (PRIMARY) HYPERTENSION	0.002
DX_F32.9_ICD_10	MAJOR DEPRESSIVE DISORDER, SINGLE EPISODE, UNSPECIFIED	0.002
PX_36415	COLLECTION VENOUS BLOOD VENIPUNCTURE	0.002
PX_99284	EMERGENCY DEPARTMENT VISIT HIGH/URGENT SEVERITY	0.002
DX_R77.8_ICD_10	OTHER SPECIFIED ABNORMALITIES OF PLASMA PROTEINS	0.002
DX_J06.9_ICD_10	ACUTE UPPER RESPIRATORY INFECTION, UNSPECIFIED	0.001
PX_J2405	INJECTION, ONDANSETRON HYDROCHLORIDE, PER 1 MG	0.001
DX_Z11.3_ICD_10	ENCNTR SCREEN FOR INFECTIONS W SEXL MODE OF TRANSMISS	0.001
DX_R05_ICD_10	COUGH	0.001
RX_78312	NARCAN	0.001
RX_02232	OXYCODONE HCL	0.001
PX_81001	URNLS DIP STICK/TABLET REAGENT AUTO MICROSCOPY	0.001
DX_Z79.899_ICD_10	OTHER LONG TERM (CURRENT) DRUG THERAPY	0.001
DX_M54.5_ICD_10	LOW BACK PAIN	0.001
PX_99223	INITIAL HOSPITAL CARE/DAY 70 MINUTES	0.001
DX_J12.89_ICD_10	OTHER VIRAL PNEUMONIA	0.001
PX_96374	THER PROPH/DX NJX IV PUSH SINGLE/1ST SBST/DRUG	0.001
DX_Z01.812_ICD_10	ENCOUNTER FOR PREPROCEDURAL LABORATORY EXAMINATION	0.001
PX_G0463	HOSPITAL OUTPATIENT CLINIC VISIT FOR ASSESSMENT	0.001
DX_Z23_ICD_10	ENCOUNTER FOR IMMUNIZATION	0.001
RX_09110	NAPROXEN	0.001
PX_80305	DRUG TEST PRSMV READ DIRECT OPTICAL OBS PR DATE	0.001
PX_87389	IAAD IA HIV-1 AG W/HIV-1 & HIV-2 ANTBDY SINGLE	0.001

DOI: http://dx.doi.org/10.5772/intechopen.99639

PX_99232	SBSQ HOSPITAL CARE/DAY 25 MINUTES	0.001
PX_71045	RADIOLOGIC EXAM CHEST SINGLE VIEW	0.001
DX_F41.9_ICD_10	ANXIETY DISORDER, UNSPECIFIED	0.001
DX_E78.5_ICD_10	HYPERLIPIDEMIA, UNSPECIFIED	0.001
PX_83735	ASSAY OF MAGNESIUM	0.001
RX_20200	CLOBAZAM	0.001
PX_70450	CT HEAD/BRAIN W/O CONTRAST MATERIAL	0.001
RX_15142	AZITHROMYCIN	0.001
RX_64310	DOXEPIN HCL	0.001
PX_80061	LIPID PANEL	0.001
PX_99233	SBSQ HOSPITAL CARE/DAY 35 MINUTES	0.001
PX_82565	CREATININE BLOOD	0.001
AGE_70_79	Age 70 – 79	0.001
PX_J7030	INFUSION, NORMAL SALINE SOLUTION , 1000 CC	0.001
PX_99291	CRITICAL CARE ILL/INJURED PATIENT INIT 30-74 MIN	0.001
PX_83690	ASSAY OF LIPASE	0.001
PX_99283	EMERGENCY DEPARTMENT VISIT MODERATE SEVERITY	0.001
DOC_P	PSYCHIATRY	0.001
PX_85610	PROTHROMBIN TIME	0.001
DX_Z01.818_ICD_10	ENCOUNTER FOR OTHER PREPROCEDURAL EXAMINATION	0.001
DX_G89.29_ICD_10	OTHER CHRONIC PAIN	0.001
DX_F41.1_ICD_10	GENERALIZED ANXIETY DISORDER	0.001
PX_94640	PRESSURIZED/NONPRESSURIZED INHALATION TREATMENT	0.001
DX_K21.9_ICD_10	GASTRO-ESOPHAGEAL REFLUX DISEASE WITHOUT ESOPHAGITIS	0.001
PX_G0480	DRUG TEST(S), DEFINITIVE, UTILIZING (1) DRUG IDE	0.001
DX_O99.89_ICD_10	OTH DISEASES AND CONDITIONS COMPL PREG/CHLDBRTH	0.001
PX_86769	ANTB SEVERE AQT RESPIR SYND SARS-COV-2 COVID-19	0.001
DX_D64.9_ICD_10	ANEMIA, UNSPECIFIED	0.001
DX_F10.139_ICD_10	ALCOHOL ABUSE WITH WITHDRAWAL, UNSPECIFIED	0.001
DX_R40.0_ICD_10	SOMNOLENCE	0.001
PX_90832	PSYCHOTHERAPY W/PATIENT 30 MINUTES	0.001
PX_G2023	SPECIMEN COLLECTION FOR SEVERE ACUTE RESPIRATORY	0.001

Table 5.
Top most important healthcare related features.

It was also interesting to see features related to COVID-19 pandemic being noted as important differentiators between the 2019 and 2020 SUD patient cohorts. The features included COVID-19 diagnosis and related symptoms: headache, cough, acute upper respiratory infection, specimen collection for severe acute respiratory condition. Procedures noting HCP in-office and tele-visits along with in-patient hospital or ER visits were also noted as important variables, further highlighting that the amount of care might have increased as a result of SUD, but also due to COVID-19 diagnoses and related symptoms. In addition, medications often used to treat viruses and infections like Azithromycin were also presented as important data elements defining the 2020 SUD patient cohort.

Furthermore, the cohorts differed on the occurrence of the comorbid conditions, such as chronic kidney condition, hypertension, hyper lipidemia, and gastro-esophagus conditions, which might inform a potential impact of a larger alcohol and other substance abuse activities during the pandemic or simply present that the patient profile changed during the pandemic, expanding the definition of the SUD patients group. There were also several data elements identifying SUD treatments such as Narcan, methadone to list a few and procedures related to drug testing, blood panels, and other related treatments, which present an increased rate of addiction testing and treatment between the two periods, confirming earlier findings of increased SUD treatment trends. The analysis also presented differences of the cohorts on a diagnoses for lower back pain and pain relieve medications use.

From the sociodemographic data elements, patients diagnosed with addiction or treated for addiction presented characteristics that can help further define the patient profiles for individuals that were likely for developing SUD during the pandemic. For example, the average age of 42 was observed for the impacted population. Ethnicity of Caucasian and Black/African American was also noted as prevalent. Patients with nicotine dependence, alcohol dependence, opioid use, and cannabis dependence were relatively more prevalent in the states of Florida and Texas. These states presented a relatively higher volume of patients with specific SUD diagnoses compared to other states. The impacted patients presented some college or achieved at least a high school diploma as well as were more likely to be associated with the lower economic status communities, with income level being less than $30 K annually. The educational and economic levels were noted by other published articles, presenting the economic impact and increased risk for COVID-19 virus within low income population [2].

5. Conclusions and study limitations

This book chapter investigated SUD and the resulting impact from the COVID-19 pandemic on the rate of diagnoses and treatment. Overall, the diagnoses rate of SUD was consistent over time in 2020 compared to 2019 (except for April and May); however, a statistically significant increase in treatment of different addiction types was noted during the pandemic. In 2020, newly diagnosed patients accounted for 62% of all SUD patients compared to 66% in 2019, but the difference was not statistically significant. Furthermore, the changes in procedures performed for addiction testing significantly declined at the beginning of the pandemic and then returned to normal levels in June of 2020, while the SUD treatment significantly increased between 2019 and 2020. In addition, patients diagnosed with addiction as well as COVID-19 represented 3% of the newly diagnosed patients and 4% of those with already a diagnosis. Patients using cannabis were found statistically significantly younger compared to the rest of the SUD population.

In 2020, a noticeable increase in alcohol consumption and drinking behaviors was observed compared to 2019, including an increase in the average gallons consumed by alcohol type: spirits, wine, and beer. Compared to the previous years, a statistically significant positive percentage change in gallons of alcohol per capita from 2017 to 2019 (a 3-year average) to 2020 was observed [22], which could be related to the increased stress levels due to the pandemic spread and prolonged lockdowns [50].

Machine learning analysis of SUD patient cohorts between 2020 and 2019 presented that the patients in the 2020 cohort who were diagnosed with SUD, were also often diagnosed with either COVID-19 or related symptoms, including headache, upper respiratory infection, and cough. Furthermore, it is likely that SUD patients with addiction to drugs and nicotine products were more likely to contract COVID-19, as a result of their weaker immune system due to lower white cells levels in the blood [51, 52]. The analysis also presented the importance of HCP in-office and tele-visits along with in-patient hospital visits that could be related to the increased level of SUD treatment, but also present the severity of COVID-19 related symptoms and the need for treatment.

Moreover, excess alcohol consumption identified as one of the important factors, differentiating between the two SUD patient cohorts could lead to immune deficiency, causing increased susceptibility to certain diseases. Prolonged alcohol abuse may cause disruptions to the digestive system and could result in liver failure. Alcohol use may also affect individual's ability to store adequate amounts of protein and nutrients. Most importantly drugs and alcohol affect white blood cells, which act as the defense system for the body. The weaker defense system can increase the risk of developing life-ending diseases [52].

Finally, based on the machine learning analysis, the SUD patient cohorts differed on occurrence of the comorbid conditions such as chronic kidney condition, hypertension, hyper lipidemia, and gastro-esophagus condition, which might present that the SUD patient profile changed during the pandemic due to the changes in the life style and increased consumption of alcohol and tobacco. Additional investigation should be conducted to further examine the patients' health history and understand the underlying reasons for the differences in the SUD patient cohort characteristics.

5.1 Study limitations

Due to the timing of writing this book chapter, not all data was available for the entire year of 2020 to allow for a comprehensive analysis. Adding the additional data for alcohol consumption, as well as data for recreational drug use by state during the pandemic could enhance the analysis in presenting the SUD population characteristics including their health, mental, and economic state. Furthermore, it might also be helpful to add COVID-19 vaccination data by state in order to understand the effects of vaccinations and COVID-19 variants on general virus trends as well as SUD impacted populations.

Additionally, the healthcare patient level claims data, comprising of prescription, medical, and hospital claims can also observe gaps in the coverage of long-term care institutions, mental health hospitals, correctional facilities, and other institutions with a limited public reporting, and result in a potential bias in the studied population when compared to the entire US population. Furthermore, the COVID-19 related symptoms' diagnoses might also skew the analysis and overestimate the impact of COVID-19 on the SUD population. The statistical results could be further enhanced and become more robust with the additional data availability and understanding of the diagnosis codes for the COVID-19 related symptoms.

Since the COVID-19 pandemic was a rare event, it became a new topic of interest for analysis. As a result, there was a limited number prior research studies conducted on this topic, which posed a challenge in creating a theoretical foundation for this book chapter's research questions and hypothesis. With little prior research, developing an entire new research typology was challenging.

The scope of the analysis can also be enhanced via adding additional data sources and having a longer timeframe to evaluate the impact of pandemic on addiction and health impact of those impacted by either condition. Furthermore, new set of advanced analytics, including deep learning and natural language processing (NLP) approaches, could be applied to create data driven evidence to confirm newly established hypothesis, research objectives, and results.

Acknowledgements

Availability of data and materials: The healthcare claims dataset that supports the findings of this study are available from Symphony Health, ICON plc Organization, but restrictions apply to the availability of these data, which were used under a license for the current study, and so they are not publicly available.

The Alcohol Consumption Dataset is available from the National institute of Alcohol Abuse and Alcoholism [Online]. https://pubs.niaaa.nih.gov/publications/surveillance-covid-19/COVSALES.htm

Funding

Authors work for Symphony Health, ICON plc Organization. The data used in the article is the property of Symphony Health, ICON plc Organization. Authors used the healthcare claims data for the sole purpose of publication of this article.

Conflict of interest

The authors declare no conflict of interest.

Notes/Thanks/Other declarations

The authors would like to thank Mike Byzon, Suzanne Rosado, Heather Valera, Lakshya Mandawat, and Koichi Iwata for their valuable feedback on earlier versions of this chapter.

Appendix

(**Tables 6–9**).

DIAG_CDE	DIAG_LONG_DESC
F12.10	CANNABIS ABUSE, UNCOMPLICATED
F12.11	CANNABIS ABUSE, IN REMISSION
F12.120	CANNABIS ABUSE WITH INTOXICATION, UNCOMPLICATED
F12.121	CANNABIS ABUSE WITH INTOXICATION DELIRIUM
F12.122	CANNABIS ABUSE WITH INTOXICATION WITH PERCEPTUAL DISTURBANCE
F12.129	CANNABIS ABUSE WITH INTOXICATION, UNSPECIFIED
F12.150	CANNABIS ABUSE WITH PSYCHOTIC DISORDER WITH DELUSIONS
F12.151	CANNABIS ABUSE WITH PSYCHOTIC DISORDER WITH HALLUCINATIONS
F12.159	CANNABIS ABUSE WITH PSYCHOTIC DISORDER, UNSPECIFIED
F12.180	CANNABIS ABUSE WITH CANNABIS-INDUCED ANXIETY DISORDER
F12.188	CANNABIS ABUSE WITH OTHER CANNABIS-INDUCED DISORDER
F12.19	CANNABIS ABUSE WITH UNSPECIFIED CANNABIS-INDUCED DISORDER
F12.20	CANNABIS DEPENDENCE, UNCOMPLICATED
F12.21	CANNABIS DEPENDENCE, IN REMISSION
F12.220	CANNABIS DEPENDENCE WITH INTOXICATION, UNCOMPLICATED
F12.221	CANNABIS DEPENDENCE WITH INTOXICATION DELIRIUM
F12.222	CANNABIS DEPENDENCE WITH INTOXICATION WITH PERCEPTUAL DISTURBANCE
F12.229	CANNABIS DEPENDENCE WITH INTOXICATION, UNSPECIFIED
F12.23	CANNABIS DEPENDENCE WITH WITHDRAWAL
F12.250	CANNABIS DEPENDENCE WITH PSYCHOTIC DISORDER WITH DELUSIONS
F12.251	CANNABIS DEPENDENCE WITH PSYCHOTIC DISORDER WITH HALLUCINATIONS
F12.259	CANNABIS DEPENDENCE WITH PSYCHOTIC DISORDER, UNSPECIFIED
F12.280	CANNABIS DEPENDENCE WITH CANNABIS-INDUCED ANXIETY DISORDER
F12.288	CANNABIS DEPENDENCE WITH OTHER CANNABIS-INDUCED DISORDER
F12.29	CANNABIS DEPENDENCE WITH UNSPECIFIED CANNABIS-INDUCED DISORDER
F12.90	CANNABIS USE, UNSPECIFIED, UNCOMPLICATED
F12.920	CANNABIS USE, UNSPECIFIED WITH INTOXICATION, UNCOMPLICATED
F12.921	CANNABIS USE, UNSPECIFIED WITH INTOXICATION DELIRIUM
F12.922	CANNABIS USE, UNSPECIFIED WITH INTOXICATION WITH PERCEPTUAL DISTURBANCE
F12.929	CANNABIS USE, UNSPECIFIED WITH INTOXICATION, UNSPECIFIED
F12.93	CANNABIS USE, UNSPECIFIED WITH WITHDRAWAL
F12.950	CANNABIS USE, UNSPECIFIED WITH PSYCHOTIC DISORDER WITH DELUSIONS
F12.951	CANNABIS USE, UNSPECIFIED WITH PSYCHOTIC DISORDER WITH HALLUCINATIONS
F12.959	CANNABIS USE, UNSPECIFIED WITH PSYCHOTIC DISORDER, UNSPECIFIED
F12.980	CANNABIS USE, UNSPECIFIED WITH ANXIETY DISORDER
F12.988	CANNABIS USE, UNSPECIFIED WITH OTHER CANNABIS-INDUCED DISORDER

F12.99	CANNABIS USE, UNSPECIFIED WITH UNSPECIFIED CANNABIS-INDUCED DISORDER
F14.10	COCAINE ABUSE, UNCOMPLICATED
F14.11	COCAINE ABUSE, IN REMISSION
F14.120	COCAINE ABUSE WITH INTOXICATION, UNCOMPLICATED
F14.121	COCAINE ABUSE WITH INTOXICATION WITH DELIRIUM
F14.122	COCAINE ABUSE WITH INTOXICATION WITH PERCEPTUAL DISTURBANCE
F14.129	COCAINE ABUSE WITH INTOXICATION, UNSPECIFIED
F14.14	COCAINE ABUSE WITH COCAINE-INDUCED MOOD DISORDER
F14.150	COCAINE ABUSE WITH COCAINE-INDUCED PSYCHOTIC DISORDER WITH DELUSIONS
F14.151	COCAINE ABUSE WITH COCAINE-INDUCED PSYCHOTIC DISORDER WITH HALLUCINATIONS
F14.159	COCAINE ABUSE WITH COCAINE-INDUCED PSYCHOTIC DISORDER, UNSPECIFIED
F14.180	COCAINE ABUSE WITH COCAINE-INDUCED ANXIETY DISORDER
F14.181	COCAINE ABUSE WITH COCAINE-INDUCED SEXUAL DYSFUNCTION
F14.182	COCAINE ABUSE WITH COCAINE-INDUCED SLEEP DISORDER
F14.188	COCAINE ABUSE WITH OTHER COCAINE-INDUCED DISORDER
F14.19	COCAINE ABUSE WITH UNSPECIFIED COCAINE-INDUCED DISORDER
F14.20	COCAINE DEPENDENCE, UNCOMPLICATED
F14.21	COCAINE DEPENDENCE, IN REMISSION
F14.220	COCAINE DEPENDENCE WITH INTOXICATION, UNCOMPLICATED
F14.221	COCAINE DEPENDENCE WITH INTOXICATION DELIRIUM
F14.222	COCAINE DEPENDENCE WITH INTOXICATION WITH PERCEPTUAL DISTURBANCE
F14.229	COCAINE DEPENDENCE WITH INTOXICATION, UNSPECIFIED
F14.23	COCAINE DEPENDENCE WITH WITHDRAWAL
F14.24	COCAINE DEPENDENCE WITH COCAINE-INDUCED MOOD DISORDER
F14.250	COCAINE DEPENDENCE WITH COCAINE-INDUCED PSYCHOTIC DISORDER WITH DELUSIONS
F14.251	COCAINE DEPENDENCE WITH COCAINE-INDUCED PSYCHOTIC DISORDER WITH HALLUCINATIONS
F14.259	COCAINE DEPENDENCE WITH COCAINE-INDUCED PSYCHOTIC DISORDER, UNSPECIFIED
F14.280	COCAINE DEPENDENCE WITH COCAINE-INDUCED ANXIETY DISORDER
F14.281	COCAINE DEPENDENCE WITH COCAINE-INDUCED SEXUAL DYSFUNCTION
F14.282	COCAINE DEPENDENCE WITH COCAINE-INDUCED SLEEP DISORDER
F14.288	COCAINE DEPENDENCE WITH OTHER COCAINE-INDUCED DISORDER
F14.29	COCAINE DEPENDENCE WITH UNSPECIFIED COCAINE-INDUCED DISORDER
F14.90	COCAINE USE, UNSPECIFIED, UNCOMPLICATED
F14.920	COCAINE USE, UNSPECIFIED WITH INTOXICATION, UNCOMPLICATED
F14.921	COCAINE USE, UNSPECIFIED WITH INTOXICATION DELIRIUM
F14.922	COCAINE USE, UNSPECIFIED WITH INTOXICATION WITH PERCEPTUAL DISTURBANCE
F14.929	COCAINE USE, UNSPECIFIED WITH INTOXICATION, UNSPECIFIED
F14.94	COCAINE USE, UNSPECIFIED WITH COCAINE-INDUCED MOOD DISORDER
F14.950	COCAINE USE, UNSPECIFIED WITH COCAINE-INDUCED PSYCHOTIC DISORDER WITH DELUSIONS

F14.951	COCAINE USE, UNSPECIFIED WITH COCAINE-INDUCED PSYCHOTIC DISORDER WITH HALLUCINATIONS
F14.959	COCAINE USE, UNSPECIFIED WITH COCAINE-INDUCED PSYCHOTIC DISORDER, UNSPECIFIED
F14.980	COCAINE USE, UNSPECIFIED WITH COCAINE-INDUCED ANXIETY DISORDER
F14.981	COCAINE USE, UNSPECIFIED WITH COCAINE-INDUCED SEXUAL DYSFUNCTION
F14.982	COCAINE USE, UNSPECIFIED WITH COCAINE-INDUCED SLEEP DISORDER
F14.988	COCAINE USE, UNSPECIFIED WITH OTHER COCAINE-INDUCED DISORDER
F14.99	COCAINE USE, UNSPECIFIED WITH UNSPECIFIED COCAINE-INDUCED DISORDER
F16.10	HALLUCINOGEN ABUSE, UNCOMPLICATED
F16.11	HALLUCINOGEN ABUSE, IN REMISSION
F16.120	HALLUCINOGEN ABUSE WITH INTOXICATION, UNCOMPLICATED
F16.121	HALLUCINOGEN ABUSE WITH INTOXICATION WITH DELIRIUM
F16.122	HALLUCINOGEN ABUSE WITH INTOXICATION WITH PERCEPTUAL DISTURBANCE
F16.129	HALLUCINOGEN ABUSE WITH INTOXICATION, UNSPECIFIED
F16.14	HALLUCINOGEN ABUSE WITH HALLUCINOGEN-INDUCED MOOD DISORDER
F16.150	HALLUCINOGEN ABUSE WITH HALLUCINOGEN-INDUCED PSYCHOTIC DISORDER WITH DELUSIONS
F16.151	HALLUCINOGEN ABUSE WITH HALLUCINOGEN-INDUCED PSYCHOTIC DISORDER WITH HALLUCINATIONS
F16.159	HALLUCINOGEN ABUSE WITH HALLUCINOGEN-INDUCED PSYCHOTIC DISORDER, UNSPECIFIED
F16.180	HALLUCINOGEN ABUSE WITH HALLUCINOGEN-INDUCED ANXIETY DISORDER
F16.183	HALLUCINOGEN ABUSE WITH HALLUCINOGEN PERSISTING PERCEPTION DISORDER (FLASHBACKS)
F16.188	HALLUCINOGEN ABUSE WITH OTHER HALLUCINOGEN-INDUCED DISORDER
F16.19	HALLUCINOGEN ABUSE WITH UNSPECIFIED HALLUCINOGEN-INDUCED DISORDER
F16.20	HALLUCINOGEN DEPENDENCE, UNCOMPLICATED
F16.21	HALLUCINOGEN DEPENDENCE, IN REMISSION
F16.220	HALLUCINOGEN DEPENDENCE WITH INTOXICATION, UNCOMPLICATED
F16.221	HALLUCINOGEN DEPENDENCE WITH INTOXICATION WITH DELIRIUM
F16.229	HALLUCINOGEN DEPENDENCE WITH INTOXICATION, UNSPECIFIED
F16.24	HALLUCINOGEN DEPENDENCE WITH HALLUCINOGEN-INDUCED MOOD DISORDER
F16.250	HALLUCINOGEN DEPENDENCE WITH HALLUCINOGEN-INDUCED PSYCHOTIC DISORDER WITH DELUSIONS
F16.251	HALLUCINOGEN DEPENDENCE WITH HALLUCINOGEN-INDUCED PSYCHOTIC DISORDER WITH HALLUCINATIONS
F16.259	HALLUCINOGEN DEPENDENCE WITH HALLUCINOGEN-INDUCED PSYCHOTIC DISORDER, UNSPECIFIED
F16.280	HALLUCINOGEN DEPENDENCE WITH HALLUCINOGEN-INDUCED ANXIETY DISORDER
F16.283	HALLUCINOGEN DEPENDENCE WITH HALLUCINOGEN PERSISTING PERCEPTION DISORDER (FLASHBACKS)
F16.288	HALLUCINOGEN DEPENDENCE WITH OTHER HALLUCINOGEN-INDUCED DISORDER
F16.29	HALLUCINOGEN DEPENDENCE WITH UNSPECIFIED HALLUCINOGEN-INDUCED DISORDER
F16.90	HALLUCINOGEN USE, UNSPECIFIED, UNCOMPLICATED
F16.920	HALLUCINOGEN USE, UNSPECIFIED WITH INTOXICATION, UNCOMPLICATED
F16.921	HALLUCINOGEN USE, UNSPECIFIED WITH INTOXICATION WITH DELIRIUM

F16.929	HALLUCINOGEN USE, UNSPECIFIED WITH INTOXICATION, UNSPECIFIED
F16.94	HALLUCINOGEN USE, UNSPECIFIED WITH HALLUCINOGEN-INDUCED MOOD DISORDER
F16.950	HALLUCINOGEN USE, UNSPECIFIED WITH HALLUCINOGEN-INDUCED PSYCHOTIC DISORDER WITH DELUSIONS
F16.951	HALLUCINOGEN USE, UNSPECIFIED WITH HALLUCINOGEN-INDUCED PSYCHOTIC DISORDER WITH HALLUCINATIONS
F16.959	HALLUCINOGEN USE, UNSPECIFIED WITH HALLUCINOGEN-INDUCED PSYCHOTIC DISORDER, UNSPECIFIED
F16.980	HALLUCINOGEN USE, UNSPECIFIED WITH HALLUCINOGEN-INDUCED ANXIETY DISORDER
F16.983	HALLUCINOGEN USE, UNSPECIFIED WITH HALLUCINOGEN PERSISTING PERCEPTION DISORDER (FLASHBACKS)
F16.988	HALLUCINOGEN USE, UNSPECIFIED WITH OTHER HALLUCINOGEN-INDUCED DISORDER
F16.99	HALLUCINOGEN USE, UNSPECIFIED WITH UNSPECIFIED HALLUCINOGEN-INDUCED DISORDER
F18.10	INHALANT ABUSE, UNCOMPLICATED
F18.11	INHALANT ABUSE, IN REMISSION
F18.120	INHALANT ABUSE WITH INTOXICATION, UNCOMPLICATED
F18.121	INHALANT ABUSE WITH INTOXICATION DELIRIUM
F18.129	INHALANT ABUSE WITH INTOXICATION, UNSPECIFIED
F18.14	INHALANT ABUSE WITH INHALANT-INDUCED MOOD DISORDER
F18.150	INHALANT ABUSE WITH INHALANT-INDUCED PSYCHOTIC DISORDER WITH DELUSIONS
F18.151	INHALANT ABUSE WITH INHALANT-INDUCED PSYCHOTIC DISORDER WITH HALLUCINATIONS
F18.159	INHALANT ABUSE WITH INHALANT-INDUCED PSYCHOTIC DISORDER, UNSPECIFIED
F18.17	INHALANT ABUSE WITH INHALANT-INDUCED DEMENTIA
F18.180	INHALANT ABUSE WITH INHALANT-INDUCED ANXIETY DISORDER
F18.188	INHALANT ABUSE WITH OTHER INHALANT-INDUCED DISORDER
F18.19	INHALANT ABUSE WITH UNSPECIFIED INHALANT-INDUCED DISORDER
F18.20	INHALANT DEPENDENCE, UNCOMPLICATED
F18.21	INHALANT DEPENDENCE, IN REMISSION
F18.220	INHALANT DEPENDENCE WITH INTOXICATION, UNCOMPLICATED
F18.221	INHALANT DEPENDENCE WITH INTOXICATION DELIRIUM
F18.229	INHALANT DEPENDENCE WITH INTOXICATION, UNSPECIFIED
F18.24	INHALANT DEPENDENCE WITH INHALANT-INDUCED MOOD DISORDER
F18.250	INHALANT DEPENDENCE WITH INHALANT-INDUCED PSYCHOTIC DISORDER WITH DELUSIONS
F18.251	INHALANT DEPENDENCE WITH INHALANT-INDUCED PSYCHOTIC DISORDER WITH HALLUCINATIONS
F18.259	INHALANT DEPENDENCE WITH INHALANT-INDUCED PSYCHOTIC DISORDER, UNSPECIFIED
F18.27	INHALANT DEPENDENCE WITH INHALANT-INDUCED DEMENTIA
F18.280	INHALANT DEPENDENCE WITH INHALANT-INDUCED ANXIETY DISORDER
F18.288	INHALANT DEPENDENCE WITH OTHER INHALANT-INDUCED DISORDER
F18.29	INHALANT DEPENDENCE WITH UNSPECIFIED INHALANT-INDUCED DISORDER
F18.90	INHALANT USE, UNSPECIFIED, UNCOMPLICATED
F18.920	INHALANT USE, UNSPECIFIED WITH INTOXICATION, UNCOMPLICATED
F18.921	INHALANT USE, UNSPECIFIED WITH INTOXICATION WITH DELIRIUM

F18.929	INHALANT USE, UNSPECIFIED WITH INTOXICATION, UNSPECIFIED
F18.94	INHALANT USE, UNSPECIFIED WITH INHALANT-INDUCED MOOD DISORDER
F18.950	INHALANT USE, UNSPECIFIED WITH INHALANT-INDUCED PSYCHOTIC DISORDER WITH DELUSIONS
F18.951	INHALANT USE, UNSPECIFIED WITH INHALANT-INDUCED PSYCHOTIC DISORDER WITH HALLUCINATIONS
F18.959	INHALANT USE, UNSPECIFIED WITH INHALANT-INDUCED PSYCHOTIC DISORDER, UNSPECIFIED
F18.97	INHALANT USE, UNSPECIFIED WITH INHALANT-INDUCED PERSISTING DEMENTIA
F18.980	INHALANT USE, UNSPECIFIED WITH INHALANT-INDUCED ANXIETY DISORDER
F18.988	INHALANT USE, UNSPECIFIED WITH OTHER INHALANT-INDUCED DISORDER
F18.99	INHALANT USE, UNSPECIFIED WITH UNSPECIFIED INHALANT-INDUCED DISORDER
F11.10	OPIOID ABUSE, UNCOMPLICATED
F11.11	OPIOID ABUSE, IN REMISSION
F11.120	OPIOID ABUSE WITH INTOXICATION, UNCOMPLICATED
F11.121	OPIOID ABUSE WITH INTOXICATION DELIRIUM
F11.122	OPIOID ABUSE WITH INTOXICATION WITH PERCEPTUAL DISTURBANCE
F11.129	OPIOID ABUSE WITH INTOXICATION, UNSPECIFIED
F11.14	OPIOID ABUSE WITH OPIOID-INDUCED MOOD DISORDER
F11.150	OPIOID ABUSE WITH OPIOID-INDUCED PSYCHOTIC DISORDER WITH DELUSIONS
F11.151	OPIOID ABUSE WITH OPIOID-INDUCED PSYCHOTIC DISORDER WITH HALLUCINATIONS
F11.159	OPIOID ABUSE WITH OPIOID-INDUCED PSYCHOTIC DISORDER, UNSPECIFIED
F11.181	OPIOID ABUSE WITH OPIOID-INDUCED SEXUAL DYSFUNCTION
F11.182	OPIOID ABUSE WITH OPIOID-INDUCED SLEEP DISORDER
F11.188	OPIOID ABUSE WITH OTHER OPIOID-INDUCED DISORDER
F11.19	OPIOID ABUSE WITH UNSPECIFIED OPIOID-INDUCED DISORDER
F11.20	OPIOID DEPENDENCE, UNCOMPLICATED
F11.21	OPIOID DEPENDENCE, IN REMISSION
F11.220	OPIOID DEPENDENCE WITH INTOXICATION, UNCOMPLICATED
F11.221	OPIOID DEPENDENCE WITH INTOXICATION DELIRIUM
F11.222	OPIOID DEPENDENCE WITH INTOXICATION WITH PERCEPTUAL DISTURBANCE
F11.229	OPIOID DEPENDENCE WITH INTOXICATION, UNSPECIFIED
F11.23	OPIOID DEPENDENCE WITH WITHDRAWAL
F11.24	OPIOID DEPENDENCE WITH OPIOID-INDUCED MOOD DISORDER
F11.250	OPIOID DEPENDENCE WITH OPIOID-INDUCED PSYCHOTIC DISORDER WITH DELUSIONS
F11.251	OPIOID DEPENDENCE WITH OPIOID-INDUCED PSYCHOTIC DISORDER WITH HALLUCINATIONS
F11.259	OPIOID DEPENDENCE WITH OPIOID-INDUCED PSYCHOTIC DISORDER, UNSPECIFIED
F11.281	OPIOID DEPENDENCE WITH OPIOID-INDUCED SEXUAL DYSFUNCTION
F11.282	OPIOID DEPENDENCE WITH OPIOID-INDUCED SLEEP DISORDER
F11.288	OPIOID DEPENDENCE WITH OTHER OPIOID-INDUCED DISORDER
F11.29	OPIOID DEPENDENCE WITH UNSPECIFIED OPIOID-INDUCED DISORDER
F11.90	OPIOID USE, UNSPECIFIED, UNCOMPLICATED

F11.920	OPIOID USE, UNSPECIFIED WITH INTOXICATION, UNCOMPLICATED
F11.921	OPIOID USE, UNSPECIFIED WITH INTOXICATION DELIRIUM
F11.922	OPIOID USE, UNSPECIFIED WITH INTOXICATION WITH PERCEPTUAL DISTURBANCE
F11.929	OPIOID USE, UNSPECIFIED WITH INTOXICATION, UNSPECIFIED
F11.93	OPIOID USE, UNSPECIFIED WITH WITHDRAWAL
F11.94	OPIOID USE, UNSPECIFIED WITH OPIOID-INDUCED MOOD DISORDER
F11.950	OPIOID USE, UNSPECIFIED WITH OPIOID-INDUCED PSYCHOTIC DISORDER WITH DELUSIONS
F11.951	OPIOID USE, UNSPECIFIED WITH OPIOID-INDUCED PSYCHOTIC DISORDER WITH HALLUCINATIONS
F11.959	OPIOID USE, UNSPECIFIED WITH OPIOID-INDUCED PSYCHOTIC DISORDER, UNSPECIFIED
F11.981	OPIOID USE, UNSPECIFIED WITH OPIOID-INDUCED SEXUAL DYSFUNCTION
F11.982	OPIOID USE, UNSPECIFIED WITH OPIOID-INDUCED SLEEP DISORDER
F11.988	OPIOID USE, UNSPECIFIED WITH OTHER OPIOID-INDUCED DISORDER
F11.99	OPIOID USE, UNSPECIFIED WITH UNSPECIFIED OPIOID-INDUCED DISORDER
F19.10	OTHER PSYCHOACTIVE SUBSTANCE ABUSE, UNCOMPLICATED
F19.11	OTHER PSYCHOACTIVE SUBSTANCE ABUSE, IN REMISSION
F19.120	OTHER PSYCHOACTIVE SUBSTANCE ABUSE WITH INTOXICATION, UNCOMPLICATED
F19.121	OTHER PSYCHOACTIVE SUBSTANCE ABUSE WITH INTOXICATION DELIRIUM
F19.122	OTHER PSYCHOACTIVE SUBSTANCE ABUSE WITH INTOXICATION WITH PERCEPTUAL DISTURBANCES
F19.129	OTHER PSYCHOACTIVE SUBSTANCE ABUSE WITH INTOXICATION, UNSPECIFIED
F19.14	OTHER PSYCHOACTIVE SUBSTANCE ABUSE WITH PSYCHOACTIVE SUBSTANCE-INDUCED MOOD DISORDER
F19.150	OTHER PSYCHOACTIVE SUBSTANCE ABUSE WITH PSYCHOACTIVE SUBSTANCE-INDUCED PSYCHOTIC DISORDER WITH DELUSIONS
F19.151	OTHER PSYCHOACTIVE SUBSTANCE ABUSE WITH PSYCHOACTIVE SUBSTANCE-INDUCED PSYCHOTIC DISORDER WITH HALLUCINATIONS
F19.159	OTHER PSYCHOACTIVE SUBSTANCE ABUSE WITH PSYCHOACTIVE SUBSTANCE-INDUCED PSYCHOTIC DISORDER, UNSPECIFIED
F19.16	OTHER PSYCHOACTIVE SUBSTANCE ABUSE WITH PSYCHOACTIVE SUBSTANCE-INDUCED PERSISTING AMNESTIC DISORDER
F19.17	OTHER PSYCHOACTIVE SUBSTANCE ABUSE WITH PSYCHOACTIVE SUBSTANCE-INDUCED PERSISTING DEMENTIA
F19.180	OTHER PSYCHOACTIVE SUBSTANCE ABUSE WITH PSYCHOACTIVE SUBSTANCE-INDUCED ANXIETY DISORDER
F19.181	OTHER PSYCHOACTIVE SUBSTANCE ABUSE WITH PSYCHOACTIVE SUBSTANCE-INDUCED SEXUAL DYSFUNCTION
F19.182	OTHER PSYCHOACTIVE SUBSTANCE ABUSE WITH PSYCHOACTIVE SUBSTANCE-INDUCED SLEEP DISORDER
F19.188	OTHER PSYCHOACTIVE SUBSTANCE ABUSE WITH OTHER PSYCHOACTIVE SUBSTANCE-INDUCED DISORDER
F19.19	OTHER PSYCHOACTIVE SUBSTANCE ABUSE WITH UNSPECIFIED PSYCHOACTIVE SUBSTANCE-INDUCED DISORDER
F19.20	OTHER PSYCHOACTIVE SUBSTANCE DEPENDENCE, UNCOMPLICATED
F19.21	OTHER PSYCHOACTIVE SUBSTANCE DEPENDENCE, IN REMISSION
F19.220	OTHER PSYCHOACTIVE SUBSTANCE DEPENDENCE WITH INTOXICATION, UNCOMPLICATED
F19.221	OTHER PSYCHOACTIVE SUBSTANCE DEPENDENCE WITH INTOXICATION DELIRIUM
F19.222	OTHER PSYCHOACTIVE SUBSTANCE DEPENDENCE WITH INTOXICATION WITH PERCEPTUAL DISTURBANCE

F19.229	OTHER PSYCHOACTIVE SUBSTANCE DEPENDENCE WITH INTOXICATION, UNSPECIFIED
F19.230	OTHER PSYCHOACTIVE SUBSTANCE DEPENDENCE WITH WITHDRAWAL, UNCOMPLICATED
F19.231	OTHER PSYCHOACTIVE SUBSTANCE DEPENDENCE WITH WITHDRAWAL DELIRIUM
F19.232	OTHER PSYCHOACTIVE SUBSTANCE DEPENDENCE WITH WITHDRAWAL WITH PERCEPTUAL DISTURBANCE
F19.239	OTHER PSYCHOACTIVE SUBSTANCE DEPENDENCE WITH WITHDRAWAL, UNSPECIFIED
F19.24	OTHER PSYCHOACTIVE SUBSTANCE DEPENDENCE WITH PSYCHOACTIVE SUBSTANCE-INDUCED MOOD DISORDER
F19.250	OTHER PSYCHOACTIVE SUBSTANCE DEPENDENCE WITH PSYCHOACTIVE SUBSTANCE-INDUCED PSYCHOTIC DISORDER WITH DELUSIONS
F19.251	OTHER PSYCHOACTIVE SUBSTANCE DEPENDENCE WITH PSYCHOACTIVE SUBSTANCE-INDUCED PSYCHOTIC DISORDER WITH HALLUCINATIONS
F19.259	OTHER PSYCHOACTIVE SUBSTANCE DEPENDENCE WITH PSYCHOACTIVE SUBSTANCE-INDUCED PSYCHOTIC DISORDER, UNSPECIFIED
F19.26	OTHER PSYCHOACTIVE SUBSTANCE DEPENDENCE WITH PSYCHOACTIVE SUBSTANCE-INDUCED PERSISTING AMNESTIC DISORDER
F19.27	OTHER PSYCHOACTIVE SUBSTANCE DEPENDENCE WITH PSYCHOACTIVE SUBSTANCE-INDUCED PERSISTING DEMENTIA
F19.280	OTHER PSYCHOACTIVE SUBSTANCE DEPENDENCE WITH PSYCHOACTIVE SUBSTANCE-INDUCED ANXIETY DISORDER
F19.281	OTHER PSYCHOACTIVE SUBSTANCE DEPENDENCE WITH PSYCHOACTIVE SUBSTANCE-INDUCED SEXUAL DYSFUNCTION
F19.282	OTHER PSYCHOACTIVE SUBSTANCE DEPENDENCE WITH PSYCHOACTIVE SUBSTANCE-INDUCED SLEEP DISORDER
F19.288	OTHER PSYCHOACTIVE SUBSTANCE DEPENDENCE WITH OTHER PSYCHOACTIVE SUBSTANCE-INDUCED DISORDER
F19.29	OTHER PSYCHOACTIVE SUBSTANCE DEPENDENCE WITH UNSPECIFIED PSYCHOACTIVE SUBSTANCE-INDUCED DISORDER
F19.90	OTHER PSYCHOACTIVE SUBSTANCE USE, UNSPECIFIED, UNCOMPLICATED
F19.920	OTHER PSYCHOACTIVE SUBSTANCE USE, UNSPECIFIED WITH INTOXICATION, UNCOMPLICATED
F19.921	OTHER PSYCHOACTIVE SUBSTANCE USE, UNSPECIFIED WITH INTOXICATION WITH DELIRIUM
F19.922	OTHER PSYCHOACTIVE SUBSTANCE USE, UNSPECIFIED WITH INTOXICATION WITH PERCEPTUAL DISTURBANCE
F19.929	OTHER PSYCHOACTIVE SUBSTANCE USE, UNSPECIFIED WITH INTOXICATION, UNSPECIFIED
F19.930	OTHER PSYCHOACTIVE SUBSTANCE USE, UNSPECIFIED WITH WITHDRAWAL, UNCOMPLICATED
F19.931	OTHER PSYCHOACTIVE SUBSTANCE USE, UNSPECIFIED WITH WITHDRAWAL DELIRIUM
F19.932	OTHER PSYCHOACTIVE SUBSTANCE USE, UNSPECIFIED WITH WITHDRAWAL WITH PERCEPTUAL DISTURBANCE
F19.939	OTHER PSYCHOACTIVE SUBSTANCE USE, UNSPECIFIED WITH WITHDRAWAL, UNSPECIFIED
F19.94	OTHER PSYCHOACTIVE SUBSTANCE USE, UNSPECIFIED WITH PSYCHOACTIVE SUBSTANCE-INDUCED MOOD DISORDER
F19.950	OTHER PSYCHOACTIVE SUBSTANCE USE, UNSPECIFIED WITH PSYCHOACTIVE SUBSTANCE-INDUCED PSYCHOTIC DISORDER WITH DELUSIONS
F19.951	OTHER PSYCHOACTIVE SUBSTANCE USE, UNSPECIFIED WITH PSYCHOACTIVE SUBSTANCE-INDUCED PSYCHOTIC DISORDER WITH HALLUCINATIONS
F19.959	OTHER PSYCHOACTIVE SUBSTANCE USE, UNSPECIFIED WITH PSYCHOACTIVE SUBSTANCE-INDUCED PSYCHOTIC DISORDER, UNSPECIFIED
F19.96	OTHER PSYCHOACTIVE SUBSTANCE USE, UNSPECIFIED WITH PSYCHOACTIVE SUBSTANCE-INDUCED PERSISTING AMNESTIC DISORDER
F19.97	OTHER PSYCHOACTIVE SUBSTANCE USE, UNSPECIFIED WITH PSYCHOACTIVE SUBSTANCE-INDUCED PERSISTING DEMENTIA
F19.980	OTHER PSYCHOACTIVE SUBSTANCE USE, UNSPECIFIED WITH PSYCHOACTIVE SUBSTANCE-INDUCED ANXIETY DISORDER
F19.981	OTHER PSYCHOACTIVE SUBSTANCE USE, UNSPECIFIED WITH PSYCHOACTIVE SUBSTANCE-INDUCED SEXUAL DYSFUNCTION

F19.982	OTHER PSYCHOACTIVE SUBSTANCE USE, UNSPECIFIED WITH PSYCHOACTIVE SUBSTANCE-INDUCED SLEEP DISORDER
F19.988	OTHER PSYCHOACTIVE SUBSTANCE USE, UNSPECIFIED WITH OTHER PSYCHOACTIVE SUBSTANCE-INDUCED DISORDER
F19.99	OTHER PSYCHOACTIVE SUBSTANCE USE, UNSPECIFIED WITH UNSPECIFIED PSYCHOACTIVE SUBSTANCE-INDUCED DISORDER
F13.10	SEDATIVE, HYPNOTIC OR ANXIOLYTIC ABUSE, UNCOMPLICATED
F13.11	SEDATIVE, HYPNOTIC OR ANXIOLYTIC ABUSE, IN REMISSION
F13.120	SEDATIVE, HYPNOTIC OR ANXIOLYTIC ABUSE WITH INTOXICATION, UNCOMPLICATED
F13.121	SEDATIVE, HYPNOTIC OR ANXIOLYTIC ABUSE WITH INTOXICATION DELIRIUM
F13.129	SEDATIVE, HYPNOTIC OR ANXIOLYTIC ABUSE WITH INTOXICATION, UNSPECIFIED
F13.14	SEDATIVE, HYPNOTIC OR ANXIOLYTIC ABUSE WITH SEDATIVE, HYPNOTIC OR ANXIOLYTIC-INDUCED MOOD DISORDER
F13.150	SEDATIVE, HYPNOTIC OR ANXIOLYTIC ABUSE WITH SEDATIVE, HYPNOTIC OR ANXIOLYTIC-INDUCED PSYCHOTIC DISORDER WITH DELUSIONS
F13.151	SEDATIVE, HYPNOTIC OR ANXIOLYTIC ABUSE WITH SEDATIVE, HYPNOTIC OR ANXIOLYTIC-INDUCED PSYCHOTIC DISORDER WITH HALLUCINATIONS
F13.159	SEDATIVE, HYPNOTIC OR ANXIOLYTIC ABUSE WITH SEDATIVE, HYPNOTIC OR ANXIOLYTIC-INDUCED PSYCHOTIC DISORDER, UNSPECIFIED
F13.180	SEDATIVE, HYPNOTIC OR ANXIOLYTIC ABUSE WITH SEDATIVE, HYPNOTIC OR ANXIOLYTIC-INDUCED ANXIETY DISORDER
F13.181	SEDATIVE, HYPNOTIC OR ANXIOLYTIC ABUSE WITH SEDATIVE, HYPNOTIC OR ANXIOLYTIC-INDUCED SEXUAL DYSFUNCTION
F13.182	SEDATIVE, HYPNOTIC OR ANXIOLYTIC ABUSE WITH SEDATIVE, HYPNOTIC OR ANXIOLYTIC-INDUCED SLEEP DISORDER
F13.188	SEDATIVE, HYPNOTIC OR ANXIOLYTIC ABUSE WITH OTHER SEDATIVE, HYPNOTIC OR ANXIOLYTIC-INDUCED DISORDER
F13.19	SEDATIVE, HYPNOTIC OR ANXIOLYTIC ABUSE WITH UNSPECIFIED SEDATIVE, HYPNOTIC OR ANXIOLYTIC-INDUCED DISORDER
F13.20	SEDATIVE, HYPNOTIC OR ANXIOLYTIC DEPENDENCE, UNCOMPLICATED
F13.21	SEDATIVE, HYPNOTIC OR ANXIOLYTIC DEPENDENCE, IN REMISSION
F13.220	SEDATIVE, HYPNOTIC OR ANXIOLYTIC DEPENDENCE WITH INTOXICATION, UNCOMPLICATED
F13.221	SEDATIVE, HYPNOTIC OR ANXIOLYTIC DEPENDENCE WITH INTOXICATION DELIRIUM
F13.229	SEDATIVE, HYPNOTIC OR ANXIOLYTIC DEPENDENCE WITH INTOXICATION, UNSPECIFIED
F13.230	SEDATIVE, HYPNOTIC OR ANXIOLYTIC DEPENDENCE WITH WITHDRAWAL, UNCOMPLICATED
F13.231	SEDATIVE, HYPNOTIC OR ANXIOLYTIC DEPENDENCE WITH WITHDRAWAL DELIRIUM
F13.232	SEDATIVE, HYPNOTIC OR ANXIOLYTIC DEPENDENCE WITH WITHDRAWAL WITH PERCEPTUAL DISTURBANCE
F13.239	SEDATIVE, HYPNOTIC OR ANXIOLYTIC DEPENDENCE WITH WITHDRAWAL, UNSPECIFIED
F13.24	SEDATIVE, HYPNOTIC OR ANXIOLYTIC DEPENDENCE WITH SEDATIVE, HYPNOTIC OR ANXIOLYTIC-INDUCED MOOD DISORDER
F13.250	SEDATIVE, HYPNOTIC OR ANXIOLYTIC DEPENDENCE WITH SEDATIVE, HYPNOTIC OR ANXIOLYTIC-INDUCED PSYCHOTIC DISORDER WITH DELUSIONS
F13.251	SEDATIVE, HYPNOTIC OR ANXIOLYTIC DEPENDENCE WITH SEDATIVE, HYPNOTIC OR ANXIOLYTIC-INDUCED PSYCHOTIC DISORDER WITH HALLUCINATIONS
F13.259	SEDATIVE, HYPNOTIC OR ANXIOLYTIC DEPENDENCE WITH SEDATIVE, HYPNOTIC OR ANXIOLYTIC-INDUCED PSYCHOTIC DISORDER, UNSPECIFIED
F13.26	SEDATIVE, HYPNOTIC OR ANXIOLYTIC DEPENDENCE WITH SEDATIVE, HYPNOTIC OR ANXIOLYTIC-INDUCED PERSISTING AMNESTIC DISORDER
F13.27	SEDATIVE, HYPNOTIC OR ANXIOLYTIC DEPENDENCE WITH SEDATIVE, HYPNOTIC OR ANXIOLYTIC-INDUCED PERSISTING DEMENTIA

F13.280	SEDATIVE, HYPNOTIC OR ANXIOLYTIC DEPENDENCE WITH SEDATIVE, HYPNOTIC OR ANXIOLYTIC-INDUCED ANXIETY DISORDER
F13.281	SEDATIVE, HYPNOTIC OR ANXIOLYTIC DEPENDENCE WITH SEDATIVE, HYPNOTIC OR ANXIOLYTIC-INDUCED SEXUAL DYSFUNCTION
F13.282	SEDATIVE, HYPNOTIC OR ANXIOLYTIC DEPENDENCE WITH SEDATIVE, HYPNOTIC OR ANXIOLYTIC-INDUCED SLEEP DISORDER
F13.288	SEDATIVE, HYPNOTIC OR ANXIOLYTIC DEPENDENCE WITH OTHER SEDATIVE, HYPNOTIC OR ANXIOLYTIC-INDUCED DISORDER
F13.29	SEDATIVE, HYPNOTIC OR ANXIOLYTIC DEPENDENCE WITH UNSPECIFIED SEDATIVE, HYPNOTIC OR ANXIOLYTIC-INDUCED DISORDER
F13.90	SEDATIVE, HYPNOTIC, OR ANXIOLYTIC USE, UNSPECIFIED, UNCOMPLICATED
F13.920	SEDATIVE, HYPNOTIC OR ANXIOLYTIC USE, UNSPECIFIED WITH INTOXICATION, UNCOMPLICATED
F13.921	SEDATIVE, HYPNOTIC OR ANXIOLYTIC USE, UNSPECIFIED WITH INTOXICATION DELIRIUM
F13.929	SEDATIVE, HYPNOTIC OR ANXIOLYTIC USE, UNSPECIFIED WITH INTOXICATION, UNSPECIFIED
F13.930	SEDATIVE, HYPNOTIC OR ANXIOLYTIC USE, UNSPECIFIED WITH WITHDRAWAL, UNCOMPLICATED
F13.931	SEDATIVE, HYPNOTIC OR ANXIOLYTIC USE, UNSPECIFIED WITH WITHDRAWAL DELIRIUM
F13.932	SEDATIVE, HYPNOTIC OR ANXIOLYTIC USE, UNSPECIFIED WITH WITHDRAWAL WITH PERCEPTUAL DISTURBANCES
F13.939	SEDATIVE, HYPNOTIC OR ANXIOLYTIC USE, UNSPECIFIED WITH WITHDRAWAL, UNSPECIFIED
F13.94	SEDATIVE, HYPNOTIC OR ANXIOLYTIC USE, UNSPECIFIED WITH SEDATIVE, HYPNOTIC OR ANXIOLYTIC-INDUCED MOOD DISORDER
F13.950	SEDATIVE, HYPNOTIC OR ANXIOLYTIC USE, UNSPECIFIED WITH SEDATIVE, HYPNOTIC OR ANXIOLYTIC-INDUCED PSYCHOTIC DISORDER WITH DELUSIONS
F13.951	SEDATIVE, HYPNOTIC OR ANXIOLYTIC USE, UNSPECIFIED WITH SEDATIVE, HYPNOTIC OR ANXIOLYTIC-INDUCED PSYCHOTIC DISORDER WITH HALLUCINATIONS
F13.959	SEDATIVE, HYPNOTIC OR ANXIOLYTIC USE, UNSPECIFIED WITH SEDATIVE, HYPNOTIC OR ANXIOLYTIC-INDUCED PSYCHOTIC DISORDER, UNSPECIFIED
F13.96	SEDATIVE, HYPNOTIC OR ANXIOLYTIC USE, UNSPECIFIED WITH SEDATIVE, HYPNOTIC OR ANXIOLYTIC-INDUCED PERSISTING AMNESTIC DISORDER
F13.97	SEDATIVE, HYPNOTIC OR ANXIOLYTIC USE, UNSPECIFIED WITH SEDATIVE, HYPNOTIC OR ANXIOLYTIC-INDUCED PERSISTING DEMENTIA
F13.980	SEDATIVE, HYPNOTIC OR ANXIOLYTIC USE, UNSPECIFIED WITH SEDATIVE, HYPNOTIC OR ANXIOLYTIC-INDUCED ANXIETY DISORDER
F13.981	SEDATIVE, HYPNOTIC OR ANXIOLYTIC USE, UNSPECIFIED WITH SEDATIVE, HYPNOTIC OR ANXIOLYTIC-INDUCED SEXUAL DYSFUNCTION
F13.982	SEDATIVE, HYPNOTIC OR ANXIOLYTIC USE, UNSPECIFIED WITH SEDATIVE, HYPNOTIC OR ANXIOLYTIC-INDUCED SLEEP DISORDER
F13.988	SEDATIVE, HYPNOTIC OR ANXIOLYTIC USE, UNSPECIFIED WITH OTHER SEDATIVE, HYPNOTIC OR ANXIOLYTIC-INDUCED DISORDER
F13.99	SEDATIVE, HYPNOTIC OR ANXIOLYTIC USE, UNSPECIFIED WITH UNSPECIFIED SEDATIVE, HYPNOTIC OR ANXIOLYTIC-INDUCED DISORDER
F15.10	OTHER STIMULANT ABUSE, UNCOMPLICATED
F15.11	OTHER STIMULANT ABUSE, IN REMISSION
F15.120	OTHER STIMULANT ABUSE WITH INTOXICATION, UNCOMPLICATED
F15.121	OTHER STIMULANT ABUSE WITH INTOXICATION DELIRIUM
F15.122	OTHER STIMULANT ABUSE WITH INTOXICATION WITH PERCEPTUAL DISTURBANCE
F15.129	OTHER STIMULANT ABUSE WITH INTOXICATION, UNSPECIFIED
F15.14	OTHER STIMULANT ABUSE WITH STIMULANT-INDUCED MOOD DISORDER
F15.150	OTHER STIMULANT ABUSE WITH STIMULANT-INDUCED PSYCHOTIC DISORDER WITH DELUSIONS

F15.151	OTHER STIMULANT ABUSE WITH STIMULANT-INDUCED PSYCHOTIC DISORDER WITH HALLUCINATIONS
F15.159	OTHER STIMULANT ABUSE WITH STIMULANT-INDUCED PSYCHOTIC DISORDER, UNSPECIFIED
F15.180	OTHER STIMULANT ABUSE WITH STIMULANT-INDUCED ANXIETY DISORDER
F15.181	OTHER STIMULANT ABUSE WITH STIMULANT-INDUCED SEXUAL DYSFUNCTION
F15.182	OTHER STIMULANT ABUSE WITH STIMULANT-INDUCED SLEEP DISORDER
F15.188	OTHER STIMULANT ABUSE WITH OTHER STIMULANT-INDUCED DISORDER
F15.19	OTHER STIMULANT ABUSE WITH UNSPECIFIED STIMULANT-INDUCED DISORDER
F15.20	OTHER STIMULANT DEPENDENCE, UNCOMPLICATED
F15.21	OTHER STIMULANT DEPENDENCE, IN REMISSION
F15.220	OTHER STIMULANT DEPENDENCE WITH INTOXICATION, UNCOMPLICATED
F15.221	OTHER STIMULANT DEPENDENCE WITH INTOXICATION DELIRIUM
F15.222	OTHER STIMULANT DEPENDENCE WITH INTOXICATION WITH PERCEPTUAL DISTURBANCE
F15.229	OTHER STIMULANT DEPENDENCE WITH INTOXICATION, UNSPECIFIED
F15.23	OTHER STIMULANT DEPENDENCE WITH WITHDRAWAL
F15.24	OTHER STIMULANT DEPENDENCE WITH STIMULANT-INDUCED MOOD DISORDER
F15.250	OTHER STIMULANT DEPENDENCE WITH STIMULANT-INDUCED PSYCHOTIC DISORDER WITH DELUSIONS
F15.251	OTHER STIMULANT DEPENDENCE WITH STIMULANT-INDUCED PSYCHOTIC DISORDER WITH HALLUCINATIONS
F15.259	OTHER STIMULANT DEPENDENCE WITH STIMULANT-INDUCED PSYCHOTIC DISORDER, UNSPECIFIED
F15.280	OTHER STIMULANT DEPENDENCE WITH STIMULANT-INDUCED ANXIETY DISORDER
F15.281	OTHER STIMULANT DEPENDENCE WITH STIMULANT-INDUCED SEXUAL DYSFUNCTION
F15.282	OTHER STIMULANT DEPENDENCE WITH STIMULANT-INDUCED SLEEP DISORDER
F15.288	OTHER STIMULANT DEPENDENCE WITH OTHER STIMULANT-INDUCED DISORDER
F15.29	OTHER STIMULANT DEPENDENCE WITH UNSPECIFIED STIMULANT-INDUCED DISORDER
F15.90	OTHER STIMULANT USE, UNSPECIFIED, UNCOMPLICATED
F15.920	OTHER STIMULANT USE, UNSPECIFIED WITH INTOXICATION, UNCOMPLICATED
F15.921	OTHER STIMULANT USE, UNSPECIFIED WITH INTOXICATION DELIRIUM
F15.922	OTHER STIMULANT USE, UNSPECIFIED WITH INTOXICATION WITH PERCEPTUAL DISTURBANCE
F15.929	OTHER STIMULANT USE, UNSPECIFIED WITH INTOXICATION, UNSPECIFIED
F15.93	OTHER STIMULANT USE, UNSPECIFIED WITH WITHDRAWAL
F15.94	OTHER STIMULANT USE, UNSPECIFIED WITH STIMULANT-INDUCED MOOD DISORDER
F15.950	OTHER STIMULANT USE, UNSPECIFIED WITH STIMULANT-INDUCED PSYCHOTIC DISORDER WITH DELUSIONS
F15.951	OTHER STIMULANT USE, UNSPECIFIED WITH STIMULANT-INDUCED PSYCHOTIC DISORDER WITH HALLUCINATIONS
F15.959	OTHER STIMULANT USE, UNSPECIFIED WITH STIMULANT-INDUCED PSYCHOTIC DISORDER, UNSPECIFIED
F15.980	OTHER STIMULANT USE, UNSPECIFIED WITH STIMULANT-INDUCED ANXIETY DISORDER
F15.981	OTHER STIMULANT USE, UNSPECIFIED WITH STIMULANT-INDUCED SEXUAL DYSFUNCTION
F15.982	OTHER STIMULANT USE, UNSPECIFIED WITH STIMULANT-INDUCED SLEEP DISORDER

F15.988	OTHER STIMULANT USE, UNSPECIFIED WITH OTHER STIMULANT-INDUCED DISORDER
F15.99	OTHER STIMULANT USE, UNSPECIFIED WITH UNSPECIFIED STIMULANT-INDUCED DISORDER
Z71.51	DRUG ABUSE COUNSELING AND SURVEILLANCE OF DRUG ABUSER
F10.10	ALCOHOL ABUSE, UNCOMPLICATED
F10.11	ALCOHOL ABUSE, IN REMISSION
F10.120	ALCOHOL ABUSE WITH INTOXICATION, UNCOMPLICATED
F10.121	ALCOHOL ABUSE WITH INTOXICATION DELIRIUM
F10.129	ALCOHOL ABUSE WITH INTOXICATION, UNSPECIFIED
F10.14	ALCOHOL ABUSE WITH ALCOHOL-INDUCED MOOD DISORDER
F10.150	ALCOHOL ABUSE WITH ALCOHOL-INDUCED PSYCHOTIC DISORDER WITH DELUSIONS
F10.151	ALCOHOL ABUSE WITH ALCOHOL-INDUCED PSYCHOTIC DISORDER WITH HALLUCINATIONS
F10.159	ALCOHOL ABUSE WITH ALCOHOL-INDUCED PSYCHOTIC DISORDER, UNSPECIFIED
F10.180	ALCOHOL ABUSE WITH ALCOHOL-INDUCED ANXIETY DISORDER
F10.181	ALCOHOL ABUSE WITH ALCOHOL-INDUCED SEXUAL DYSFUNCTION
F10.182	ALCOHOL ABUSE WITH ALCOHOL-INDUCED SLEEP DISORDER
F10.188	ALCOHOL ABUSE WITH OTHER ALCOHOL-INDUCED DISORDER
F10.19	ALCOHOL ABUSE WITH UNSPECIFIED ALCOHOL-INDUCED DISORDER
F10.20	ALCOHOL DEPENDENCE, UNCOMPLICATED
F10.21	ALCOHOL DEPENDENCE, IN REMISSION
F10.220	ALCOHOL DEPENDENCE WITH INTOXICATION, UNCOMPLICATED
F10.221	ALCOHOL DEPENDENCE WITH INTOXICATION DELIRIUM
F10.229	ALCOHOL DEPENDENCE WITH INTOXICATION, UNSPECIFIED
F10.230	ALCOHOL DEPENDENCE WITH WITHDRAWAL, UNCOMPLICATED
F10.231	ALCOHOL DEPENDENCE WITH WITHDRAWAL DELIRIUM
F10.232	ALCOHOL DEPENDENCE WITH WITHDRAWAL WITH PERCEPTUAL DISTURBANCE
F10.239	ALCOHOL DEPENDENCE WITH WITHDRAWAL, UNSPECIFIED
F10.24	ALCOHOL DEPENDENCE WITH ALCOHOL-INDUCED MOOD DISORDER
F10.250	ALCOHOL DEPENDENCE WITH ALCOHOL-INDUCED PSYCHOTIC DISORDER WITH DELUSIONS
F10.251	ALCOHOL DEPENDENCE WITH ALCOHOL-INDUCED PSYCHOTIC DISORDER WITH HALLUCINATIONS
F10.259	ALCOHOL DEPENDENCE WITH ALCOHOL-INDUCED PSYCHOTIC DISORDER, UNSPECIFIED
F10.26	ALCOHOL DEPENDENCE WITH ALCOHOL-INDUCED PERSISTING AMNESTIC DISORDER
F10.27	ALCOHOL DEPENDENCE WITH ALCOHOL-INDUCED PERSISTING DEMENTIA
F10.280	ALCOHOL DEPENDENCE WITH ALCOHOL-INDUCED ANXIETY DISORDER
F10.281	ALCOHOL DEPENDENCE WITH ALCOHOL-INDUCED SEXUAL DYSFUNCTION
F10.282	ALCOHOL DEPENDENCE WITH ALCOHOL-INDUCED SLEEP DISORDER
F10.288	ALCOHOL DEPENDENCE WITH OTHER ALCOHOL-INDUCED DISORDER
F10.29	ALCOHOL DEPENDENCE WITH UNSPECIFIED ALCOHOL-INDUCED DISORDER
F10.920	ALCOHOL USE, UNSPECIFIED WITH INTOXICATION, UNCOMPLICATED
F10.921	ALCOHOL USE, UNSPECIFIED WITH INTOXICATION DELIRIUM

F10.929	ALCOHOL USE, UNSPECIFIED WITH INTOXICATION, UNSPECIFIED
F10.94	ALCOHOL USE, UNSPECIFIED WITH ALCOHOL-INDUCED MOOD DISORDER
F10.950	ALCOHOL USE, UNSPECIFIED WITH ALCOHOL-INDUCED PSYCHOTIC DISORDER WITH DELUSIONS
F10.951	ALCOHOL USE, UNSPECIFIED WITH ALCOHOL-INDUCED PSYCHOTIC DISORDER WITH HALLUCINATIONS
F10.959	ALCOHOL USE, UNSPECIFIED WITH ALCOHOL-INDUCED PSYCHOTIC DISORDER, UNSPECIFIED
F10.96	ALCOHOL USE, UNSPECIFIED WITH ALCOHOL-INDUCED PERSISTING AMNESTIC DISORDER
F10.97	ALCOHOL USE, UNSPECIFIED WITH ALCOHOL-INDUCED PERSISTING DEMENTIA
F10.980	ALCOHOL USE, UNSPECIFIED WITH ALCOHOL-INDUCED ANXIETY DISORDER
F10.981	ALCOHOL USE, UNSPECIFIED WITH ALCOHOL-INDUCED SEXUAL DYSFUNCTION
F10.982	ALCOHOL USE, UNSPECIFIED WITH ALCOHOL-INDUCED SLEEP DISORDER
F10.988	ALCOHOL USE, UNSPECIFIED WITH OTHER ALCOHOL-INDUCED DISORDER
F10.99	ALCOHOL USE, UNSPECIFIED WITH UNSPECIFIED ALCOHOL-INDUCED DISORDER
G62.1	ALCOHOLIC POLYNEUROPATHY
G72.1	ALCOHOLIC MYOPATHY
I42.6	ALCOHOLIC CARDIOMYOPATHY
K29.20	ALCOHOLIC GASTRITIS WITHOUT BLEEDING
K29.21	ALCOHOLIC GASTRITIS WITH BLEEDING
K70.0	ALCOHOLIC FATTY LIVER
K70.10	ALCOHOLIC HEPATITIS WITHOUT ASCITES
K70.11	ALCOHOLIC HEPATITIS WITH ASCITES
K70.2	ALCOHOLIC FIBROSIS AND SCLEROSIS OF LIVER
K70.30	ALCOHOLIC CIRRHOSIS OF LIVER WITHOUT ASCITES
K70.31	ALCOHOLIC CIRRHOSIS OF LIVER WITH ASCITES
K70.40	ALCOHOLIC HEPATIC FAILURE WITHOUT COMA
K70.41	ALCOHOLIC HEPATIC FAILURE WITH COMA
K70.9	ALCOHOLIC LIVER DISEASE, UNSPECIFIED

Table 6.
Substance abuse disorder diagnosis codes.

PRCDR_CDE	PRCDR_DESC
H0001	ALCOHOL AND/OR DRUG ASSESSMENT
H0002	BEHAVIORAL HEALTH SCREENING TO DETERMINE ELIGIBI
H0003	ALCOHOL AND/OR DRUG SCREENING; LABORATORY ANALYS
H0005	ALCOHOL AND/OR DRUG SERVICES; GROUP COUNSELING B
H0006	ALCOHOL AND/OR DRUG SERVICES; CASE MANAGEMENT
H0007	ALCOHOL AND/OR DRUG SERVICES; CRISIS INTERVENTIO
H0008	ALCOHOL AND/OR DRUG SERVICES; SUB-ACUTE DETOXIFI
H0009	ALCOHOL AND/OR DRUG SERVICES; ACUTE DETOXIFICATI
H0010	ALCOHOL AND/OR DRUG SERVICES; SUB-ACUTE DETOXIFI
H0011	ALCOHOL AND/OR DRUG SERVICES; ACUTE DETOXIFICATI
H0012	ALCOHOL AND/OR DRUG SERVICES; SUB-ACUTE DETOXIFI
H0013	ALCOHOL AND/OR DRUG SERVICES; ACUTE DETOXIFICATI
H0014	ALCOHOL AND/OR DRUG SERVICES; AMBULATORY DETOXIF
H0015	ALCOHOL AND/OR DRUG SERVICES; INTENSIVE OUTPATIE
H0016	ALCOHOL AND/OR DRUG SERVICES; MEDICAL/SOMATIC (M
H0020	ALCOHOL AND/OR DRUG SERVICES; METHADONE ADMINIST
H0021	ALCOHOL AND/OR DRUG TRAINING SERVICE (FOR STAFF
H0022	ALCOHOL AND/OR DRUG INTERVENTION SERVICE (PLANNE
H0026	ALCOHOL AND/OR DRUG PREVENTION PROCESS SERVICE,
H0027	ALCOHOL AND/OR DRUG PREVENTION ENVIRONMENTAL SER
H0028	ALCOHOL AND/OR DRUG PREVENTION PROBLEM IDENTIFIC
H0029	ALCOHOL AND/OR DRUG PREVENTION ALTERNATIVES SERV
H0047	ALCOHOL AND/OR OTHER DRUG ABUSE SERVICES, NOT OT
H0048	ALCOHOL AND/OR OTHER DRUG TESTING: COLLECTION AN
H0049	ALCOHOL AND/OR DRUG SCREENING
H0050	ALCOHOL AND/OR DRUG SERVICES, BRIEF INTERVENTION
99408	ALCOHOL/SUBSTANCE SCREEN & INTERVEN 15-30 MIN
99409	ALCOHOL/SUBSTANCE SCREEN & INTERVENTION >30 MIN
H0049	ALCOHOL AND/OR DRUG SCREENING
H0050	ALCOHOL AND/OR DRUG SERVICES, BRIEF INTERVENTION

Table 7.
Substance abuse disorder procedure codes.

DRUG_NAME	GENERIC_NAME	NDC12
BUNAVAIL	BUPRENORPHINE HCL/NALOXONE HCL	593850001201
BUNAVAIL	BUPRENORPHINE HCL/NALOXONE HCL	593850001230
BUNAVAIL	BUPRENORPHINE HCL/NALOXONE HCL	593850001401
BUNAVAIL	BUPRENORPHINE HCL/NALOXONE HCL	593850001430
BUNAVAIL	BUPRENORPHINE HCL/NALOXONE HCL	593850001601
BUNAVAIL	BUPRENORPHINE HCL/NALOXONE HCL	593850001630
BUPRENORPHINE-NALOXONE	BUPRENORPHINE HCL/NALOXONE HCL	003780876816
BUPRENORPHINE-NALOXONE	BUPRENORPHINE HCL/NALOXONE HCL	003780876893
BUPRENORPHINE-NALOXONE	BUPRENORPHINE HCL/NALOXONE HCL	007810724906
BUPRENORPHINE-NALOXONE	BUPRENORPHINE HCL/NALOXONE HCL	007810724964
BUPRENORPHINE-NALOXONE	BUPRENORPHINE HCL/NALOXONE HCL	435980058101
BUPRENORPHINE-NALOXONE	BUPRENORPHINE HCL/NALOXONE HCL	435980058130
BUPRENORPHINE-NALOXONE	BUPRENORPHINE HCL/NALOXONE HCL	477810035803
BUPRENORPHINE-NALOXONE	BUPRENORPHINE HCL/NALOXONE HCL	524270071203
BUPRENORPHINE-NALOXONE	BUPRENORPHINE HCL/NALOXONE HCL	524270071211
BUPRENORPHINE-NALOXONE	BUPRENORPHINE HCL/NALOXONE HCL	007810721606
BUPRENORPHINE-NALOXONE	BUPRENORPHINE HCL/NALOXONE HCL	007810721664
BUPRENORPHINE-NALOXONE	BUPRENORPHINE HCL/NALOXONE HCL	435980057901
BUPRENORPHINE-NALOXONE	BUPRENORPHINE HCL/NALOXONE HCL	435980057930
BUPRENORPHINE-NALOXONE	BUPRENORPHINE HCL/NALOXONE HCL	477810035503
BUPRENORPHINE-NALOXONE	BUPRENORPHINE HCL/NALOXONE HCL	524270069203
BUPRENORPHINE-NALOXONE	BUPRENORPHINE HCL/NALOXONE HCL	524270069211
BUPRENORPHINE-NALOXONE	BUPRENORPHINE HCL/NALOXONE HCL	000540018813
BUPRENORPHINE-NALOXONE	BUPRENORPHINE HCL/NALOXONE HCL	000930572056
BUPRENORPHINE-NALOXONE	BUPRENORPHINE HCL/NALOXONE HCL	002280315403
BUPRENORPHINE-NALOXONE	BUPRENORPHINE HCL/NALOXONE HCL	002280315473
BUPRENORPHINE-NALOXONE	BUPRENORPHINE HCL/NALOXONE HCL	004060192303
BUPRENORPHINE-NALOXONE	BUPRENORPHINE HCL/NALOXONE HCL	004060800503
BUPRENORPHINE-NALOXONE	BUPRENORPHINE HCL/NALOXONE HCL	422910017430
BUPRENORPHINE-NALOXONE	BUPRENORPHINE HCL/NALOXONE HCL	502680014411
BUPRENORPHINE-NALOXONE	BUPRENORPHINE HCL/NALOXONE HCL	502680014415
BUPRENORPHINE-NALOXONE	BUPRENORPHINE HCL/NALOXONE HCL	503830029493
BUPRENORPHINE-NALOXONE	BUPRENORPHINE HCL/NALOXONE HCL	557000018430
BUPRENORPHINE-NALOXONE	BUPRENORPHINE HCL/NALOXONE HCL	604290058630
BUPRENORPHINE-NALOXONE	BUPRENORPHINE HCL/NALOXONE HCL	604290058633
BUPRENORPHINE-NALOXONE	BUPRENORPHINE HCL/NALOXONE HCL	621750045232
BUPRENORPHINE-NALOXONE	BUPRENORPHINE HCL/NALOXONE HCL	627560096983
BUPRENORPHINE-NALOXONE	BUPRENORPHINE HCL/NALOXONE HCL	651620041603
BUPRENORPHINE-NALOXONE	BUPRENORPHINE HCL/NALOXONE HCL	007810722706
BUPRENORPHINE-NALOXONE	BUPRENORPHINE HCL/NALOXONE HCL	007810722764

BUPRENORPHINE-NALOXONE	BUPRENORPHINE HCL/NALOXONE HCL	435980058001
BUPRENORPHINE-NALOXONE	BUPRENORPHINE HCL/NALOXONE HCL	435980058030
BUPRENORPHINE-NALOXONE	BUPRENORPHINE HCL/NALOXONE HCL	477810035603
BUPRENORPHINE-NALOXONE	BUPRENORPHINE HCL/NALOXONE HCL	524270069403
BUPRENORPHINE-NALOXONE	BUPRENORPHINE HCL/NALOXONE HCL	524270069411
BUPRENORPHINE-NALOXONE	BUPRENORPHINE HCL/NALOXONE HCL	003780876716
BUPRENORPHINE-NALOXONE	BUPRENORPHINE HCL/NALOXONE HCL	003780876793
BUPRENORPHINE-NALOXONE	BUPRENORPHINE HCL/NALOXONE HCL	007810723806
BUPRENORPHINE-NALOXONE	BUPRENORPHINE HCL/NALOXONE HCL	007810723864
BUPRENORPHINE-NALOXONE	BUPRENORPHINE HCL/NALOXONE HCL	435980058201
BUPRENORPHINE-NALOXONE	BUPRENORPHINE HCL/NALOXONE HCL	435980058230
BUPRENORPHINE-NALOXONE	BUPRENORPHINE HCL/NALOXONE HCL	477810035703
BUPRENORPHINE-NALOXONE	BUPRENORPHINE HCL/NALOXONE HCL	524270069803
BUPRENORPHINE-NALOXONE	BUPRENORPHINE HCL/NALOXONE HCL	524270069811
BUPRENORPHINE-NALOXONE	BUPRENORPHINE HCL/NALOXONE HCL	000540018913
BUPRENORPHINE-NALOXONE	BUPRENORPHINE HCL/NALOXONE HCL	000930572156
BUPRENORPHINE-NALOXONE	BUPRENORPHINE HCL/NALOXONE HCL	002280315503
BUPRENORPHINE-NALOXONE	BUPRENORPHINE HCL/NALOXONE HCL	002280315567
BUPRENORPHINE-NALOXONE	BUPRENORPHINE HCL/NALOXONE HCL	002280315573
BUPRENORPHINE-NALOXONE	BUPRENORPHINE HCL/NALOXONE HCL	004060192403
BUPRENORPHINE-NALOXONE	BUPRENORPHINE HCL/NALOXONE HCL	004060802003
BUPRENORPHINE-NALOXONE	BUPRENORPHINE HCL/NALOXONE HCL	422910017530
BUPRENORPHINE-NALOXONE	BUPRENORPHINE HCL/NALOXONE HCL	502680014511
BUPRENORPHINE-NALOXONE	BUPRENORPHINE HCL/NALOXONE HCL	502680014515
BUPRENORPHINE-NALOXONE	BUPRENORPHINE HCL/NALOXONE HCL	503830028793
BUPRENORPHINE-NALOXONE	BUPRENORPHINE HCL/NALOXONE HCL	545690640800
BUPRENORPHINE-NALOXONE	BUPRENORPHINE HCL/NALOXONE HCL	604290058730
BUPRENORPHINE-NALOXONE	BUPRENORPHINE HCL/NALOXONE HCL	604290058733
BUPRENORPHINE-NALOXONE	BUPRENORPHINE HCL/NALOXONE HCL	621750045832
BUPRENORPHINE-NALOXONE	BUPRENORPHINE HCL/NALOXONE HCL	627560097083
BUPRENORPHINE-NALOXONE	BUPRENORPHINE HCL/NALOXONE HCL	651620041503
SUBOXONE	BUPRENORPHINE HCL/NALOXONE HCL	124960121201
SUBOXONE	BUPRENORPHINE HCL/NALOXONE HCL	124960121203
SUBOXONE	BUPRENORPHINE HCL/NALOXONE HCL	124960120201
SUBOXONE	BUPRENORPHINE HCL/NALOXONE HCL	124960120203
SUBOXONE	BUPRENORPHINE HCL/NALOXONE HCL	124960128302
SUBOXONE	BUPRENORPHINE HCL/NALOXONE HCL	165900066630
SUBOXONE	BUPRENORPHINE HCL/NALOXONE HCL	499990039507
SUBOXONE	BUPRENORPHINE HCL/NALOXONE HCL	499990039515
SUBOXONE	BUPRENORPHINE HCL/NALOXONE HCL	499990039530
SUBOXONE	BUPRENORPHINE HCL/NALOXONE HCL	529590074930
SUBOXONE	BUPRENORPHINE HCL/NALOXONE HCL	545690549600

SUBOXONE	BUPRENORPHINE HCL/NALOXONE HCL	548680575000
SUBOXONE	BUPRENORPHINE HCL/NALOXONE HCL	636290402801
SUBOXONE	BUPRENORPHINE HCL/NALOXONE HCL	638740108503
SUBOXONE	BUPRENORPHINE HCL/NALOXONE HCL	680710151003
SUBOXONE	BUPRENORPHINE HCL/NALOXONE HCL	682580299903
SUBOXONE	BUPRENORPHINE HCL/NALOXONE HCL	124960120401
SUBOXONE	BUPRENORPHINE HCL/NALOXONE HCL	124960120403
SUBOXONE	BUPRENORPHINE HCL/NALOXONE HCL	124960120801
SUBOXONE	BUPRENORPHINE HCL/NALOXONE HCL	124960120803
SUBOXONE	BUPRENORPHINE HCL/NALOXONE HCL	545690639900
SUBOXONE	BUPRENORPHINE HCL/NALOXONE HCL	557000014730
SUBOXONE	BUPRENORPHINE HCL/NALOXONE HCL	124960130601
SUBOXONE	BUPRENORPHINE HCL/NALOXONE HCL	124960130602
SUBOXONE	BUPRENORPHINE HCL/NALOXONE HCL	353560000407
SUBOXONE	BUPRENORPHINE HCL/NALOXONE HCL	353560000430
SUBOXONE	BUPRENORPHINE HCL/NALOXONE HCL	430630018407
SUBOXONE	BUPRENORPHINE HCL/NALOXONE HCL	430630018430
SUBOXONE	BUPRENORPHINE HCL/NALOXONE HCL	529590030430
SUBOXONE	BUPRENORPHINE HCL/NALOXONE HCL	545690573900
SUBOXONE	BUPRENORPHINE HCL/NALOXONE HCL	545690573901
SUBOXONE	BUPRENORPHINE HCL/NALOXONE HCL	545690573902
SUBOXONE	BUPRENORPHINE HCL/NALOXONE HCL	548680570700
SUBOXONE	BUPRENORPHINE HCL/NALOXONE HCL	548680570701
SUBOXONE	BUPRENORPHINE HCL/NALOXONE HCL	548680570702
SUBOXONE	BUPRENORPHINE HCL/NALOXONE HCL	548680570703
SUBOXONE	BUPRENORPHINE HCL/NALOXONE HCL	548680570704
SUBOXONE	BUPRENORPHINE HCL/NALOXONE HCL	550450378403
SUBOXONE	BUPRENORPHINE HCL/NALOXONE HCL	636290403401
SUBOXONE	BUPRENORPHINE HCL/NALOXONE HCL	636290403402
SUBOXONE	BUPRENORPHINE HCL/NALOXONE HCL	636290403403
SUBOXONE	BUPRENORPHINE HCL/NALOXONE HCL	638740108403
SUBOXONE	BUPRENORPHINE HCL/NALOXONE HCL	663360001630
SUBOXONE	BUPRENORPHINE HCL/NALOXONE HCL	680710138003
ZUBSOLV	BUPRENORPHINE HCL/NALOXONE HCL	541230090730
ZUBSOLV	BUPRENORPHINE HCL/NALOXONE HCL	541230091430
ZUBSOLV	BUPRENORPHINE HCL/NALOXONE HCL	541230011430
ZUBSOLV	BUPRENORPHINE HCL/NALOXONE HCL	541230092930
ZUBSOLV	BUPRENORPHINE HCL/NALOXONE HCL	541230095730
ZUBSOLV	BUPRENORPHINE HCL/NALOXONE HCL	541230098630
BUPRENORPHINE HCL	BUPRENORPHINE HCL	000540017613
BUPRENORPHINE HCL	BUPRENORPHINE HCL	000930537856
BUPRENORPHINE HCL	BUPRENORPHINE HCL	002280315603

BUPRENORPHINE HCL	BUPRENORPHINE HCL	003780092393
BUPRENORPHINE HCL	BUPRENORPHINE HCL	353560055530
BUPRENORPHINE HCL	BUPRENORPHINE HCL	428580050103
BUPRENORPHINE HCL	BUPRENORPHINE HCL	503830092493
BUPRENORPHINE HCL	BUPRENORPHINE HCL	557000030230
BUPRENORPHINE HCL	BUPRENORPHINE HCL	627560045983
BUPRENORPHINE HCL	BUPRENORPHINE HCL	683080020230
BUPRENORPHINE HCL	BUPRENORPHINE HCL	000540017713
BUPRENORPHINE HCL	BUPRENORPHINE HCL	000930537956
BUPRENORPHINE HCL	BUPRENORPHINE HCL	002280315303
BUPRENORPHINE HCL	BUPRENORPHINE HCL	003780092493
BUPRENORPHINE HCL	BUPRENORPHINE HCL	353560055630
BUPRENORPHINE HCL	BUPRENORPHINE HCL	428580050203
BUPRENORPHINE HCL	BUPRENORPHINE HCL	430630066706
BUPRENORPHINE HCL	BUPRENORPHINE HCL	430630075306
BUPRENORPHINE HCL	BUPRENORPHINE HCL	503830093093
BUPRENORPHINE HCL	BUPRENORPHINE HCL	557000030330
BUPRENORPHINE HCL	BUPRENORPHINE HCL	627560046083
BUPRENORPHINE HCL	BUPRENORPHINE HCL	683080020830
PROBUPHINE	BUPRENORPHINE HCL	524400010014
PROBUPHINE	BUPRENORPHINE HCL	582840010014
SUBLOCADE	BUPRENORPHINE	124960010001
SUBLOCADE	BUPRENORPHINE	124960010005
SUBLOCADE	BUPRENORPHINE	124960030001
SUBLOCADE	BUPRENORPHINE	124960030005
SUBUTEX	BUPRENORPHINE HCL	124960127802
SUBUTEX	BUPRENORPHINE HCL	499990063830
SUBUTEX	BUPRENORPHINE HCL	124960131002
SUBUTEX	BUPRENORPHINE HCL	499990063930
SUBUTEX	BUPRENORPHINE HCL	638740117303
DISKETS	METHADONE HCL	000540453825
DOLOPHINE HCL	METHADONE HCL	000020168702
DOLOPHINE HCL	METHADONE HCL	000020168712
DOLOPHINE HCL	METHADONE HCL	000020107202
DOLOPHINE HCL	METHADONE HCL	000540421725
DOLOPHINE HCL	METHADONE HCL	000540421925
DOLOPHINE HCL	METHADONE HCL	000020168201
DOLOPHINE HCL	METHADONE HCL	000020168225
DOLOPHINE HCL	METHADONE HCL	000540121811
DOLOPHINE HCL	METHADONE HCL	000540121842
DOLOPHINE HCL	METHADONE HCL	000020106402
DOLOPHINE HCL	METHADONE HYDROCHLORIDE	000020106404

DOLOPHINE HCL	METHADONE HCL	000540421625
DOLOPHINE HCL	METHADONE HCL	000540421825
METHADONE	METHADONE HCL	000540355467
METHADONE	METHADONE HCL	548680285403
METHADONE	METHADONE HCL	681150057100
METHADONE	METHADONE HCL	000540355367
METHADONE	METHADONE HCL	510790069439
METHADONE	METHADONE HCL	666890069430
METHADONE	METHADONE HCL	666890069439
METHADONE	METHADONE HCL	666890069479
METHADONE	METHADONE HCL	663360017060
METHADONE	METHADONE HCL	681150057200
METHADONE HCL	METHADONE HCL	000190151056
METHADONE HCL	METHADONE HCL	000190151057
METHADONE HCL	METHADONE HCL	000190151059
METHADONE HCL	METHADONE HCL	000190151061
METHADONE HCL	METHADONE HCL	000540975085
METHADONE HCL	METHADONE HCL	000540975088
METHADONE HCL	METHADONE HCL	004060151056
METHADONE HCL	METHADONE HCL	004060151057
METHADONE HCL	METHADONE HCL	004060151059
METHADONE HCL	METHADONE HCL	004060151061
METHADONE HCL	METHADONE HCL	387790010403
METHADONE HCL	METHADONE HCL	387790010404
METHADONE HCL	METHADONE HCL	387790010405
METHADONE HCL	METHADONE HCL	494520455301
METHADONE HCL	METHADONE HCL	494520455302
METHADONE HCL	METHADONE HCL	494520455303
METHADONE HCL	METHADONE HCL	510790068155
METHADONE HCL	METHADONE HCL	515520072801
METHADONE HCL	METHADONE HCL	515520072802
METHADONE HCL	METHADONE HCL	515520072804
METHADONE HCL	METHADONE HCL	515520072806
METHADONE HCL	METHADONE HCL	519270101700
METHADONE HCL	METHADONE HCL	523720079601
METHADONE HCL	METHADONE HCL	523720079602
METHADONE HCL	METHADONE HCL	523720079603
METHADONE HCL	METHADONE HCL	629910140801
METHADONE HCL	METHADONE HCL	629910140802
METHADONE HCL	METHADONE HCL	629910140803
METHADONE HCL	METHADONE HCL	629910140805
METHADONE HCL	METHADONE HCL	632750910004

METHADONE HCL	METHADONE HCL	632750910005
METHADONE HCL	METHADONE HCL	640190075088
METHADONE HCL	METHADONE HCL	666890068155
METHADONE HCL	METHADONE HCL	000540457125
METHADONE HCL	METHADONE HCL	000540855411
METHADONE HCL	METHADONE HCL	000540855424
METHADONE HCL	METHADONE HCL	003780327201
METHADONE HCL	METHADONE HCL	004060577101
METHADONE HCL	METHADONE HCL	004060577123
METHADONE HCL	METHADONE HCL	004060577162
METHADONE HCL	METHADONE HCL	009040653060
METHADONE HCL	METHADONE HCL	009040653061
METHADONE HCL	METHADONE HCL	105440037808
METHADONE HCL	METHADONE HCL	105440037828
METHADONE HCL	METHADONE HCL	105440037830
METHADONE HCL	METHADONE HCL	105440037860
METHADONE HCL	METHADONE HCL	131070008901
METHADONE HCL	METHADONE HCL	165900067007
METHADONE HCL	METHADONE HCL	165900067045
METHADONE HCL	METHADONE HCL	165900067060
METHADONE HCL	METHADONE HCL	165900067071
METHADONE HCL	METHADONE HCL	165900067072
METHADONE HCL	METHADONE HCL	165900067082
METHADONE HCL	METHADONE HCL	165900067083
METHADONE HCL	METHADONE HCL	165900067090
METHADONE HCL	METHADONE HCL	234900587703
METHADONE HCL	METHADONE HCL	234900587706
METHADONE HCL	METHADONE HCL	234900587707
METHADONE HCL	METHADONE HCL	234900587709
METHADONE HCL	METHADONE HCL	317220094701
METHADONE HCL	METHADONE HCL	353560083401
METHADONE HCL	METHADONE HCL	353560083430
METHADONE HCL	METHADONE HCL	353560083460
METHADONE HCL	METHADONE HCL	353560083490
METHADONE HCL	METHADONE HCL	425490057802
METHADONE HCL	METHADONE HCL	425490057808
METHADONE HCL	METHADONE HCL	425490057828
METHADONE HCL	METHADONE HCL	425490057830
METHADONE HCL	METHADONE HCL	425490057856
METHADONE HCL	METHADONE HCL	425490057860
METHADONE HCL	METHADONE HCL	428060031801
METHADONE HCL	METHADONE HCL	499990083901

METHADONE HCL	METHADONE HCL	499990083930
METHADONE HCL	METHADONE HCL	499990083960
METHADONE HCL	METHADONE HCL	499990083990
METHADONE HCL	METHADONE HCL	529590038602
METHADONE HCL	METHADONE HCL	529590038630
METHADONE HCL	METHADONE HCL	529590038660
METHADONE HCL	METHADONE HCL	529590038690
METHADONE HCL	METHADONE HCL	548680285400
METHADONE HCL	METHADONE HCL	548680494800
METHADONE HCL	METHADONE HCL	548680494801
METHADONE HCL	METHADONE HCL	548680494802
METHADONE HCL	METHADONE HCL	548680494803
METHADONE HCL	METHADONE HCL	548680494805
METHADONE HCL	METHADONE HCL	548680494806
METHADONE HCL	METHADONE HCL	548680494807
METHADONE HCL	METHADONE HCL	552890081430
METHADONE HCL	METHADONE HCL	552890081460
METHADONE HCL	METHADONE HCL	552890081490
METHADONE HCL	METHADONE HCL	552890081493
METHADONE HCL	METHADONE HCL	552890081498
METHADONE HCL	METHADONE HCL	552890081499
METHADONE HCL	METHADONE HCL	558870020060
METHADONE HCL	METHADONE HCL	558870020082
METHADONE HCL	METHADONE HCL	558870020090
METHADONE HCL	METHADONE HCL	578660707001
METHADONE HCL	METHADONE HCL	578660707002
METHADONE HCL	METHADONE HCL	578660707003
METHADONE HCL	METHADONE HCL	578660707006
METHADONE HCL	METHADONE HCL	636290377101
METHADONE HCL	METHADONE HCL	636290377102
METHADONE HCL	METHADONE HCL	636290377103
METHADONE HCL	METHADONE HCL	636290377104
METHADONE HCL	METHADONE HCL	636290377105
METHADONE HCL	METHADONE HCL	636290377106
METHADONE HCL	METHADONE HCL	637390000610
METHADONE HCL	METHADONE HCL	663360017130
METHADONE HCL	METHADONE HCL	663360017142
METHADONE HCL	METHADONE HCL	663360017156
METHADONE HCL	METHADONE HCL	663360017160
METHADONE HCL	METHADONE HCL	663360017162
METHADONE HCL	METHADONE HCL	663360017190
METHADONE HCL	METHADONE HCL	663360017194

METHADONE HCL	METHADONE HCL	663360017198
METHADONE HCL	METHADONE HCL	666890081010
METHADONE HCL	METHADONE HCL	678770011601
METHADONE HCL	METHADONE HCL	680840073801
METHADONE HCL	METHADONE HCL	680840073811
METHADONE HCL	METHADONE HCL	684620080101
METHADONE HCL	METHADONE HCL	000540355663
METHADONE HCL	METHADONE HCL	000540854916
METHADONE HCL	METHADONE HCL	666890071216
METHADONE HCL	METHADONE HCL	242000028363
METHADONE HCL	METHADONE HCL	000540039168
METHADONE HCL	METHADONE HCL	000540039268
METHADONE HCL	METHADONE HCL	640190055367
METHADONE HCL	METHADONE HCL	640190055467
METHADONE HCL	METHADONE HCL	666890069579
METHADONE HCL	METHADONE HCL	615530014940
METHADONE HCL	METHADONE HCL	615530014978
METHADONE HCL	METHADONE HCL	174780038020
METHADONE HCL	METHADONE HCL	664790053002
METHADONE HCL	METHADONE HCL	665910081551
METHADONE HCL	METHADONE HCL	674570021720
METHADONE HCL	METHADONE HCL	000020215302
METHADONE HCL	METHADONE HCL	000540454725
METHADONE HCL	METHADONE HCL	000540854725
METHADONE HCL	METHADONE HCL	234900779801
METHADONE HCL	METHADONE HCL	234900779803
METHADONE HCL	METHADONE HCL	510790089840
METHADONE HCL	METHADONE HCL	558870013460
METHADONE HCL	METHADONE HCL	558870013490
METHADONE HCL	METHADONE HCL	578660708101
METHADONE HCL	METHADONE HCL	578660708102
METHADONE HCL	METHADONE HCL	640190053825
METHADONE HCL	METHADONE HCL	666890089840
METHADONE HCL	METHADONE HCL	680840097732
METHADONE HCL	METHADONE HCL	680840097733
METHADONE HCL	METHADONE HCL	000540355563
METHADONE HCL	METHADONE HCL	000540457025
METHADONE HCL	METHADONE HCL	000540855311
METHADONE HCL	METHADONE HCL	000540855324
METHADONE HCL	METHADONE HCL	003780326001
METHADONE HCL	METHADONE HCL	004060575501
METHADONE HCL	METHADONE HCL	004060575523

METHADONE HCL	METHADONE HCL	004060575562
METHADONE HCL	METHADONE HCL	105440037702
METHADONE HCL	METHADONE HCL	105440037728
METHADONE HCL	METHADONE HCL	131070008801
METHADONE HCL	METHADONE HCL	165900068945
METHADONE HCL	METHADONE HCL	165900068960
METHADONE HCL	METHADONE HCL	165900068972
METHADONE HCL	METHADONE HCL	165900068990
METHADONE HCL	METHADONE HCL	234900587801
METHADONE HCL	METHADONE HCL	234900587802
METHADONE HCL	METHADONE HCL	234900587803
METHADONE HCL	METHADONE HCL	234900587809
METHADONE HCL	METHADONE HCL	317220094601
METHADONE HCL	METHADONE HCL	353560083530
METHADONE HCL	METHADONE HCL	353560083560
METHADONE HCL	METHADONE HCL	353560083590
METHADONE HCL	METHADONE HCL	425490057702
METHADONE HCL	METHADONE HCL	425490057728
METHADONE HCL	METHADONE HCL	428060031701
METHADONE HCL	METHADONE HCL	430630022260
METHADONE HCL	METHADONE HCL	430630022290
METHADONE HCL	METHADONE HCL	430630022293
METHADONE HCL	METHADONE HCL	430630022298
METHADONE HCL	METHADONE HCL	499990096330
METHADONE HCL	METHADONE HCL	499990096360
METHADONE HCL	METHADONE HCL	499990096390
METHADONE HCL	METHADONE HCL	529590043530
METHADONE HCL	METHADONE HCL	548680570100
METHADONE HCL	METHADONE HCL	548680570101
METHADONE HCL	METHADONE HCL	548680570102
METHADONE HCL	METHADONE HCL	548680570103
METHADONE HCL	METHADONE HCL	558870009082
METHADONE HCL	METHADONE HCL	558870009090
METHADONE HCL	METHADONE HCL	578660395001
METHADONE HCL	METHADONE HCL	578660395002
METHADONE HCL	METHADONE HCL	578660395003
METHADONE HCL	METHADONE HCL	606870021401
METHADONE HCL	METHADONE HCL	606870021411
METHADONE HCL	METHADONE HCL	636290378801
METHADONE HCL	METHADONE HCL	663360017030
METHADONE HCL	METHADONE HCL	663360017062
METHADONE HCL	METHADONE HCL	663360017090

METHADONE HCL	METHADONE HCL	663360017094
METHADONE HCL	METHADONE HCL	684620080001
METHADONE HCL	METHADONE HCL	242000028149
METHADONE HCL	METHADONE HCL	000540854816
METHADONE HCL	METHADONE HCL	666890071116
METHADONE HCL-0.9% NACL	METHADONE HCL IN 0.9 % NACL	242000027503
METHADONE HCL-0.9% NACL	METHADONE IN 0.9 % SOD.CHLORID	615530012078
METHADONE HCL-0.9% NACL	METHADONE IN 0.9 % SOD.CHLORID	615530013490
METHADONE HYDROCHLORIDE	METHADONE HCL	004060254001
METHADONE INTENSOL	METHADONE HCL	000540355344
METHADOSE	METHADONE HCL	004060345434
METHADOSE	METHADONE HCL	499990084030
METHADOSE	METHADONE HCL	499990084060
METHADOSE	METHADONE HCL	548680285401
METHADOSE	METHADONE HCL	548680285402
METHADOSE	METHADONE HCL	578660318701
METHADOSE	METHADONE HCL	578660318702
METHADOSE	METHADONE HCL	000190052705
METHADOSE	METHADONE HCL	004060052705
METHADOSE	METHADONE HCL	004060052710
METHADOSE	METHADONE HCL	004060872510
METHADOSE	METHADONE HCL	004060054034
METHADOSE	METHADONE HCL	499990084130
METHADOSE	METHADONE HCL	499990084160
METHADOSE	METHADONE HCL	578660318801
METHADOSE	METHADONE HCL	578660318802
METHADOSE	METHADONE HCL	606870020932
METHADOSE	METHADONE HCL	606870020933
METHADOSE	METHADONE HCL	004060697434
METHADOSE	METHADONE HCL	548680440800
METHADOSE	METHADONE HCL	548680440801
DEPADE	NALTREXONE HCL	004060009201
DEPADE	NALTREXONE HCL	004060009203
NALTREXONE HCL	NALTREXONE HCL	001850003901
NALTREXONE HCL	NALTREXONE HCL	004060117001
NALTREXONE HCL	NALTREXONE HCL	004060117003
NALTREXONE HCL	NALTREXONE HCL	005550090201
NALTREXONE HCL	NALTREXONE HCL	005550090202
NALTREXONE HCL	NALTREXONE HCL	167290008101
NALTREXONE HCL	NALTREXONE HCL	167290008110
NALTREXONE HCL	NALTREXONE HCL	422910063230

NALTREXONE HCL	NALTREXONE HCL	430630059115
NALTREXONE HCL	NALTREXONE HCL	473350032683
NALTREXONE HCL	NALTREXONE HCL	473350032688
NALTREXONE HCL	NALTREXONE HCL	500900286600
NALTREXONE HCL	NALTREXONE HCL	504360010501
NALTREXONE HCL	NALTREXONE HCL	512240020630
NALTREXONE HCL	NALTREXONE HCL	512240020650
NALTREXONE HCL	NALTREXONE HCL	548680557400
NALTREXONE HCL	NALTREXONE HCL	636290104601
NALTREXONE HCL	NALTREXONE HCL	636290104701
NALTREXONE HCL	NALTREXONE HCL	680840029111
NALTREXONE HCL	NALTREXONE HCL	680840029121
NALTREXONE HCL	NALTREXONE HCL	680940085362
NALTREXONE HYDROCHLORIDE	NALTREXONE HCL	001850003930
NALTREXONE HYDROCHLORIDE	NALTREXONE HCL	521520010502
NALTREXONE HYDROCHLORIDE	NALTREXONE HCL	521520010504
NALTREXONE HYDROCHLORIDE	NALTREXONE HCL	521520010530
NALTREXONE HYDROCHLORIDE	NALTREXONE HCL	656940010003
NALTREXONE HYDROCHLORIDE	NALTREXONE HCL	656940010010
NALTREXONE HYDROCHLORIDE	NALTREXONE HCL	681150068030
REVIA	NALTREXONE HCL	000560001122
REVIA	NALTREXONE HCL	000560001130
REVIA	NALTREXONE HCL	000560001170
REVIA	NALTREXONE HCL	000560001176
REVIA	NALTREXONE HCL	000560007950
REVIA	NALTREXONE HCL	000560008050
REVIA	NALTREXONE HCL	512850027501
REVIA	NALTREXONE HCL	512850027502
VIVITROL	NALTREXONE MICROSPHERES	634590030042
VIVITROL	NALTREXONE MICROSPHERES	657570030001
ANTABUSE	DISULFIRAM	000460080981
ANTABUSE	DISULFIRAM	512850052302
ANTABUSE	DISULFIRAM	545690179000
ANTABUSE	DISULFIRAM	545690179001
ANTABUSE	DISULFIRAM	545690179002
ANTABUSE	DISULFIRAM	548680503400
ANTABUSE	DISULFIRAM	548680503401
ANTABUSE	DISULFIRAM	548680503402
ANTABUSE	DISULFIRAM	654730070601
ANTABUSE	DISULFIRAM	000460081050

ANTABUSE	DISULFIRAM	000460081091
ANTABUSE	DISULFIRAM	512850052402
ANTABUSE	DISULFIRAM	654730070701
DISULFIRAM	DISULFIRAM	387790197102
DISULFIRAM	DISULFIRAM	387790197105
DISULFIRAM	DISULFIRAM	387790197108
DISULFIRAM	DISULFIRAM	387790197109
DISULFIRAM	DISULFIRAM	494520264501
DISULFIRAM	DISULFIRAM	515520109505
DISULFIRAM	DISULFIRAM	519270312100
DISULFIRAM	DISULFIRAM	000540035613
DISULFIRAM	DISULFIRAM	000540035625
DISULFIRAM	DISULFIRAM	000930503501
DISULFIRAM	DISULFIRAM	001500118060
DISULFIRAM	DISULFIRAM	001570066301
DISULFIRAM	DISULFIRAM	001820053201
DISULFIRAM	DISULFIRAM	001820053210
DISULFIRAM	DISULFIRAM	003020231001
DISULFIRAM	DISULFIRAM	003040080101
DISULFIRAM	DISULFIRAM	003490846701
DISULFIRAM	DISULFIRAM	003640033601
DISULFIRAM	DISULFIRAM	003780414001
DISULFIRAM	DISULFIRAM	004050436301
DISULFIRAM	DISULFIRAM	005360376701
DISULFIRAM	DISULFIRAM	005370600401
DISULFIRAM	DISULFIRAM	005800119101
DISULFIRAM	DISULFIRAM	005910537601
DISULFIRAM	DISULFIRAM	005910537604
DISULFIRAM	DISULFIRAM	006030343121
DISULFIRAM	DISULFIRAM	006030343321
DISULFIRAM	DISULFIRAM	006770100101
DISULFIRAM	DISULFIRAM	007190132010
DISULFIRAM	DISULFIRAM	007190132013
DISULFIRAM	DISULFIRAM	007790037825
DISULFIRAM	DISULFIRAM	007810106001
DISULFIRAM	DISULFIRAM	008140262514
DISULFIRAM	DISULFIRAM	008140262708
DISULFIRAM	DISULFIRAM	008140262714
DISULFIRAM	DISULFIRAM	008390128606
DISULFIRAM	DISULFIRAM	008390128616
DISULFIRAM	DISULFIRAM	009040118060
DISULFIRAM	DISULFIRAM	009040118061

DISULFIRAM	DISULFIRAM	170220390302
DISULFIRAM	DISULFIRAM	354700012801
DISULFIRAM	DISULFIRAM	472020247201
DISULFIRAM	DISULFIRAM	477810060730
DISULFIRAM	DISULFIRAM	496480080101
DISULFIRAM	DISULFIRAM	497270090302
DISULFIRAM	DISULFIRAM	498840015301
DISULFIRAM	DISULFIRAM	498840015305
DISULFIRAM	DISULFIRAM	501110033101
DISULFIRAM	DISULFIRAM	501110033103
DISULFIRAM	DISULFIRAM	516550023224
DISULFIRAM	DISULFIRAM	517280053801
DISULFIRAM	DISULFIRAM	524460017721
DISULFIRAM	DISULFIRAM	584690376730
DISULFIRAM	DISULFIRAM	604290019601
DISULFIRAM	DISULFIRAM	604290019630
DISULFIRAM	DISULFIRAM	649800017101
DISULFIRAM	DISULFIRAM	649800017103
DISULFIRAM	DISULFIRAM	000540035713
DISULFIRAM	DISULFIRAM	000540035725
DISULFIRAM	DISULFIRAM	000930503601
DISULFIRAM	DISULFIRAM	001500118151
DISULFIRAM	DISULFIRAM	001820053301
DISULFIRAM	DISULFIRAM	001820053305
DISULFIRAM	DISULFIRAM	003040080250
DISULFIRAM	DISULFIRAM	003490846850
DISULFIRAM	DISULFIRAM	003640033750
DISULFIRAM	DISULFIRAM	003780414101
DISULFIRAM	DISULFIRAM	005360376805
DISULFIRAM	DISULFIRAM	005360376806
DISULFIRAM	DISULFIRAM	005370600505
DISULFIRAM	DISULFIRAM	005370600550
DISULFIRAM	DISULFIRAM	005800157501
DISULFIRAM	DISULFIRAM	005910536800
DISULFIRAM	DISULFIRAM	005910536801
DISULFIRAM	DISULFIRAM	005910536803
DISULFIRAM	DISULFIRAM	006030343221
DISULFIRAM	DISULFIRAM	007190132110
DISULFIRAM	DISULFIRAM	007190132112
DISULFIRAM	DISULFIRAM	007790037925
DISULFIRAM	DISULFIRAM	007810107001
DISULFIRAM	DISULFIRAM	007810107050

DISULFIRAM	DISULFIRAM	008390128706
DISULFIRAM	DISULFIRAM	008390128716
DISULFIRAM	DISULFIRAM	009040118151
DISULFIRAM	DISULFIRAM	009040118160
DISULFIRAM	DISULFIRAM	472020248501
DISULFIRAM	DISULFIRAM	496480080250
DISULFIRAM	DISULFIRAM	497270090402
DISULFIRAM	DISULFIRAM	498840015401
DISULFIRAM	DISULFIRAM	498840015403
DISULFIRAM	DISULFIRAM	498840015405
DISULFIRAM	DISULFIRAM	501110033201
DISULFIRAM	DISULFIRAM	501110033202
DISULFIRAM	DISULFIRAM	501110033203
DISULFIRAM	DISULFIRAM	517280053901
DISULFIRAM	DISULFIRAM	524460017821
DISULFIRAM	DISULFIRAM	550840090550
DISULFIRAM	DISULFIRAM	584690376830
DISULFIRAM	DISULFIRAM	649800017201
DISULFIRAM	DISULFIRAM	649800017203
ACAMPROSATE CALCIUM	ACAMPROSATE CALCIUM	000930535286
ACAMPROSATE CALCIUM	ACAMPROSATE CALCIUM	002580400060
ACAMPROSATE CALCIUM	ACAMPROSATE CALCIUM	003780633380
ACAMPROSATE CALCIUM	ACAMPROSATE CALCIUM	101350063632
ACAMPROSATE CALCIUM	ACAMPROSATE CALCIUM	422910010418
ACAMPROSATE CALCIUM	ACAMPROSATE CALCIUM	510790024101
ACAMPROSATE CALCIUM	ACAMPROSATE CALCIUM	510790024106
ACAMPROSATE CALCIUM	ACAMPROSATE CALCIUM	606870012125
ACAMPROSATE CALCIUM	ACAMPROSATE CALCIUM	606870012195
ACAMPROSATE CALCIUM	ACAMPROSATE CALCIUM	683820056928
ACAMPROSATE CALCIUM	ACAMPROSATE CALCIUM	684620043518
CAMPRAL	ACAMPROSATE CALCIUM	004560333001
CAMPRAL	ACAMPROSATE CALCIUM	004560333060
CAMPRAL	ACAMPROSATE CALCIUM	004560333063
CAMPRAL	ACAMPROSATE CALCIUM	545690576700
CAMPRAL	ACAMPROSATE CALCIUM	548680529300

Table 8.
Substance abuse disorder treatment codes.

Code Name	Code
Confirmed Diagnoses of COVID 19	U07.1
Personal history of COVID-19	Z86.16

Table 9.
COVID-19 diagnoses codes.

Author details

Ewa J. Kleczyk[1,2*], Jill Bana[3] and Rishabh Arora[1]

1 Symphony Health, ICON plc Organization, Blue Bell, PA, USA

2 School of Economics, The University of Maine, Orono, ME, USA

3 Symphony Health, ICON plc Organization, Phoenix, AZ, USA

*Address all correspondence to: ewa.kleczyk@symphonyhealth.com

References

[1] SAMHSA. Leveraging Existing Health and Disease Management Programs to Provide Mental Health and Substance Use Disorder Resources During the COVID-19 Public Health Emergency (PHE). June 2020. [Online] https://www.cms.gov/CCIIO/Programs-and-Initiatives/Health-Insurance-Marketplaces/Downloads/Mental-Health-Substance-Use-Disorder-Resources-COVID-19.pdf. Accessed on July 22, 2021.

[2] GBD 2016 Alcohol and drug use collaborators the global burden of disease attributable to alcohol and drug use in 195 countries and territories, 1990-2016: A systematic analysis for the global burden of disease study 2016. Lancet Psychiatr. 2018;5:987–1012.

[3] SAMHSA. 2007. Results from the 2006 National Survey on Drug Use and Health: National Findings. (DHHS Publication no. SMA 07–4293, NSDUH series H-32) Office of Applied Studies: Rockville, MD.

[4] Feltenstein, M.W. and See, R.E. The neurocircuitry of addiction: an overview. British Journal of Pharmacology. 2008 154: 261-274. [Online] DOI:10.1038/bjp.2008.5. Accessed on July 15, 2021.

[5] Pedersen T. How Substance Use Disorders (SUD) are Treated? Psych Central. May 2021. [Online] https://psychcentral.com/addictions/substance-use-disorders-treatment#basic-principles. Accessed on July 15, 2021.

[6] Baumgartner, J. C. and Radley, D. C. The Spike in Drug Overdose Deaths During the COVID-19 Pandemic and Policy Options to Move Forward. March 2021. [Online] https://www.commonwealthfund.org/blog/2021/spike-drug-overdose-deaths-during-covid-19-pandemic-and-policy-options-move-forward. Accessed on July 15, 2021.

[7] Dubey S., Biswas P., Ghosh R., Chatterjee S., Dubey M.J., Chatterjee S. Psychosocial impact of COVID-19. Diabetes Metab Syndrome. 2020 DOI: 10.1016/j.dsx.2020.05.035.

[8] Ornell F., Moura H.F., Scherer J.N., Pechansky F., Kessler F., von Diemen L. The COVID-19 pandemic and its impact on substance use: Implications for prevention and treatment. Psychiatr Res. 2020;289:113096.

[9] Columb D., Hussain R., O'Gara C. Addiction Psychiatry and COVID-19 – Impact on patients and service provision. Ir J Psychol Med. 2020 May 21:1–15. DOI:10.1017/ipm.2020.47.

[10] Hefler M., Gartner C.E. The tobacco industry in the time of COVID-19: Time to shut it down? Tobac Contr. 2020;29: 245–246.

[11] The Times of India. 2020. How to use lockdown as an opportunity to overcome alcohol addiction. [Online] https://timesofindia.indiatimes.com/life-style/health-fitness/health-news/how-to-use-lockdown-to-de-addict-yourself-and-ways-to-manage-withdrawal-symptoms/articleshow/75494592.cms. Accessed on February 1, 2021.

[12] News18. 2020. Amid coronavirus lockdown, states across India witness surge in suicide cases due to alcohol withdrawal symptoms. [Online] https://www.news18.com/news/india/amid-coronavirus-lockdown-states-across-india-witness-surge-in-deaths-due-to-alcohol-withdrawal-symptoms-2561191.html. Accessed on February 1, 2021.

[13] Rani S., Sahoo S., Parveen S., Mehra A., Subodh B.N., Grover S. Alcohol-related self-harm due to COVID-19 pandemic: Might be an emerging crisis in the near future: A case report. Indian J Psychiatr. 2020;62:333–335.

[14] Sun Y., Bao Y., Kosten T., Strang J., Shi J., Lu L. Editorial: Challenges to opioid use disorders during COVID-19. Am J Addict. 2020;29:174–175.

[15] Becker W.C., Fiellin D.A. When epidemics collide: Coronavirus disease 2019 (COVID-19) and the opioid crisis. Ann Intern Med. 2020 Apr 2:M20–M1210. DOI:10.7326/M20-1210.

[16] Vecchio S., Ramella R., Drago A., Carraro D., Littlewood R., Somaini L. COVID19 pandemic and people with opioid use disorder: Innovation to reduce risk. Psychiatr Res. 2020;289: 113047.

[17] Håkansson A., Fernández-Aranda F., Menchón J.M., Potenza M.N., Jiménez-Murcia S. Gambling during the COVID-19 crisis – A cause for concern? J Addiction Med. 2020 May 18 DOI: 10.1097/ADM.0000000000000690.

[18] Schalkwyk M.C., Cheetham D., Reeves A., Petticrew M. Covid-19: we must take urgent action to avoid an increase in problem gambling and gambling related harms. BMJ Opinion. 2020. [Online] https://blogs.bmj.com/bmj/2020/04/06/covid-19-we-must-take-urgent-action-to-avoid-an-increase-in-problem-gambling-and-gambling-related-harms. Accessed on February 1, 2021.

[19] Touyz S., Lacey H., Hay P. Eating disorders in the time of COVID-19. Version 2. J Eat Disord. 2020;8:19.

[20] Watanabe M. 2020. Beyond retail therapy the case against pandemic shopping. [Online] https://www.bitchmedia.org/article/compulsive-online-shopping-COVID-19. Accessed on February 1, 2021.

[21] Integrated Dataverse (IDV®). [Online] https://symphonyhealth.prahs.com/what-we-do/view-health-data. Accessed on October 1, 2020.

[22] National institute of Alcohol Abuse and Alcoholism. [Online] https://pubs.niaaa.nih.gov/publications/surveillance-covid-19/COVSALES.htm. Accessed on March 1, 2021.

[23] David A. Freedman (2009). Statistical models: Theory and practice. Cambridge university press. p. 26. "a simple regression equation has on the right hand side an intercept and an explanatory variable with a slope coefficient. A multiple regression e right hand side, Each with its Own Slope Coefficient."

[24] Hilary L. Seal (1967). "The historical development of the gauss linear model". Biometrika. 54 (1/2): 1–24. DOI: 10.1093/biomet/54.1-2.1. JSTOR 2333849.

[25] Sarker, I.H. Machine Learning: Algorithms, real-world applications and research directions. SN COMPUT. SCI. 2, 160. 2021. [online] DOI:10.1007/s42979-021-00592-x. Accessed on July 15, 2021.

[26] Hastie, T., Tibshirani, R., And Friedman, J. Overview of Supervised Learning. The Elements of Statistical Learning. Springer. (2009). Pp. 9–39. Alpaydın, E. (2014).

[27] Introduction to machine learning. Cambridge, MA: MIT Press. Hosmer, D. W., Lemeshow, S. Applied Logistic Regression. New York: Wiley. (2013). ISBN 978-0-470-58247-3.

[28] Ballantyne Draelos, R.L. Best Use of Train/Val/Test Splits, with Tips for Medical Data. Glass Box Machine Learning and Medicine. [Online] https://glassboxmedicine.com/2019/09/15/best-use-of-train-val-test-splits-with-tips-for-medical-data. Accessed on October 5, 2020.

[29] Simeone, O. A very brief introduction to machine learning with applications to communication systems.

arXiv preprint arXiv:1808.02342v4. (2018).

[30] Hinton, G., Sejnowski, T. Unsupervised Learning: Foundations of Neural Computation. MIT Press. (1999). ISBN 978-0262581684.

[31] Friedman, J.H. Greedy function approximation: A gradient boosting machine. The Annals of Statistics 29: 1189-1232. (2001). [Online] DOI: 10.1214/aos/1013203451. Accessed on October 1, 2020.

[32] Extreme Gradient Boosting. [Online] https://xgboost.readthedocs.io/en/latest/tutorials/model.html. Accessed October 1, 2020.

[33] Hastie, T., Tibshirani, R., Friedman, J. H. '10. Boosting and Additive Trees'. The Elements of Statistical Learning (2nd ed.). New York: Springer. (2009). pp. 337–384.

[34] Cochran, W.G. The chi-square test of goodness of fit. The Annals of Mathematical Statistics 23(3): 315–345. (1952).

[35] Ho, Tin Kam (1995). Random Decision Forests (PDF). Proceedings of the 3rd International Conference on Document Analysis and Recognition, Montreal, QC, 14–16 August 1995. pp. 278–282. Archived from the original (PDF) on 17 April 2016. Retrieved 5 June 2016.

[36] Ho TK (1998). "The random subspace method for constructing decision forests" (PDF). IEEE Transactions on Pattern Analysis and Machine Intelligence. 20 (8): 832–844. DOI:10.1109/34.709601.

[37] On the interpretation of $\chi 2$ from contingency tables, and the calculation of p. Journal of the Royal Statistical Society 85(1): 87-94. (1922). [Online] DOI:10.2307/2340521. Accessed on July 15, 2021.

[38] Manning, C.D., Raghavan, P., and Schütze, H. Introduction to Information Retrieval. Feature Selection, Chi-Square Feature Selection Cambridge University Press. (2008).

[39] Prescription Sedative Misuse and Abuse. [Online] https://www.ncbi.nlm.nih.gov/pmc/articles/PMC4553644/. Accessed on March 1, 2021.

[40] Centers for Disease Control and Prevention; Coping with stress. [Online] https://www.cdc.gov/coronavirus/2019-ncov/daily-life-coping/managing-stress-anxiety.html. Accessed on March 1, 2021.

[41] Narasimha V.L., Shukla L., Mukherjee D., Menon J., Huddar S., Panda U.K. Complicated alcohol withdrawal-an unintended consequence of COVID-19 lockdown. Alcohol Alcohol. 2020 May 13 agaa042.

[42] Varma R.P. Alcohol withdrawal management during the Covid-19 lockdown in Kerala. Indian J Med Ethics. 2020; V:105–106.

[43] List of alcohol laws of the United States. [Online] https://en.wikipedia.org/wiki/List_of_alcohol_laws_of_the_United_States

[44] Bhattacharyya, I. Feature Selection (Boruta/Light GBM/Chi Square)-Categorical Feature Selection. [Online] https://medium.com/@indreshbhattacharyya/feature-selection-categorical-feature-selection-boruta-light-gbm-chi-square-bf47e94e2558. Accessed on March 1, 2021.

[45] Random Forest Algorithm. [Online] https://www.stat.berkeley.edu/~breiman/RandomForests/cc_home.htm; https://www.ibm.com/cloud/learn/random-forest; https://builtin.com/data-science/random-forest-algorithm. Accessed on March 1, 2021.

[46] XGBoost Algorithm. [Online] https://www.mygreatlearning.com/

blog/xgboost-algorithm/. Accessed on March 1, 2021.

[47] Hyper Tunning [Online] https://xgboost.readthedocs.io/en/latest/parameter.html, https://scikit-learn.org/stable/modules/generated/sklearn.ensemble.RandomForestClassifier.html. Accessed on March 1, 2021.

[48] MedlinePlus. [Online] https://medlineplus.gov/druginfo/meds/a682602.html. Accessed on March 1, 2021.

[49] HCPCS. Codes https://hcpcs.codes/g-codes/G2067/. Accessed on March 1, 2021.

[50] Alcohol Consumption during the COVID-19 Pandemic: A Cross-Sectional Survey of US Adults. [Online] https://www.ncbi.nlm.nih.gov/pmc/articles/PMC7763183/. Accessed on March 1, 2021.

[51] Effect of alcohol on immune system [Online] https://vertavahealth.com/blog/drugs-alcohol-affect-immune-system. Accessed on March 1, 2021.

[52] COVID-19 and People who Use Drugs [Online] https://www.cdc.gov/coronavirus/2019-ncov/need-extra-precautions/other-at-risk-populations/people-who-use-drugs/QA.html. Accessed on March 1, 2021.

Section 2

Addiction Treatment

Chapter 5

Revisiting 12-Step Approaches: An Evidence-Based Perspective

Dorothy Greene

Abstract

Alcoholics Anonymous (AA) is the longest-running mutual aid group for people with alcohol use disorders, and AA turned 85 years old in 2020. Though there has been much criticism regarding AA and other 12-step programs, there has been an equal amount of evidence to support their efficacy. This chapter explores the history of AA and other 12-step approaches, the foundational philosophy of the 12-steps, the key elements that support recovery, cultural considerations for special populations, and a review of the criticisms as well as strengths of 12-step approaches. The chapter concludes with recommendations for the integration of the approach into clinical practice.

Keywords: 12-steps, alcoholics anonymous, narcotics anonymous, substance use disorders, addiction, mutual aid groups, efficacy

1. Introduction

In 2020, the most rigorous scientific study to date regarding the efficacy of Alcoholics Anonymous (AA) and other 12 step approaches were published [1]. Soon after, a sweeping review of scientific studies relative to Narcotics Anonymous (NA) was released [2]. Outcomes gleaned from these publications suggests substantial benefit to members of AA and NA both as an adjunct to professional treatment and as a stand-alone intervention for substance use disorder (SUD). Although valid criticisms exist regarding 12-step approaches, for those whom 12-step approaches work, they appear to work quite well. While alternatives to 12-step approaches are increasing, scientific information is limited. Thus, this chapter focuses primarily on 12 step-approaches.

The chapter begins with an introduction presenting demographic data, history of 12-step programs, and the fundamental philosophy of the 12-steps. Because AA and NA are the largest and most studied 12-step programs, most of this discussion is drawn from literature specific to these two programs. Additionally, there is a dearth of scientific literature pertaining to 12-step approaches and behavioral addictions. At present, there is only one behavioral disorder included in the DSM's classification of Substance-related and Addictive Disorders [3], gambling disorder, so the chapter's focus is 12-step approaches relative to substance use disorders. An introduction to the most common 12-step programs associated with behavioral addictions is also presented.

Substance use disorder mutual aid recovery has an intricate and complex history. Many mark the year 1935 as the birth of the mutual aid recovery movement as that is the year Alcoholics Anonymous was formed. According to White [4], the mutual aid recovery movement began centuries before in the late 1700s with Native American Recovery Circles. Section II presents a brief survey of the history of mutual aid groups, followed by a more pointed examination of the histories of AA and NA. A concise overview of common 12-step offshoots follows. The section concludes with a look at how 12-step approaches became integrated into professional addiction treatment services.

In section III, the philosophical underpinnings of the 12 steps and recovery-related activities associated with 12-step mutual aid recovery are described. According to research, those who participate in 12-step activities such as sponsorship, regular meeting attendance, and service have better outcomes regarding sustained abstinence [5–9].

Section IV presents the evidence surrounding 12-step mutual aid recovery. Beginning with an examination of several core elements that appear to support recovery, the section explores the efficacy and strengths of 12-step approaches as well as its criticisms and limitations.

The discussion continues in section V with a consideration of culture as it relates to 12-step approaches. One size does not fit all, and the spiritual or religious undertone of the 12 steps is likely the most cited barrier for those who prefer a secular approach to addiction recovery. In contrast, many are attracted to 12-step programs because of the emphasis on spirituality and a Higher Power. This and several additional cultural influences are explored.

Before the chapter concludes, recommendations are offered for integrating 12-step approaches into professional treatment services.

2. Demographics of 12-step membership

In 2011, there were 54 different 12-step programs [10]. Alcoholics Anonymous and Narcotics Anonymous are by far the largest. A strength of 12-step programs is their wide availability across the globe. Estimated membership in Alcoholics Anonymous is 2,077,374 individual members and 125,557 groups as of 2019 [11].

A 2014 AA membership survey [12] reported the following demographic information. Sixty-two percent of membership identified as male and 38% identified as female. A large majority of membership identified as white, 89%, 4% black, 3% Hispanic, 1% Native American, 1% Asian, and 2% identified as other. The average age of AA members is estimated at 50 years.

Members are introduced to AA from a variety of sources. Thirty two percent of members are introduced to AA by an AA member, and another 32% are introduced by a treatment facility. Thirty percent of AA members report being self-motivated to attend, and 27% are referred by a family member. Other referrals come through the criminal justice system (14%), and medical and behavioral health professionals (17%). Less common referrals include Al-anon/Alateen member, AA literature, employer, or colleague, newspaper/magazine/radio/tv, clergy, and the internet. The survey reported the average length of sobriety is 10 years, with a range between less than one year (27%) and over 20 years (22%). On average, members attend 2.5 meetings per week, and 82% reported having a sponsor.

Narcotics Anonymous released a membership survey more recently [13]. They report 77,000 meetings weekly in 144 countries across the globe. Compared to AA, NA's membership is more diverse, with 70% identifying as White, 13% Black, 7% Hispanic, 4% multiracial, 2% Asian, 1% Indigenous, and 1% as other. In terms of gender, 58% identified as male and 42% as female. The average age of NA members is 46 years, with a range between less than 21 (1%) and over 60 (15%). The mean number of years clean is 8.32 years, with a range between less than 1 year (8%) and over 20 years (25%).

Most members are referred through other NA members (49%) and treatment of counseling services (45%). Other referral sources include family members, NA literature or an NA service effort, and AA members.

NA members reported using a variety of substances. Alcohol was the most common substance reported (73%), followed by cannabis (62%), cocaine (52%), opiates (38%), stimulants (38%), crack (31%), opioids (26%), tranquilizers (25%), hallucinogens (25%), prescribed medications (23%), ecstasy (17%), methadone or buprenorphine (14%), inhalants (11%), and other (14%).

It is important to note that these two surveys are *membership* surveys and not designed for research. The purpose is to provide a snapshot of current membership rather than the general population of people with SUDs. Nonetheless, there exists important challenges to researchers who seek to study recovery via 12-step mutual aid programs. This is explored further in section 8.

3. History of mutual aid groups and 12-step programs

According to the addiction field's leading historian, William White, the history of abstinence-based mutual aid recovery groups begins with the Native American recovery circles [4]. Between 1737 and 1840, Indigenous leaders such as Handsome Lake, Wagomend, and Paounhan had transformational experiences leading to sobriety. These transformations led to cultural and religious reformations, which included the rejection of alcohol. Spawned by the temperance movement, the 1800s saw a variety of mutual aid societies begin and end. These included the Washingtonians, The Red Ribbon Reform Club, the Drunkard's Club, and several others. White further explicates that for those whose goal was moderation rather than abstinence, other groups formed such as Businessman's Moderation Society in 1879. European temperance societies formed in the 1800s as well. For example, in 1851 the Order of Good Templars formed, and in 1877 Switzerland founded the Blue Cross. White also states that European culture, like American culture, formed mutual aid groups founded on moderate drinking rather than abstinence such as the German Order of Temperance, French Temperance Society, and the Irish New Ross Temperance Society.

In the early 1900s, many American mutual aid and treatment organizations failed, and this was partly influenced by prohibition. According to White, the absence of mutual aid groups in the early decades of the 20th century is notable, but in 1935, an historic meeting occurred between two self-defined hopeless alcoholics that revolutionized the treatment for people with alcohol use disorders and a host of other addictive behaviors across the globe [14]. Today, AA is the largest and longest running mutual aid group for alcohol use disorders in the world. Such a profound impact has been made by AA, that its co-founder, Bill Wilson, was recognized by Time Magazine as one of the most influential people of the Millennium [15]. A brief history of AA is provided next.

3.1 AA's beginning

From the book Alcoholics Anonymous [16], affectionately known as the *Big Book* because of its over 500 pages, and the Alcoholics Anonymous' website [17], Bill W.'s story follows.

In 1934, Bill W. sat alone drinking at his kitchen table when the telephone rang. He was greeted by an old high school friend and drinking buddy, named Ebby T., whom he had not spoken to in quite some time. He had heard his old friend was institutionalized due to chronic alcoholism. Ebby T. asked if he could visit Bill, and later that day the two men sat reminiscing about old times. Bill offered Ebby a drink, but he refused and told Bill that he *got religion*. Ebby shared his experience with spiritual principles and a process of change that required surrender to the alcoholic condition and acceptance of guidance from a Higher Power. Because Bill balked at the idea of organized religion and God, Ebby informed Bill that he could formulate his own conception of this power. The spiritual process described by Ebby also included a process of self-inventory, confession, and making amends to those whom he had harmed. Bill recognized a difference in his friend – something had changed. Though Bill did not stop drinking at this point, he opened his mind to the ideas presented by his friend for nothing else had helped him overcome the compulsion to drink.

According to Alcoholics Anonymous [16], the process described by Ebby T. was the foundation of the Oxford group. A mostly non-alcoholic, non-denominational, Christian group. Its fundamental principles and beliefs were later expanded and revised into what are now known as the 12-steps of Alcoholics Anonymous.

After that fateful meeting with Ebby T., Bill went on yet another drinking binge that eventually landed him in Towns Hospital in New York with delirium tremens. Remembering his friend's spiritual directions, he proceeded to take the steps as outlined by Ebby T. In Towns Hospital, 1934, Bill W. experienced his famous white light experience, never to drink again.

What happened in the following six months formalizes the beginning of AA. Upon release from Towns Hospital, Bill joined the Oxford Group. He and Ebby embarked on a mission to share this spiritual process with as many alcoholics as possible. A profound lesson was learned, which is the bedrock of AA.

After several month, Bill W. became very disheartened because although they had shared the message of recovery with with every alcoholic they met, none were able to maintain sobriety. Bill was ready to abandon their effort when Ebby emphasized that even though none of their recruits remained sober, he and Bill did. This is the crux of AA - *we can only keep what we have by giving it away*. Through helping other alcoholics, one could remain sober.

About six months after Bill's spiritual experience in Towns Hospital, he went on a business trip to Akron Ohio, alone for the first time in his newfound sobriety. Bill walked through the lobby of the hotel, immediately spotting the hotel lounge. The old memories of drink ensued, and the familiar craving took root. He went to the lobby phone booth and found a church directory where he began frantically calling churches to see if one knew of an alcoholic with whom he could speak. At the end of the church directory, he found a possibility. A meeting was arranged by the wife of an Akron surgeon to speak with her husband as he was dying of alcoholism. Dr. Bob Smith had been a member of the Oxford Group where he had sought help for his alcoholism, but to no avail.

On June 10th, 1935, Bill W. and Dr. Bob Smith met for the first time. Bill shared his experience with a chronic and seemingly hopeless alcoholic condition (what it used to be like), the spiritual process that transformed him (what happened), and how his life unfolded moving forward (what it's like now). The two men spoke for hours and agreed to work together to share their experience with other alcoholics who still suffered. From this point forward, Bill W. and Dr. Bob dedicated the rest of their lives to carrying the message of AA's 12-steps to other alcoholics. After 2 and a half years of sobriety, in 1937 Ebby T. relapsed. He did regain sobriety and died sober in 1966.

With the publication of AA's Big Book in 1939 and a flurry of articles published thereafter, AA's growth blossomed. A defining moment in AA's growth trajectory occurred in 1941 when Jack Alexander's article, *"Alcoholics Anonymous: Freed Slaves of Drink, Now They Free Others,"* was published in the Saturday Evening Post. The AA office received countless inquiries after its publication, and by 1950 AA's membership had reached over 100,000. The tireless dedication of Bill W. and Dr. Bob has resulted in millions of people helped worldwide, revolutionizing the way people with substance use disorders are treated.

3.2 Narcotics Anonymous

Because the only requirement for membership in AA is a desire to stop drinking, and drug addicts were often shunned by AA, Narcotics Anonymous was formed. Unlike AA's beginnings, NA's first few decades were tumultuous, experiencing several starts and stops, and more than one version of the program [18].

Addicts Anonymous held its first meeting in 1947, but the Narcotics Anonymous we know today began in earnest in 1953, but nearly died in 1959 [18]. When this happened, Jimmy K. and two others started what became today's NA with the *mother group*, Architects of Adversity [18]. Though many members came and went, Jimmy K. was the mainstay in the early days of NA. Jimmy K's tireless effort to keep NA alive in those tenuous times is why he is credited as the founding member of NA [18].

In his historical presentation of NA, William White [4] describes Jimmy K.'s addiction as one that progressed from sneaking tastes of paregoric and alter wine as a child to binging on whiskey and pills in adulthood. According to White, Jimmy K.'s addiction "left him bankrupt physically, mentally, and spiritually, and an abject failure as a man, a husband, and a father" [4], p. 335. As a result, he began attending AA in 1950, introducing himself as an alcoholic and addict. He had a passion for helping those with multiple addictions. Jimmy befriended Dorothy S. in AA, who like Jimmy, had multiple addictions. Together, with the help from Danny C in New York, they worked to establish the NA we know today.

Narcotics Anonymous utilizes the same 12 steps and 12 traditions developed by AA, with several adaptations specific to *addiction* rather than *alcoholism*. For example, AA states: The only requirement for membership is the desire to stop drinking, and NA substitutes the word *using* for the word *drinking*. Additionally, AA's first step reads *We admitted we were powerless over alcohol—that our lives had become unmanageable*, whereas NA states *we were powerless over our addiction*.

Another point from which NA diverges from AA is that NA is a program of abstinence from all drugs [19], and NA does not differentiate between substances of misuse. Further, NA clearly considers alcohol a drug. Though for some, this may be a barrier to participation in NA. In nearly every NA meeting this section from the NA Basic Text is read:

> *The only way to keep from returning to active addiction is not to take that first drug. If you are like us, you know that one is too many and a thousand never enough. We put great emphasis on this, for we know that when we use drugs in any form, or substitute one for another, we release our addiction all over again.*
>
> *Thinking of alcohol as different from other drugs has caused a great many addicts to relapse. Before we came to NA, many of us viewed alcohol separately, but we cannot afford to be confused about this. Alcohol is a drug. We are people with the disease of addiction who must abstain from all drugs in order to recover. [19]*

Alcoholics Anonymous and Narcotics Anonymous also have offshoots for family members. Al-Anon, Alateen, and Nar-anon operate under the 12 steps and 12 traditions but are designed for those who love people with substance use disorders.

Though Alcoholics Anonymous and Narcotics Anonymous are by far the largest of the 12 step fellowships, numerous other groups have formed modeled after the AA prototype. The following section briefly introduces a few of its more common descendants.

4. Other 12-step programs

Many twelve step programs have formed to treat both substance use disorders and behavioral addictions. In addition to AA and NA, several substance specific 12 step programs have followed: for example, Cocaine Anonymous, Heroin Anonymous, Marijuana Anonymous, and Nicotine Anonymous. Each AA derivative substitutes the word alcohol in the 12-step language for the substance or behavior the program addresses.

Although behavioral addiction is an unscientific term, many groups have formed to address a variety of compulsive behaviors. Gambling use disorder is the only exception and is classified in the DSM 5 as a Substance-Related or Other Addictive Disorder [3]. Gamblers Anonymous is one of the largest of the behavioral addiction 12 step programs. Gamblers Anonymous began in 1957 and "is a fellowship of men and women who share their experience, strength, and hope with each other that they may solve their common problem and help others to recovery from a gambling problem" [20].

Overeaters Anonymous formed to address a variety of compulsive eating behaviors. It is "a community of people who support each other in order to recover from compulsive eating and food behaviors. We welcome everyone who feels they have a problem with food" [21]. Overeaters Anonymous was founded in 1960 and currently has over 6500 groups in 75 countries, and an estimated 60,000 members worldwide.

Another well-known 12 step program is Codependents Anonymous program. "Codependents Anonymous (CoDA) is a 12 Step Fellowship for people seeking loving and healthy relationships" [22]. The concept of co-dependency has come under fire by feminist scholars. For example, Anderson [23] argued that the concept pathologizes and blames women. Yet, Melody Beattie's 1986 bestseller, *Co-dependent No More,* has sold more than 5 million copies [24].

5. 12-step integration into professional treatment

The Minnesota Model, known as the fundamental philosophy of the well-known Hazelden Betty Ford Center, was born in 1949. It was one of the first facilities to provide therapeutic and human treatment for alcoholics and addicts [25]. Borrowing principles from Wilmar State Hospital and Alcoholics Anonymous, the model was replicated across the globe. So popular was the 12-step movement that by 1989, an estimated 90% of treatment facilities followed the Minnesota Model [26]. The core practices of the Minnesota Model included patient education on the 12 steps and the idea that addiction is a physical, mental, and spiritual disease [25]. Moreover, the model integrates the notion that alcoholics and addicts can stay sober best by helping one another as did Bill W. and Dr. Bob, the AA co-founders; thus, the beginnings of utilizing recovering alcoholics as lay counselors.

Before this section concludes, it is important to acknowledge one of the most utilized evidence-based models for addiction treatment, Twelve Step Facilitation Therapy or TSF. In the largest clinical trial of its kind, Project Match examined three of the most common evidence-based models for alcohol use disorder: cognitive behavioral therapy, motivational enhancement therapy, and TSF [27]. The purpose of the study was to learn if certain patients would have better outcomes with a specific therapeutic model compared to another. Overall, the study found that patient matching did not change outcomes and that all models were equally effective. Two exceptions should be noted. First, those with low levels of psychiatric comorbidities treated with TSF, experienced higher rates of days completely abstinent. Second, those who received TSF had higher rates of complete abstinence at year one. The next section will explore the 12-step philosophy, principles, and practices more fully.

6. 12 step philosophy

When describing 12-step philosophy several core elements are emphasized: the 12-steps, 12 traditions, sponsorship, meeting attendance, service, and spirituality.

No discussion on the application of 12-step principles is complete without the perspective of those with lived experience. In addition to the author's voice, this section integrates the voices of those who identify as persons in recovery. The section begins with the 12-steps and 12 traditions of the program.

6.1 The 12 steps

1. We admitted we were powerless over alcohol—that our lives had become unmanageable.

2. Came to believe that a Power greater than ourselves could restore us to sanity.

3. Made a decision to turn our will and our lives over to the care of God as we understood Him.

4. Made a searching and fearless moral inventory of ourselves.

5. Admitted to God, to ourselves, and to another human being the exact nature of our wrongs.

6. Were entirely ready to have God remove all these defects of character.

7. Humbly asked Him to remove our shortcomings.

8. Made a list of all persons we had harmed and became willing to make amends to them all.

9. Made direct amends to such people wherever possible, except when to do so would injure them or others.

10. Continued to take personal inventory and when we were wrong promptly admitted it.

11. Sought through prayer and meditation to improve our conscious contact with God as we understood Him, praying only for knowledge of His will for us and the power to carry that out.

12. Having had a spiritual awakening as the result of these steps, we tried to carry this message to alcoholics, and to practice these principles in all our affairs [28].

The program is described as "a set of principles written so simply that we can follow them in our daily lives" [19], p. 9. A simple translation of the 12-step process is provided by a woman who attends both AA and NA:

> *For me, steps 1-3 are about developing a relationship with a power greater than myself, steps 4-7 are about healing the relationship with myself, and steps 8-12 are about healing and supporting my relationships with others. I don't do this by myself. My sponsor's main role is to guide and support me through working the steps. (Anonymous 12-step group member, personal communication, November 23, 2020).*

6.2 The 12 traditions

Eddy G., a long-time member of NA, describes the purpose of the 12-traditions this way.

> *If the 12-steps are how the program works, the 12-traditions are why the program works. The traditions keep the focus of the fellowship on helping each other. They teach us how to help each other while maintaining the integrity of the fellowship and the principles that drive it. (Eddy G., personal communication, December 30, 2020)*

1. Our common welfare should come first; personal recovery depends upon A.A. unity.

2. For our group purpose there is but one ultimate authority—a loving God as He may express Himself in our group conscience. Our leaders are but trusted servants; they do not govern.

3. The only requirement for A.A. membership is a desire to stop drinking.

4. Each group should be autonomous except in matters affecting other groups or A.A. as a whole.

5. Each group has but one primary purpose—to carry its message to the alcoholic who still suffers.

6. An A.A. group ought never endorse, finance, or lend the A.A. name to any related facility or outside enterprise, lest problems of money, property, and prestige divert us from our primary purpose.

7. Every A.A. group ought to be fully self-supporting, declining outside contributions.

8. Alcoholics Anonymous should remain forever nonprofessional, but our service centers may employ special workers.

9. A.A., as such, ought never be organized; but we may create service boards or committees directly responsible to those they serve.

10. Alcoholics Anonymous has no opinion on outside issues; hence the A.A. name ought never be drawn into public controversy.

11. Our public relations policy is based on attraction rather than promotion; we need always maintain personal anonymity at the level of press, radio, and films.

12. Anonymity is the spiritual foundation of all our Traditions, ever reminding us to place principles before personalities [28].

6.3 Sponsorship

Sponsorship and carrying the message to the person who still suffers (step 12) are fundamental practices in 12-step communities. Sponsorship is the tradition of a more experienced, sober member of the program supporting a newer member along their recovery journey. "The heart of NA beats when two addicts share their recovery" [29].

Though the following sponsorship guidelines are not required, they are suggested. In general, sponsors and sponsees should be same sexed as to avoid romantic distraction. A limitation here is the assumption that all members are heterosexual. There is not an established guideline for those who identify as LGBTQ. Additionally, the sponsor should have experience in working the steps and have attained stable recovery. There is not a written standard in terms of length of sobriety or how far along in the step process a sponsor should be.

Dekkers, Vos, and Vanderplasschen [30] discovered mutual understanding facilitates connection, and connection was identified as a key theme supporting recovery in their qualitative study of NA members. A large study of over 1800 veterans showed that having a sponsor was one element that helped mediate positive outcomes among participants of 12-step programs [7]. According to NA, "the two-way street of sponsorship is a loving, spiritual, and compassionate relationship that helps both the sponsor and sponsee" [29]. Sponsorship may be considered analogous to the therapeutic alliance [31]. Contact with a sponsor and a strong sponsorship relationship contribute to increased 12-step participation and abstinence.

6.4 Meeting attendance

One often hears the maxim, *90 meetings in 90 days,* suggested to newcomers in the program. A substantial scholarly literature shows that regular 12-step meeting attendance supports positive substance use outcomes [5, 6, 8, 9, 29]. For example, results from a large National Institute of Drug Abuse funded project show that weekly or more frequent attendance at 12-step groups support alcohol and other drug (AOD) abstinence [32]. Similar findings are reported bey Greene and colleagues in a national sample of recovering addiction professionals [6]. Those attending meetings weekly had the lowest rates of relapse compared to those who attended less frequently.

The value of meeting attendance is best described by an anonymous member of AA and NA.

> *The 12-step fellowship provides immediate access to a pro-recovery support system. All my friends were using buddies. I didn't have anyone in my life that didn't use drugs and alcohol, and I was young when I entered recovery. I needed a social network. I never would have been able to stay sober had I not attended so many meetings. (Anonymous 12-step member, personal communication, November 29, 2020)*

It is important to note that research also indicates 12-step meeting attendance alone may be insufficient for the maintenance of recovery. Participation in activities such as sponsorship, service work, working the steps, etc. appears to increase positive benefits compared to meeting attendance alone. In a study of 303 young adults, 12 step meeting attendance and *active* participation in the program lead to positive substance use outcomes [33]. Interestingly, for meeting attendance alone positive effects diminished over time, but positive effects increased over time with active involvement.

6.5 Service

As noted in the previous section, positive recovery outcomes increase with the addition of other recovery activities to meeting attendance, and service is one of the foundational elements of 12-step programs.

One long-term NA member described service in NA as follows.

> *Service in NA, in the beginning, is a way for me become accountable to a group of people that I've come to trust, and it allows me to build trust within the group. Later in recovery, it becomes a way to reverse self-centered fear because the opposite of self-centered fear is selfless service. It's pure volunteer. I don't get paid for any of it. Now that I've been given the gift of recovery, it's my responsibility to give it back. It's the 12th step. The only way I can keep the gift of recovery is to give it away. (NA member, personal communication, November 28, 2020)*

Service work in 12 step programs encompasses a variety of activities. The more common tasks, other than sponsorship, include, opening and closing the meeting; setting up and putting away chairs; making coffee; holding positions such as group chairperson, treasurer, or secretary. Service may also include activities such as taking meetings into facilities where clients are unable to attend in the community. Treatment centers, jail and prison facilities are the most common. Service commitments might extend all the way to the level of world service. In keeping with the fundamental tenets of the program, all service positions are unpaid. According to the traditions of the 12-step programs, there are no dues or fees for memberships, there are no leaders, groups are self-supporting and autonomous, and 12 step mutual aid groups do not accept outside contributions. So entrenched are these principles, that guests attending an NA group are often explicitly asked not to contribute when the donation basket is passed at the meeting.

Why is service such an important component of 12-step programs? Two theoretical ideas are proposed: the helper therapy principle and the wounded healer archetype [34]. These theories suggest that one's experience with addiction might be reduced through helping others. Further, by having addiction oneself, it may render the individual with special knowledge and insight that can be shared to help a person still struggling with addiction. This provides a logical segue into the final section of 12-step philosophy, spirituality.

7. Spirituality and 12-step programs

While religion tends to be associated with an organized set of beliefs, practices, rules, and doctrines [35], 12-step programs' clearly state the program "should remain forever non-professional... ought never be organized" [19], pp. 69–70, and is "not connected with any sect, denomination, politics, organization or institution" [36]. Yet, 12-step programs are unapologetically spiritual in nature. A common axiom cited in AA and NA meetings asserts *there is no chemical solution to a spiritual problem.*

An entire chapter in AA Big Book is devoted to those who may struggle with organized religion and the concept of God – it is titled *We Agnostics* [16]. The fundamental premise is that spirituality is subjective and defined by each member individually. Written in 1952, a companion text to the original AA Big Book, *The Twelve Steps and Twelve Traditions*, says AA does not demand that you believe anything ... I must quickly assure that AAs tread innumerable paths in their quest for faith ... You can if you wish, make AA itself your 'higher power' ... [37], pp. 25-27. The AA Big Book encourages readers to develop their own conception of God, and further states "don't let any prejudice you may have against spiritual terms deter you from asking yourself what they mean to you" [16], p. 47.

If 12 step programs are not religious but rather *spiritual* programs, what exactly is spirituality and how does it support recovery? Spirituality is described as a creative and universal part of the human experience. Subjective in nature, it is about one's connection to self, others, social groups, communities, and traditions. It can be experienced as an inner and/or transcendent personal relationship, which may exist beyond the self. Fundamental to this definition is the notion that spirituality is concerned with human values, truth, and experiences that provide meaning and purpose in life. Given the earlier discussion of 12-step philosophy's core elements, its fit within this definition of spirituality is undeniable [38].

No academic endeavor is complete, however, without a critical examination. The next section will do just that.

8. Strengths and limitations of 12-step programs

While millions of people worldwide have found recovery from addiction through 12-step programs, millions more have found the program unhelpful. The science of addiction and recovery provides empirical evidence of the efficacy of 12-step approaches, but it equally shows there are multiple efficacious paths to recovery. One size does not fit all.

This section begins with the counterargument to the last section on spirituality. Likely the most frequently cited criticism to 12-step programs is its religious undertone. As noted in the history section of the chapter, AA and the 12-steps were birthed from a non-denominational Christian organization, the Oxford Group. Osten and Switzer argue that for those who identify as atheist, agnostic, or a non-Christian faith, 12-step programs might be challenging [39]. For example, multiple references to God, using the male pronoun, are found in the in 12-step literature. Step 3 of the 12-steps suggests *we turned our will and our lives over to the care of God as we understood Him.* Further, the recitation of the Lord's Prayer is common in many AA meetings, and many, if not most, 12-step meetings are held in churches.

Building on this criticism, feminist writers have named several barriers to accepting the 12-step path for women and people of color [40, 41]. Not the least of which is the reference to God using the male pronoun in steps 3, 7, and 11, and throughout the AA literature. For women, there is a long and painful history of patriarchy, oppression, and subjugation. Thus, the idea of turning one's life over to a male God may feel reminiscent of this history for some. Additionally, concepts of surrender, powerlessness, and turning one's life over are not only difficult for some women to accept but may also be challenging for ethnic minorities. For groups who have experienced the horrors of genocide and slavery, such as Native Americans and African Americans, these ideas may be particularly difficult.

One anonymous 12-step member, a middle-aged woman in long-term recovery, understands this criticism and has experienced discrimination and oppression in a male-dominated, patriarchal society, but states she has not experienced the 12-step community as such (Anonymous NA member, personal communication, December 1st, 2020). She shared that the terms *powerless* and *surrender* are not used in the same context as oppression and subjugation associated with slavery and a discriminatory and patriarchal culture. In fact, the 12-step process of recovery is experienced by many as an empowering process that leads to freedom from dependence on substances [42]. Alcoholics Anonymous asserts that through dependence upon a power greater than oneself, an individual becomes more personally independent [37]. Yet, it is important to acknowledge the era in which the original texts were written. Alcoholics Anonymous was founded by White, middle-class men in 1935, so the language of the time may create a barrier for many. Though the literature has been slightly updated, Alcoholics Anonymous has not conducted a major revision to the original literature for historical reasons. The biased language in AA's primary texts, written in 1939 and 1952, may impede AA's growth, particularly for women [43] and people of color.

Another criticism regarding language in AA and NA is related to stigma. Critics say that the tradition of introducing oneself in meetings as an "addict" or "alcoholic" places a negative label on the individual and perpetuates stigma and stereotypical views of people who have SUDs. Additionally, identifying oneself as their disorder is contradictory to strength-based and person-centered philosophies. A differing perspective is offered in Greene's article:

> *In some marginalized groups, words that were historically pejorative have been reclaimed as a label of power, pride, and history—for example, the use of the term queer in some LGBTQ communities. Speaking for myself as a person in long-term recovery, the labels of "alcoholic" or "addict" serve, in a sense, as a badge of honor because I have survived a potentially fatal illness—and also thrive as a result. I feel a sense of pride and gratitude when I say, "Hi, my name is ____, and I'm an alcoholic." [44], p 11-12*

For those who have difficulty adapting to the language in AA's original literature, NA language may be more relevant to the present day, particularly newer NA publications and the latest edition of the NA Basic Text. However, the language of the 12-steps remains as originally written. Substitutes can be made in the language. For example, the male pronoun used in reference to God, may be substituted by a gender-neutral term. For example, dropping the male pronoun in the 11th step reads as follows: *We sought through prayer and meditation to improve our conscious contact with God as we understood God, praying only for knowledge of God's will for us and the power to carry that out.*

For those who do not identify as Christian, the word God may be substituted with Allah, Jehovah, Yahweh, the generic phrase Higher Power, or whatever is true for the individual. It is important to understand that 12-tep programs do not require a belief in God. In fact, many agnostic and atheist AA groups exist and are growing rapidly. In AA, one might hear GOD referred to as a Group Of Drunks, while a group of sober alcoholics might be considered a higher power for whom to turn to for help. An interesting finding by Tonigan and colleagues found that belief in God is not necessary to experience benefit from AA, but those who identify as atheist or agnostic are less likely to attend meetings [45].

Another criticism should be highlighted. Some have found the language of the 12-steps reflects a tearing down rather than a building up process that emphasizes moral inventory and examination of one's character flaws. Steps 4 through 7 best show this critique. These steps recommend critical self-examination, admission to the exact nature of wrongs to God and another person, followed by a willingness to let go of, and have God remove, such character defects and shortcomings. When asked about these criticisms, an NA member had this to say.

> *Well, I can certainly understand the criticisms because when you look at the steps as written without further guidance and instruction from a sponsor, it looks that way. It's important to understand a foundation is laid in steps 1-3, with the guidance of a sponsor, in preparation for working steps 4-7. Another important process to understand is that it's not only about wrongs committed, but also an inventory of assets and liabilities. We must self-examine in order to know what qualities and behaviors we want to nurture and what behavior patterns are unhealthy and need to be eliminated. If we don't change in a positive direction, we're likely to continue using. (NA member, personal communication, December 4, 2020)*

A major criticism is related to research. The tradition of anonymity in 12-step mutual aid recovery groups is an important aspect that attracts many to the program who otherwise may not attend. However, the lack of organization, anonymity, and the voluntary participation of members create methodological barriers to research. Additionally, survey research has inherent methodological flaws, particularly when studying members of 12-step programs. Self-selection bias is unavoidable, and this is particularly problematic as the voices of those who have not done well via 12-step mutual aid recovery may be missing and the voices of those doing well may be over-represented. Twelve-step attendees often come and go many times before they commit to sobriety or leave permanently. When evaluating the research literature, this criticism should not be overlooked.

Although 12-step meetings are more plentiful than alternative mutual aid recovery groups, availability is variable depending on geographic location. Meetings may be scant in rural areas and in some countries other than the U.S. Additionally, specialty meetings such as gender specific groups, LGBT groups, groups for adolescents, and groups for those who identify as atheist or agnostic are not available in all areas.

Depending upon which lens through which one views 12-step programs (member or researcher), the program's 12 traditions are both strengths and limitations. From a members' perspectives the traditions, as Eddy G. noted uphold the integrity of the program. But for researchers, anonymity, group autonomy, lack of professionalism and organizational structure, and their commitment to hold no opinion on outside issues, makes studying the program difficult. There is tremendous variability in how groups run and how one works the steps, for example.

This section ends with two additional strengths of 12-step programs – the first is cost. Membership in 12-step mutual aid programs is free. There are no membership dues or fees, no professionals, and the only requirement for membership is a desire to stop drinking or using [19]. The program is totally self-supported by its members' contributions collected at each meeting. A dollar or two is typical, but not required. Newcomers and those who do not identify as members are usually asked not to contribute. Finally, healthcare costs are substantially reduced for those who participate in 12-step programs. In their systematic review, Kelley and colleagues demonstrated higher healthcare cost savings for individuals treated with AA or Twelve Step Facilitation (TSF) compared to those treated in an outpatient facility utilizing CBT, or no AA/TSF exposure [1]. Further, for those with a poor prognosis, AA/TSF had higher cost savings compared to Motivational Enhancement Therapy.

The final and maybe most important strength of the program discussed here concerns science. Several 12-step activities are supported by research. Though provision of a comprehensive review is not possible here, two empirically supported activities are highlighted. The first, helping others, is the primary purpose of the 12-step programs and is underscored in Tradition five, “Each group has but one primary purpose—to carry its message to the alcoholic who still suffers.” Supported by a substantial scientific literature, personal well-being is enhanced by helping behaviors [46–49], and 12-step mutual aid recovery is founded on the principle of service. A common evidence-based practice for SUDs, contingency management [50], where rewards and incentives are provided to help reinforce abstinence and other health promoting behaviors, is exemplified in nearly every 12-step meeting. Through the chip system in AA or the key tag system often used in NA, members are recognized with a different colored chip or key tag for each marker of recovery, typically followed by a round of applause from the group. For example, if an NA member achieves 30 days of continued abstinence, they receive an orange key tag, 60 days is green, 90 days is red, blue is for 6-months, green for 9-months, and a glow in the dark key tag is awarded for one year clean. For members who attain multiple years of recovery, they often receive a special medallion.

9. Cultural considerations and the 12-steps

Culture has been defined as “a community or society. It structures the way people view the world. It involves the particular set of beliefs, norms, and values concerning the nature of relationships, the way people live their lives, and the way people organize their environments” [51], p.11. Additionally, culture includes the many cultural identities one holds in terms of ethnicity, gender, sexual orientation, age, socioeconomic status, geographic region, etc. Narcotics Anonymous is one of the most culturally diverse mutual aid programs, and this seems to be generalizable across the globe [2]. An important question to consider is this: Are there cultural considerations relative to 12-step philosophy and who may, and may not, fare well with the approach?

9.1 Spirituality as a cultural element

A key element of cultural beliefs, values, and norms is spirituality. In addition to examining spirituality as cultural element, this discussion provides a contradictory view of a primary criticism of 12-step programs, the religious and spiritual undertones. Abraham Maslow, noted psychologist and theorist, said “the spiritual life is part of the human essence. It is a defining characteristic of human nature, without which human nature is not fully human.” In a large survey conducted by the Pew Research Center, nearly 90% of survey respondents reported belief in God or a Universal Spirit [52]. Spirituality and religion seem to be in the fabric of many cultures. Based on data from the Higher Power Project, Dossett suggests that helping professionals need not be wary of referring individuals and families to 12-step programs, and in fact may want to consider supporting individuals and families in seeking recovery through 12-step programs [53]. Participants in the

HHP consistently report the notion of "autonomous and personal construction of a Higher Power which works for them" [53], p. 380. Koenig [35] underscores the importance of allowing individuals to define spirituality for themselves. Findings consistently show that those who attend 12-step meetings regularly and actively participate in the program have better substance use and quality of life outcomes [53, 54].

While much of the criticism of 12-step programs surrounds language that may be interpreted as oppressive, a substantial literature exists that contradicts the criticisms. Though a comprehensive cultural review is not possible here, the following discussion highlights several population groups that have historically experienced oppression or may experience unique issues in terms of SUD recovery. The author would be remiss to fail to mention that culture is subjectively experienced, and there are substantial differences within groups as well as between groups. Maintaining cultural humility [55] is always recommended. The discussion that follows highlights several special population groups and associated findings relative to 12-step recovery: African Americans, Native Americans, women, adolescents, and LGBTQ populations.

9.2 African Americans and 12-step models

In general, African American communities highly value spirituality and religion. Consequently, the topic of spirituality provides a smooth transition into the examination of the African American culture relative to 12-step programs. Peavy, Garret, Doyle, and Donovan compared outcomes of 12-step facilitation treatment between African American and Caucasian stimulant users and found treatment was equally effective for both groups [56]. One study found that African Americans were just as likely to attend and benefit from 12-step group attendance as their White counterparts and were slightly more likely to remain abstinent [57]. Another study explored spirituality among African American men attending a methadone maintenance program. The group of 25 men all reported a group focused on spirituality would be preferable to treatment as usual [58]. Given the spiritual foundation of 12-step programs, African American individuals with SUDs may derive great benefit from AA/NA.

9.3 Women and 12-step models

While valid criticisms exist relative to women and 12-step programs, there is also substantial literature to support the efficacy of 12-step approaches for women. As highlighted in the introduction, women make up approximately 42% of NA membership and 38% of AA's membership. According to some authors, 12-step programs are equally effective for women and people of color compared to their European-Male counterparts. For example, Hillhouse and Fiorentine found that women were just as likely to attend 12-step groups and recover as their White male counterparts [57]. Data were analyzed from the Los Angeles Target Cities Evaluation Project (n = 356), inclusive of 26 outpatient programs. Participants were followed for 2-years. At each of three follow-up points in the study, over 50% of participants identified as female, and no statistically significant differences were found between men and women. Moreover, approximately 35% of women reported weekly attendance at a 12-step meeting, and 30% of men reported weekly attendance. Men and women were equally likely to be abstinent at the 2-year follow-up, but women were slightly more likely to be abstinent from alcohol than were men; however, this finding was not statistically significant. Further, women and men were equally likely to dropout, 33.1% and 33.2% respectively. As a bridge into the next section, gender difference was compared among a sample of urban Native American individuals with SUDs as well, and none were found. Men and women in this sample experienced AA-related benefits equally, and 12-step meeting attendance helped to explain increased abstinence for both groups. For those who prefer gender specific 12-step meetings, there is availability in many areas.

9.4 Native Americans and 12-step models

There are more than 566 recognized Native American tribes in the U.S., and as a cultural group, Native Americans have experienced significant historical trauma and harms relative substance use and addiction. Some of the highest rates of substance use disorders are found among this population group. For example, SAMHSA reports that American Indian/Native Alaskans have the highest rates of alcohol misuse compared to other cultural groups [51]. Because a frequently cited value of this community is spirituality, 12-step mutual aid groups may be effective for Native Americans with SUDs [26]. However, research is quite limited specific to the efficacy of 12-step programs among Indigenous populations.

Although there has been speculation that cultural factors may render 12-step programs less effective for Native Americans, some studies have contradicted that assumption. One study, longitudinal in design, compared 12-step group attendance, attrition, and abstinence outcomes between urban Native Americans and White Americans [59]. The authors found no significant differences between meeting attendance and abstinence outcomes at 3-, 6-, and 9-month follow-ups. Decreased drinking intensity and increased abstinence was associated with greater meeting attendance for both groups. Interestingly, Native American participants were less likely to decrease meeting attendance. A more recent study relative to benefits experienced by urban Native Americans who attended AA also found benefit for those who attended 12-step groups relative to positive drinking outcomes [60].

Before concluding this section, the Wellbriety Movement deserves mention. It is described as "a sustainable grassroots movement that provides culturally based healing for the next seven generations of Indigenous people" [61]. Though an oversimplification, Wellbriety is an integration of traditional 12-step philosophy and Native cultural practices, such as the Medicine Wheel. Currently, an estimated 175 Wellbriety meetings exist in the U.S.

9.5 Adolescents and 12-step models

As a cultural group, adolescents with SUDs likely have the strongest need for social connection, and one benefit of 12-step program involvement is just that - mutual aid group communities provide instant access to sober social support. Multiple studies show that adolescents benefit from 12-step program involvement [5, 33, 62–64]. Because teens are more susceptible to peer influence and identification, they appear to benefit more from youth-focused 12-step groups, and like adults, teens seem to have improved SUD outcomes with increased participation in 12-step-activities [64, 65]. There are several barriers for adolescents noted in the literature: lack of transportation, resistance to the 12-steps, and the idea of powerlessness [65]. Kingston, Knight, Williams, and Gordon build on ideas set forth by Nash: adolescents may not only reject the notion of powerlessness but also the idea of a Higher Power [66]. Overall, however, there is substantial research to support the consideration of 12-step models for treating adolescents with SUDs [1, 2, 65, 67].

9.6 LGBTQ populations

Given the fact that as a cultural group, sexual minorities have high rates of substance misuse and SUDs, it is surprising that so little research exists specific to this population and 12 step recovery programs. In fact, SAMHSA suggests this cultural group has about a 30% prevalence rate of SUDs [68]. As a cultural group, sexual minorities tend to be highly stigmatized, which may contribute to higher rates of SUDs. For this reason, 12-step groups specific to the LGBTQ population are steadily increasing. For clients wishing to attend an LGBTQ specific AA group, Gay and Lesbian AA (GaL-AA) is an excellent resource and provides a meeting list for all LGBTQ AA meetings nationwide [69]. Narcotics Anonymous does not have an equivalent resource, but an internet search will locate LGBTQ NA meetings.

9.7 Co-occurring disorders and 12-step groups

Nearly half of people with an SUD also have a co-morbid psychiatric condition [70]. According to SAMHSA, people with SUDs are twice as likely than the general population to experience mood and anxiety disorders, and anti-social and conduct disorders [71]. Further, about 50% of those diagnosed with schizophrenia will develop an SUD over their lifetime. So, how do those with co-occurring disorders fare in 12-step programs? According to Project Match, those with more psychiatric severity did less well in 12-step approaches compared to cognitive behavioral interventions [27].

Mutual aid groups utilizing the 12-step framework and specific to those with co-occurring SUDs and mental health disorders are becoming more common. One such group, Double Trouble in Recovery (DTR), seems to provide an extra layer of comfort and emotional safety for members when sharing about both conditions, SUD, and mental illness [72–74]. Dual Recovery Anonymous (DRA) is a similar program that also follows the 12-steps. There are meetings located in each of the United States as well as Australia, Canada, Iceland, India, and New Zealand [75]; yet there is an absence of scholarly literature relative to its efficacy. The factors that appear to support recovery via 12-step affiliation for those with co-morbid conditions are identification, emotional safety, social support, and increased abstinence [72–74]. Because this group tends to have higher rates of relapse [76], referral to these specialty groups in addition to traditional 12-step groups is suggested.

10. Recommendations for integrating 12-step mutual aid programs

With such a strong literature supporting the efficacy of 12-step programs for individuals with SUDs, inclusion of 12-step approaches in the menu of therapeutic options for clients is warranted. From their comprehensive review on Narcotics Anonymous, White and colleagues underscore three salient findings [2]:

1. Much like Duncan and colleagues describe allegiance to a therapeutic model as an important factor influencing therapeutic outcomes [77], clinicians' beliefs regarding 12-step recovery matters, and may influence client participation and outcomes.

2. Successful linkage is crucial. Utilize assertive connection strategies rather than passive ones.

3. When clients are linked with 12-step groups while in treatment, their post-treatment attendance and participation increases.

10.1 Eight recommendations for integrating 12-step approaches

1. Integrate 12-step recovery as a topic for psychoeducation in group or individual sessions.

2. Clinicians should educate themselves about 12-step programs, not just via academic literature, but attendance at *several* 12-step groups and via interviews with those in long-term recovery.

3. Reach out to local AA and NA communities and coordinate to bring a meeting to your facility, or to locate individual members willing to come in and speak to clients and patients at your facility.

4. Place 12-step literature and meetings lists in the waiting area of your facility or in your office.

5. As appropriate, integrate 12-step group attendance into the change plan.

6. Utilize Twelve Step Facilitation (TSF) in your agency among other evidence-based models.

7. Monitor mutual aid group attendance as a relapse prevention technique rather than a punitive strategy.

8. With individuals for whom 12-step approaches are not a good fit, refer to alternative mutual aid groups (SMART, Women for Sobriety, Moderation Management, Dharma Recovery, and many others). Though the empirical evidence is still lacking for 12-step alternatives, similar mechanisms of action are likely at work.

11. Conclusion

As the chapter closes, it ends where it began, with the most rigorous scientific studies to date, and the main findings are presented here. Kelley and colleagues [1] examined 12-step mutual aid groups and professional therapeutic models based on 12-step philosophy, such as Twelve Step Facilitation (TSF), and their impact on SUD-related outcomes: "abstinence, reduced drinking intensity, reduced alcohol-related consequences, alcohol addiction severity, and healthcare cost offset" [1], p. 1. Twenty-seven studies and 10,536 study participants are included in the review.

The main findings for manualized AA/TSF intervention groups follow. Compared to the clinical intervention groups (e.g., CBT), AA/TSF participants demonstrated higher rates of complete abstinence, and this effect held over time. Further, AA/TSF interventions performed equally to the clinical intervention relative to percentage of days abstinent, but at 24 months performed better. AA/TSF appears to be equally effective to comparison groups in terms of longest period of abstinence. Another equal comparison was shown regarding intensity of drinking and number of drinks per drinking day. For alcohol-related consequences, AA/TSF does just as well as comparison groups, and may also perform equally in terms of reducing alcohol use severity, with one study showing better outcomes for AA/TSF.

Findings for non-manualized 12-step interventions are just as good. At 3 to 9 months follow-up, AA/TSF appears to perform as well as comparison groups in terms of the proportion of individuals completely abstinent but may perform

DOI: http://dx.doi.org/10.5772/intechopen.95985

slightly better than the clinical intervention for percentage of days abstinent. Regarding drinking intensity and percentage of heavy drinking days, AA/TSF also performed as well as the clinical intervention.

The review conducted by White and colleagues asked, "what is known about Narcotics Anonymous from the standpoint of science?" [2], p. 3. Included in their review were 232 studies. Though the scientific literature on NA needs more rigorous and methodologically sound study, so far it appears to mirror the evidence of AA's efficacy. Researchers from this review concluded that participation in NA contributes to increased abstinence and decreased substance use. Physical, mental, and spiritual health is improved, and improvement in overall social functioning seems to occur for many members. Decreased healthcare costs, increased self-esteem, improved coping, increased pro-recovery social networks, and decreased depression and anxiety are also benefits experienced by some NA members. Additionally, participation in activities such as reading NA literature, working the steps, service, and sponsorship appear to extend the benefits. According to the review, diverse sub-groups of people with SUDs may also benefit from NA; in particular, people of color, women, adolescents, and those with co-occurring mental health conditions.

The evidence for the efficacy of 12-step interventions is compelling. Not only is the research compelling, but 12-step programs also have an interesting history. Millions of individuals have experienced addiction recovery through 12-step pathways and have intimately experienced its transformational power. Organizations are unsustainable without leaders, structure, organization, funding, profits, or grants. Yet, the 12 traditions include ideas such as these: the program should have no leaders, no initiation dues, or fees; the program should remain forever non-professional; and, the program ought never be organized. Even so, and for over 85 years, 12-step programs across the globe have helped millions of people achieve recovery. It is unfathomable the 12-step movement has thrived without a traditional organizational structure. The 12-step organizational structure is built on spiritual principles, 12-steps, and the fundamental idea of one addict/alcoholic helping another. The 12-step movement revolutionized professional treatment services and has been tested across numerous populations. Scientific literature consistently demonstrates 12-step interventions to be equal in efficacy compared to common evidence-based models, and sometimes they perform even better than the intervention for which they are compared. 12-step groups can serve as an adjunctive service to professional addiction treatment to extend treatment benefits; and for some, 12-step groups may be the primary mode of intervention. In addition to its demonstrated efficacy, 12-step meetings are abundant, making accessibility a minimal concern. Finally, because 12-step meetings are free, it is quite cost-effective. In closing, clinicians should consider adding 12-step interventions to their clinical toolbox if they have not already done so. The science is out.

Author details

Dorothy Greene
East Tennessee State University, Johnson City Tennessee, United States

*Address all correspondence to: greeneds@etsu.edu

References

[1] Kelly JF, Humphreys K, Ferri M. Alcoholics Anonymous and other 12-step programs for alcohol use disorder. Cochrane Database of Systematic Reviews [Internet]. Wiley; 2017 Nov 21; Available from: http://dx.doi.org/10.1002/14651858.cd012880

[2] White, W, Galanter, M, Humphreys, K, Kelly, J. We do recover: Scientific studies on Narcotics Anonymous. Selected Papers of William White [Internet]. 2020. Available from http://www.williamwhitepapers.com/pr/dlm_uploads/2020-Review-of-Scientific-Studies-on-NA.pdf

[3] American Psychiatric Association. Diagnostic and Statistical Manual of Mental Health Disorders. 5th ed. Washington, DC: APA, 2013. 945 p.

[4] White, W. Slaying the Dragon: The history of addiction treatment and recovery in America. (2nd ed.). Bloomington: Chestnut Health Systems; 2014. 557 p.

[5] Chi FW, Sterling S, Campbell CI, Weisner C. 12-Step Participation and Outcomes Over 7 Years Among Adolescent Substance Use Patients With and Without Psychiatric Comorbidity. Substance Abuse [Internet]. Informa UK Limited; 2013 Jan;34(1):33-42. DOI: org/10.1080/08897077.2012.691780

[6] Greene, D, Yaffe, J, Kopack, A. Relapse among Recovering Addiction Professionals: Prevalence and Predictors, Journal of Social Work Practice in the Addictions. 2019; 19:4, 323-344, DOI: 10.1080/1533256X.2019.1653718

[7] Johnson JE, Finney JW, Moos RH. End-of-treatment outcomes in cognitive-behavioral treatment and 12-step substance use treatment programs: Do they differ and do they predict 1-year outcomes? J Subst Abuse Treat. 2006; 31: 41-50. DOI: 10.1016/j.jsat.2006.03.008. PMID: 16814009.

[8] Kelly, JF, Moos, R. Dropout from 12-step self-help groups: Prevalence, predictors, and counteracting treatment influences. Journal of Substance Abuse Treatment [Internet]. Elsevier BV; 2003 Apr;24(3):241-50. Available from: http://dx.doi.org/10.1016/s0740-5472(03)00021-7

[9] Vederhus J-K, Kristensen Ø. High effectiveness of self-help programs after drug addiction therapy. BMC Psychiatry [Internet]. Springer Science and Business Media LLC; 2006 Aug 23;6(1). Available from: http://dx.doi.org/10.1186/1471-244x-6-35

[10] SoberNation. List of 12-step programs. [Internet]. 2020. Available from: https://sobernation.com/list-of-12-step-programs/

[11] Alcoholics Anonymous. Estimated worldwide A.A. individual and group membership. [Internet]. 2019. Available from: https://www.aa.org/assets/en_US/smf-132_en.pdf

[12] Alcoholics Anonymous. 2014 Membership Survey. [Internet]. 2014. Available from: https://www.aa.org/assets/en_US/p-48_membershipsurvey.pdf

[13] Narcotics Anonymous. 2018 Narcotics Anonymous Membership Survey. [Internet]. 2018. Available from: https://www.na.org/admin/include/spaw2/uploads/pdf/pr/2301_MS_2018.pdf

[14] White WL. Addiction recovery mutual aid groups: an enduring international phenomenon. Addiction [Internet]. Wiley; 2004 May;99(5):532-8. Available from: http://dx.doi.org/10.1111/j.1360-0443.2004.00684.x

[15] Cheever, S. Bill W.: The Helper. Time. [Internet]. 1999. June 14. Available from: http://content.time.com/time/magazine/article/0,9171,991266,00.html

[16] Alcoholics Anonymous World Services, Inc. Alcoholics Anonymous (3rd ed.). NY: Author; 1976. 575 p.

[17] Alcoholics Anonymous. Archives and History. [Internet]. 2020. Available from: https://www.aa.org/pages/en_US/archives-and-history

[18] White, W, Budnick, C, Pickard, B. Narcotics Anonymous: Its history and culture. [Internet]. 2011. Available from: http://www.williamwhitepapers.com/pr/2011%20Narcotics%20Anonymous%20History%20and%20Culture.pdf

[19] Narcotics Anonymous World Services, Inc. Narcotics Anonymous. 5th ed. Van Nuys, CA: Narcotics Anonymous, Inc. 2003, 286 p.

[20] Gamblers Anonymous. [Internet]. Available from: http://www.gamblersanonymous.org/ga/node/1

[21] Overeaters Anonymous. [Internet]. 2020. Available from: https://oa.org/

[22] Co-dependents Anonymous. [Internet]. Available from: https://coda.org/

[23] Anderson, SC. Critical Analysis of the Concept of Codependency. Social Work [Internet]. Oxford University Press (OUP); 1994 Nov; Available from: http://dx.doi.org/10.1093/sw/39.6.677

[24] Beatty, M. Codependent No More: How to stop controlling others and start caring for yourself. Center City: Hazelden Foundation. 1986. 229 p.

[25] Hazelden Betty Ford Foundation. Hazelden Betty Ford Foundation History. [Internet].Available from: https://www.hazeldenbettyford.org/about-us/history

[26] van Wormer, K, Davis, D. Addiction Treatment: A strengths Perspective. 4th ed. Boston: Cengage; 2018. 632 p.

[27] National Institute of Alcohol Abuse and Alcoholism. NIAAA Reports Project MATCH Main Findings. [Internet]. 1996. Available from: https://www.niaaa.nih.gov/news-events/news-releases/niaaa-reports-project-match-main-findings

[28] Alcoholics Anonymous. The Twelve Steps of Alcoholics Anonymous. [Internet]. 2016. Available from: https://www.aa.org/assets/en_US/smf-121_en.pdf

[29] Narcotics Anonymous. IP No. 11 Sponsorship. Revised. [Internet]. 2004. Available from: https://www.na.org/admin/include/spaw2/uploads/pdf/litfiles/us_english/IP/EN3111.pdf

[30] Dekkers A, Vos S, Vanderplasschen W. "Personal recovery depends on NA unity": an exploratory study on recovery-supportive elements in Narcotics Anonymous Flanders. Substance Abuse Treatment, Prevention, and Policy [Internet]. Springer Science and Business Media LLC; 2020 Jul 31;15(1). Available from: http://dx.doi.org/10.1186/s13011-020-00296-0

[31] Kelly JF, Greene MC, Bergman BG. Recovery benefits of the "therapeutic alliance" among 12-step mutual-help organization attendees and their sponsors. Drug and Alcohol Dependence [Internet]. Elsevier BV; 2016 May;162:64-71. Available from: http://dx.doi.org/10.1016/j.drugalcdep.2016.02.028

[32] Witbrodt J, Ye Y, Bond J, Chi F, Weisner C, Mertens J. Alcohol and

drug treatment involvement, 12-step attendance and abstinence: 9-year cross-lagged analysis of adults in an integrated health plan. Journal of Substance Abuse Treatment [Internet]. Elsevier BV; 2014 Apr;46(4):412-9. Available from: http://dx.doi.org/10.1016/j.jsat.2013.10.015

[33] Kelly JF, Stout RL, Slaymaker V. Emerging adults' treatment outcomes in relation to 12-step mutual-help attendance and active involvement. Drug and Alcohol Dependence [Internet]. Elsevier BV; 2013 Apr;129(1-2):151-7. Available from: http://dx.doi.org/10.1016/j.drugalcdep.2012.10.005

[34] Pagano ME, White WL, Kelly JF, Stout RL, Tonigan JS. The 10-Year Course of Alcoholics Anonymous Participation and Long-Term Outcomes: A Follow-Up Study of Outpatient Subjects in Project MATCH. Substance Abuse [Internet]. Informa UK Limited; 2013 Jan;34(1):51-9. Available from: http://dx.doi.org/10.1080/08897077.2012.691450

[35] Koenig, HG. Religion, spirituality, and health: A review and update. Advances in Mind - Body Medicine. 2015; 29, 19-26. Available from: https://login.iris.etsu.edu:3443/login?url=https://www.proquest.com/magazines/religion-spirituality-health-review-update/docview/1698024209/se-2?accountid=10771

[36] Alcoholics Anonymous. Preamble. [Internet]. 2020. Available from: https://www.aa.org/assets/en_US/aa-literature/smf-92-aa-preamble

[37] Alcoholics Anonymous. World Services, Inc. Twelve steps and twelve traditions. NY: Author. 1952, 192 p.

[38] Allen, J, Nieuwsma, JA, Pollitt, MJ, & Blazer, D. Recovery on Higher Ground: Spirituality in the Treatment of Substance Abuse: Considering Spirituality and Religion during Recovery Can Enhance Treatment Outcomes. Current psychiatry. 2014;13: 24-40

[39] Examining the Components of a 12-Step Program: The Benefits and Criticisms. Integrating 12-Steps and Psychotherapy: Helping Clients Find Sobriety and Recovery [Internet]. SAGE Publications, Inc.; 27-42. Available from: http://dx.doi.org/10.4135/9781483387611.n2

[40] Sanders JM. Feminist Perspectives on 12-Step Recovery: A Comparative Descriptive Analysis of Women in Alcoholics Anonymous and Narcotics Anonymous. Alcoholism Treatment Quarterly [Internet]. Informa UK Limited; 2011 Sep 30;29(4):357-78. Available from: http://dx.doi.org/10.1080/07347324.2011.608595

[41] Whitaker, H. The patriarchy of Alcoholics Anonymous. The New York Times. [Internet]. 2019. Available from: https://www.nytimes.com/2019/12/27/opinion/alcoholics-anonymous-women.html

[42] Brigham GS. 12-Step Participation as a Pathway to Recovery: The Maryhaven Experience and Implications for Treatment and Research. Science & Practice Perspectives [Internet]. NIDA/RTI International; 2003 Aug;2(1):43-51. Available from: http://dx.doi.org/10.1151/spp032143

[43] Peele, S. AA's Male Culture: Does the dominance of men and male thinking in AA hurt women? Psychology Today. 2014, May 21. Available from: https://www.psychologytoday.com/us/blog/addiction-in-society/201405/aa-s-male-culture

[44] Greene, DS. 85 years old and going strong: Revisiting AA's place in a social worker's toolbox. Intersections in Practice. National Association of Social Workers; 2020 (14): 11-12. Available from: https://www.socialworkers.org/

Careers/Specialty-Practice-Sections/Intersections-in-Practice-Public

[45] Tonigan JS, Miller WR, Schermer C. Atheists, agnostics and Alcoholics Anonymous. Journal of Studies on Alcohol [Internet]. Alcohol Research Documentation, Inc.; 2002 Sep;63(5):534-41. Available from: http://dx.doi.org/10.15288/jsa.2002.63.534

[46] Hanniball KB, Aknin LB, Douglas KS, Viljoen JL. Does helping promote well-being in at-risk youth and ex-offender samples? Journal of Experimental Social Psychology [Internet]. 2019 May [cited 2021 Jan 1];82:307-17. Available from: https://search.ebscohost.com/login.aspx?direct=true&AuthType=ip,shib&db=psyh&AN=2018-59421-001&site=ehost-live&scope=site

[47] Schwartz CE, Keyl PM, Marcum JP, Bode R. Helping others shows differential benefits on health and well-being for male and female teens. Journal of Happiness Studies: An Interdisciplinary Forum on Subjective Well-Being [Internet]. 2009 Aug [cited 2021 Jan 1];10(4):431-48. Available from: https://search.ebscohost.com/login.aspx?direct=true&AuthType=ip,shib&db=psyh&AN=2009-10842-004&site=ehost-live&scope=site

[48] Grayman-Simpson N, Mattis JS. Doing good and feeling good among African Americans: Subjective religiosity, helping, and satisfaction. Journal of Black Psychology [Internet]. 2013 Aug [cited 2021 Jan 1];39(4):411-27. Available from: https://search.ebscohost.com/login.aspx?direct=true&AuthType=ip,shib&db=psyh&AN=2013-26043-004&site=ehost-live&scope=site

[49] Curry OS, Rowland LA, Van Lissa CJ, Zlotowitz S, McAlaney J, Whitehouse H. Happy to help? A systematic review and meta-analysis of the effects of performing acts of kindness on the well-being of the actor. Journal of Experimental Social Psychology [Internet]. 2018,76:320-9. Available from: https://search.ebscohost.com/login.aspx?direct=true&AuthType=ip,shib&db=psyh&AN=2018-12418-001&site=ehost-live&scope=site

[50] NIDA. Contingency Management Interventions/Motivational Incentives (Alcohol, Stimulants, Opioids, Marijuana, Nicotine). National Institute on Drug Abuse website. https://www.drugabuse.gov/publications/principles-drug-addiction-treatment-research-based-guide-third-edition/evidence-based-approaches-to-drug-addiction-treatment/behavioral-therapies/contingency-management-interventions-motivational-incentives. June 1, 2020 Accessed December 31, 2020.

[51] Substance Abuse and Mental Health Services Administration (SAMHSA). Improving Cultural Competence. Treatment Improvement Protocol (TIP) Series No. 59. HHS Publication No. (SMA) 14-4849. Rockville, MD: Substance Abuse and Mental Health Services Administration, 2014, 329 p. Available from: https://store.samhsa.gov/product/TIP-59-Improving-Cultural-Competence/SMA15-4849

[52] Pew Research Center. Key findings about America's belief in God. [Internet]. 2018, April 18. Available from: https://www.pewresearch.org/fact-tank/2018/04/25/key-findings-about-americans-belief-in-god/

[53] Dossett W. Addiction, spirituality, and 12-step programmes. International Social Work [Internet]. SAGE Publications; 2013 Apr 29;56(3):369-83. Available from: http://dx.doi.org/10.1177/0020872813475689

[54] Kaskutas LA. Alcoholics Anonymous Effectiveness: Faith

Meets Science. Journal of Addictive Diseases [Internet]. Informa UK Limited; 2009 Apr 2;28(2):145-57. Available from: http://dx.doi.org/10.1080/10550880902772464

[55] Tervalon M, Murray-García J. Cultural Humility Versus Cultural Competence: A Critical Distinction in Defining Physician Training Outcomes in Multicultural Education. Journal of Health Care for the Poor and Underserved [Internet]. Project Muse; 1998;9(2):117-25. Available from: http://dx.doi.org/10.1353/hpu.2010.0233

[56] Peavy KM, Garrett S, Doyle S, Donovan D. A comparison of African American and Caucasian stimulant users in 12-step facilitation treatment. Journal of Ethnicity in Substance Abuse [Internet]. Informa UK Limited; 2016 Jun 13;16(3):380-99. Available from: http://dx.doi.org/10.1080/15332640.2016.1185657

[57] Hillhouse MP, Fiorentine R. 12-Step Program Participation and Effectiveness: Do Gender and Ethnic Differences Exist? Journal of Drug Issues [Internet]. SAGE Publications; 2001 Jul;31(3):767-80. Available from: http://dx.doi.org/10.1177/002204260103100313

[58] Heinz AJ, Disney ER, Epstein DH, Glezen LA, Clark PI, Preston KL. A Focus-Group Study on Spirituality and Substance-User Treatment. Substance Use & Misuse [Internet]. Informa UK Limited; 2009 Dec 21;45(1-2):134-53. Available from: http://dx.doi.org/10.3109/10826080903035130

[59] Tonigan JS, Martinez-Papponi B, Hagler KJ, Greenfield BL, Venner KL. Longitudinal Study of Urban American Indian 12-Step Attendance, Attrition, and Outcome. Journal of Studies on Alcohol and Drugs [Internet]. Alcohol Research Documentation, Inc.; 2013 Jul;74(4):514-20. Available from: http://dx.doi.org/10.15288/jsad.2013.74.514

[60] Muñoz RE, Tonigan JS. Alcoholics Anonymous-Related Benefit for Urban Native Americans: Does Urban Native American Gender Moderate AA Engagement and Outcomes? Alcoholism Treatment Quarterly [Internet]. Informa UK Limited; 2016 Dec 12;35(1):34-45. Available from: http://dx.doi.org/10.1080/07347324.2016.1256715

[61] White Bison. Wellbriety Movement. [Internet]. 2020. Available from: https://wellbriety.com/about-us/

[62] Bekkering GE, Mariën D, Parylo O, Hannes K. The Effectiveness of Self-Help Groups for Adolescent Substance Misuse: A Systematic Review. Journal of Child & Adolescent Substance Abuse [Internet]. Informa UK Limited; 2016 Mar 2;25(3):229-44. Available from: http://dx.doi.org/10.1080/1067828x.2014.981772

[63] Kelly JF, Myers MG, Brown SA. Do adolescents affiliate with 12-step groups? A multivariate process model of effects. Journal of Studies on Alcohol [Internet]. Alcohol Research Documentation, Inc.; 2002 May;63(3):293-304. Available from: http://dx.doi.org/10.15288/jsa.2002.63.293

[64] Kelly JF, Bergman BG, Fallah-Sohy N. Mechanisms of Behavior Change in 12-Step Approaches to Recovery in Young Adults. Current Addiction Reports [Internet]. Springer Science and Business Media LLC; 2018 Apr 26;5(2):134-45. Available from: http://dx.doi.org/10.1007/s40429-018-0203-1

[65] Nash AJ. The Twelve Steps and Adolescent Recovery: A Concise Review. Substance Abuse: Research and Treatment [Internet]. SAGE Publications; 2020 Jan;14:117822182090439. Available from: http://dx.doi.org/10.1177/1178221820904397

[66] Kingston S, Knight E, Williams J, Gordon H. How do Young Adults View 12-Step Programs? A Qualitative Study. Journal of Addictive Diseases [Internet]. Informa UK Limited; 2015 Aug 17;34(4):311-22. Available from: http://dx.doi.org/10.1080/10550887.2015.1074506

[67] Sussman S. A Review of Alcoholics Anonymous/ Narcotics Anonymous Programs for Teens. Evaluation & the Health Professions [Internet]. SAGE Publications; 2010 Feb 17;33(1):26-55. Available from: http://dx.doi.org/10.1177/0163278709356186

[68] Substance Abuse and Mental Health Services Administration. Center for Substance Abuse Treatment. A Provider's Introduction to Substance Abuse Treatment for Lesbian, Gay, Bisexual, and Transgender Individuals. [Internet]. 2012, 197 p. Available from

[69] Gays and Lesbians in AA (GaL-AA). Available from: http://gal-aa.org/meetings/meeting-listing/)

[70] Miller, W, Forechimes,A, Zweben, A. Treating addiction: A guide for professionals. 2nd ed. NY: Guilford. 2019; 520 p.

[71] Substance Abuse and Mental Health Services Administration. Substance Use Disorder Treatment for People With Co-Occurring Disorders. Treatment Improvement Protocol (TIP) Series, No. 42. SAMHSA Publication No. PEP20-02-01-004. Rockville, MD: Substance Abuse and Mental Health Services Administration, 2020.

[72] Magura S. Effectiveness of Dual Focus Mutual Aid for Co-Occurring Substance Use and Mental Health Disorders: A Review and Synthesis of the "Double Trouble" in Recovery Evaluation. Substance Use & Misuse [Internet]. Informa UK Limited; 2008 Oct;43(12-13):1904-26. Available from: http://dx.doi.org/10.1080/10826080802297005

[73] Vogel HS, Knight E, Laudet AB, Magura S. Double trouble in recovery: Self-help for people with dual diagnoses. Psychiatric Rehabilitation Journal [Internet]. American Psychological Association (APA); 1998;21(4):356-64. Available from: http://dx.doi.org/10.1037/h0095288

[74] Aase DM, Jason LA, Robinson WL. 12-step participation among dually-diagnosed individuals: A review of individual and contextual factors. Clinical Psychology Review [Internet]. Elsevier BV; 2008 Oct;28(7):1235-48. Available from: http://dx.doi.org/10.1016/j.cpr.2008.05.002

[75] Dual Recovery Anonymous. [Internet]. 2009. Available from: http://www.draonline.org/

[76] Kushner MG, Abrams K, Thuras P, Hanson KL, Brekke M, Sletten S. Follow-up Study of Anxiety Disorder and Alcohol Dependence in Comorbid Alcoholism Treatment Patients. Alcoholism: Clinical & Experimental Research [Internet]. Wiley; 2005 Aug;29(8):1432-43. Available from: http://dx.doi.org/10.1097/01.alc.0000175072.17623.f8

[77] Duncan BL, Miller SD., Wampolod BE, and Hubble MA. (2009). *The heart and soul of change: Delivering what works in therapy*. (2nd ed.). Washington, DC: American Psychological Association

Chapter 6

Assessment and Treatment of Addictions in Community Corrections

Jacob D. Armstrong, Amy Bauman, Krystal J. Moroney and C. Brendan Clark

Abstract

This chapter discusses the treatment of substance use disorders within community corrections populations. The history of substance abuse treatment within correctional populations is outlined to provide context for the current diversion and rehabilitation models currently in use. Common systems where treatment is provided such as mental health court, drug court, and TASC are described. Common forms of therapy including Cognitive Behavioral Therapy, Mindfulness, social skills training, pharmacotherapy, and smoking cessation are discussed. This chapter focuses on their effectiveness as well as how these forms of therapy differ in community corrections as compared to other populations. Finally, recommendations and future directions for research are provided.

Keywords: Community Corrections, Criminal Justice, TASC, Drug Court, Mental Health Court

1. Introduction

The United States (U.S.) incarcerates a higher proportion of its citizens than any other country in the world [1], approximately two-thirds of whom are supervised under community corrections [2]. In the substance abuse and mental health literatures, community corrections is a broadly inclusive term intended to categorize a variety of supervision models where individuals are subjected to legal supervision while being permitted to remain in the community. Both the BJS [3] and the National Institute of Justice [4] restrict definitions of community corrections to individuals under probation (i.e., being supervised in the community for a crime that does not warrant detainment in jail or prison) or parole (i.e., community supervision post detainment before one's sentence has expired). In the grey literature, this term is much more loosely defined, varies considerably across jurisdictions, and may be restricted to defining specific models that are not considered parole or probation. For the purposes of this chapter, community corrections will refer to any criminal offender being supervised in the community outside of jail or prison. Those supervised under community corrections tend to be low-risk offenders (i.e., drug offenders) and are often awaiting trial and sentencing. Individuals supervised under community corrections as well as the correctional population in general tend to have high rates of substance misuse [5], mental illness [6, 7], traumatic brain injury [8], and suicidality [9]. These multiple comorbidities likely contribute to the high rates of recidivism (i.e., 45-65%) observed for correctional populations [10, 11]. Historically, the correctional system has not emphasized rehabilitation but has instead focused on longer and more severe sentencing in an effort to deter future crime. The increased incarceration rates and high recidivism rates are evidence that this approach has not worked. Over the past twenty years, the U.S. correctional system has shifted its focus toward a diversion rehabilitation model. The goals of this model are to identify the needs of low-risk offenders and provide treatment while diverting them from jail and prison into community supervision. Virtually all treatment models focus on addiction due to the high rates of substance misuse observed in these populations, but different treatment modalities also include psychotherapy, social skill training, vocational rehabilitation, and education, all of which have been shown to reduce crime and recidivism [12–14]. These efforts have been largely successful and have led to reductions in the recidivism rate for the first time in decades [2]. The goal of this chapter is to explain how treatment in corrections has evolved over time and what models and techniques are being used today. We will explain the more popular models of service delivery in community-based supervision (i.e., TASC, Drug Court, Mental Health Court) as well as different therapies utilized in community corrections which have been either popularly employed (Cognitive Behavioral Therapy, mindfulness, Social Skills training) or call for increased use (pharmacotherapy, smoking cessation).

2. History of substance abuse treatment in corrections

Historically, the U.S. government's approach to reducing illicit substance abuse has been to impose harsher sentencing while offering minimal treatment opportunities to the incarcerated. Harsher and more severe sentencing was enacted to deter future crime. More prominent examples of such legislation include Nixon's "war on drugs," the zero tolerance policies of the 1980s, and the three strikes laws of the 1990s. Collectively, these and similar laws led to higher conviction rates as well as longer and mandatory sentencing requirements for substance offenders [15]. Starting in the early 1990s, crime, especially violent crime, began to decrease [16]; however, the arrest and conviction rates for drug offenses continued to increase. These rates remained high for years and propped up a continually increasing incarceration rate that remains high to this day [17]. These steadily increasing incarceration rates for substance-related offenses indicate that these policies were not effective at deterring future crime; however, lawmakers repeatedly doubled down on these efforts to impose harsher laws. Conversely, as sentencing was increased for substance related offenders, minimal funding was provided for treatment efforts aimed at rehabilitating these offenders. Early treatment efforts such as Transcendental Meditation showed promise, but these efforts were poorly funded. A prominent review was published in 1974 examining the effectiveness of different treatment modalities on incarcerated populations, and the author famously concluded that "nothing works" [18]. The article was credited with debunking the idea that criminals could be rehabilitated and had a tremendous impact not just on the scientific literature, but on policy makers and the correctional system itself for the next 25 years [19]. Thus, individuals abusing substances were being arrested at higher and higher rates, no genuine efforts were made to rehabilitate these offenders during most of the 20th century.

Today diversion and rehabilitation models, which divert individuals from jail and prison and provide a variety of therapies, are reducing recidivism for the first time in decades. The most influential and prominent of which is the

Risk-Need-Responsivity (RNR) model [12]. The RNR model was developed in Canada, but due to its success it was quickly adapted across the U.S. and has become the dominant model used in community corrections to reduce recidivism. The RNR model has three main components: identifying individuals who could benefit from services, identifying the needs of the offender, and tailoring treatment to meet those needs. The model assesses eight factors, which have been strongly linked to criminal behavior and recidivism (i.e., antisocial behavior, antisocial personality patterns, procriminal condition, antisocial associates, substance abuse, family/marital relationships, school/work, and lack of prosocial recreational activities), then diverts individuals to the appropriate level of community-based supervision and prescribes treatment recommendations based on these factors. The treatment recommendations provided by the model vary from program to program, but therapy tends to be far more comprehensive than typical psychotherapies due largely to the severity of symptoms and multiple comorbidities typically observed in criminal justice populations. These needs are assessed through the Level of Service Inventory–Revised (LSI-R; [20]), a standardized measure which provides specific recommendations. The RNR model has grown in popularity since its inception and remains the most popular and influential diversion rehabilitation model today.

3. Models of Treatment Delivery

The TASC program, originally known as "Treatment alternatives to street crime," was developed in 1972 by the federal government to address the connection between drug abuse and criminal activity [21]. Today, the acronym represents a variety of different programs. The original goals of TASC were to decrease the possession, manufacturing, and distribution of illegal drugs and to derail the cycle of drug dependent individuals committing "street crimes" by diverting offenders with substance use issues to the appropriate community-based treatment programs [21]. Today TASC programs, known by several names including Treatment Accountability for Safer Communities and Treatment Alternatives for Safe Communities, represent a variety of diverse and tailored services based on the needs of client populations and surrounding communities, but each maintains the same overarching goals. TASC is not a direct treatment provider but instead acts as a link between the criminal justice system and community-based treatment programs. This separation of corrections and treatment maintains the confidentiality of the client and is a key component in promoting honesty, trust, and recovery. TASC's common objectives are to assess offenders' need for substance abuse treatment (regardless of their crime), direct qualifying individuals to the appropriate treatment programs and ancillary services, and to monitor offenders' progress throughout the program. In addition to substance abuse treatment, offenders in the TASC program may be referred to programs that aid in providing mental health treatment, medical treatment, housing assistance, education, and vocational skills training [22]. Federal funding for TASC programs was largely reduced in the 1980s due to the rising popularity of substances, such as cocaine, for which there were few treatment programs at the time [13]. Currently, most programs rely on local funds, grants, fees, and donations.

Evaluations of the TASC program have shown it to be a cost-effective alternative to incarceration [13] and largely successful in effectively identifying offenders in need of substance abuse treatment and making appropriate referrals. Offenders enrolled in TASC programs are more likely to complete substance abuse treatment compared to those with no legal involvement [23] and remain in the community longer without rearrest compared to offenders who drop out [22, 24]. Successful completion of TASC may require completion of ancillary service programs unique to each offender (e.g., GED, vocational rehabilitation, mental health treatment) in addition to substance abuse treatment. TASC has been influential in the development of similar programs for offenders throughout the U.S. [23, 25], with numerous adapted programs, as well as distinct programs that provide comparable services, such as "Breaking the Cycle" (BTC), "Drug Treatment Alternatives to Prison" (DTAP), and California's "Proposition 36" [26].

Although TASC has been successful in linking offenders with appropriate interventions and overall reducing recidivism, there remain populations of offenders with substance abuse issues for which TASC has been less successful. Individuals who experience more instability in their living conditions and employment, as well as marital instability at the beginning of treatment tend to fail in TASC programs more rapidly, as do those who were arrested for non-drug related crimes [9]. Drug of choice is also impactful, in that offenders who abuse more addictive substances such as crack/cocaine and opioids tend to fail the TASC program more quickly, and those who do complete the program are quicker to be rearrested [9, 26]. Although TASC is available to offenders arrested for a variety of offenses, it might be most valuable for offenders arrested for drug crimes. Additionally, given that instability and preferred substances also impact the likelihood of success, TASC programs might consider implementing aftercare, which has shown to reduce the likelihood of substance use, relapse, and rearrest beyond treatment [27].

Drug court is a term typically used to refer to courtrooms dedicated solely to providing judicially-monitored and enforced drug treatment, testing, and services for non-violent drug offenders. The first drug court was established in 1989, in Miami, Florida, to address the high rates of substance abuse related recidivism observed by judges in Dade County. By 1997, there were approximately 275 jurisdictions across the country with operating drug courts [28]. By the late 1990's university and government researchers began publishing the first efficacy and effectiveness studies on the drug court model more broadly [29–32]. In one such critical review, Dr. Belenko summarized research on the model as follows:

> *"The study found drug courts provide closer, more comprehensive supervision and much more frequent drug testing and monitoring during the program, than other forms of community supervision. More importantly, drug use and criminal behavior are substantially reduced while offenders are participating in drug court ([8], p. 2)."*

Drug offenders are selected for participation in a drug court program by prosecutors based upon their eligibility (i.e., severity and nature of their crime) and typically participate for between 12 and 18 months. The drug court model emphasizes collaboration between the varying components of the criminal justice system (i.e., judge, prosecutor, defense attorney, probation official, etc.) and the substance abuse treatment system (i.e., mental healthcare providers, medical providers, social services, etc.) in order to promote prosocial and treatment seeking behavior and reduce recidivism [33]. The successes of the first drug court program led to the proliferation of drug courts in the United States. In 1999, there were over 425 in operation across the country [34]. In 2020, the U.S. Department of Justice places the approximate number of drug courts in the United States at over 3000 (See [35]).

Like modern TASC programs, drug court programs are united by a key set of goals. There is a high degree of heterogeneity in drug court components and practices, as their operation is not only subject to differences in state laws and state funding, but also the preferences of the individual judges presiding over each drug court. In 1997, a report on drug courts compiled by the U.S. General Accounting Office concluded that, in addition to the huge variability observed among bona fide drug courts, some programs were observed to be drug courts only by name, displaying no emphasis on judicial oversight of treatment delivery observed in the traditional drug courts described in this chapter. The variance in adherence to the drug court model represents a major limitation in the current drug court literature [36, 37].

In 1997, the Drug Court Standards Committee, part of the National Association of Drug Court Professionals, published a document detailing the ten key components of drug court. These key components concern early identification of eligible participants, referral to treatment and community services, ongoing participation in drug court status hearings, required completion of substance abuse treatment, regular random drug screening, positive reinforcement for continued compliance, rapid sanctions for noncompliance, and typically dismissal of charges upon completion of the program [38]. Due to differences in court structure, community context, and availability of local resources, drug courts differ in their adherence to these key components [39].

The literature has demonstrated drug courts to be significantly more effective at breaking the cycle of recidivism seen in substance abuse populations than traditional courts, with an average effect of reducing recidivism ranging from 50% to 38% [40, 41]. However, the literature has also demonstrated that not all drug courts exhibit the same levels of success. The results of studies examining the effectiveness of DWI courts and juvenile courts have been mixed, and structural components of drug court procedure, such as how participants are admitted to the court, have also shown to have an impact. There is also evidence suggesting the drug court model is more effective for participants with certain individual characteristics, such as being older and more educated [42]. Current research focuses on examining drug court outcomes utilizing disparate models in service of differing populations in order to identify which components of the drug court model are responsible for successful outcomes and how individual characteristics may impact successful completion of the program [39].

In addition to TASC programs and drug courts, mental health courts also serve as a system where offenders within community corrections with substance use issues may receive services. Popularized in the 1990s, mental health courts are part of the court system that intends to divert people with mental illness from prisons and jails by using a model that is problem-solving oriented as opposed to punishment oriented. Beginning in the 1960s, state hospitals began closing due to poor treatment within facilities. Government budget cuts of community-based mental health care resulted in numerous individuals with mental illness not receiving necessary treatment and instead being retained in prisons and jails. Mental health courts are, in part, a response to the overrepresentation of offenders with mental illness within correctional facilities. There is significant comorbidity between externalizing disorders (e.g., drug use disorders), internalizing disorders (e.g., bipolar disorder), and criminal behavior within community corrections populations. Offenders with comorbid substance use and internalizing disorders are also at higher risk of reoffending should they remain untreated, further indicating a need for treatment options within the community. The amount of mental health courts in the U.S. has grown rapidly in the past few decades. Currently, there are more than 300 mental health courts for both juvenile and adult offenders with various levels of enrollment size and approved target participants (e.g., severely mentally ill, misdemeanor) [43]. Mental health courts divert offenders with mental illness to various be behavioral health services based on individual needs including individual therapy, group therapy, psychopharmacology, and assessment [44].

Mental health courts vary in how they are structured, as there is not a national standardized protocol [45], and offenders are usually given the choice of whether to participate. Mental health courts consist of a collaborative team made up of a judge, prosecution and defense attorneys, and a mental health professional. These courts may have incentives, such as a decreased sentence for compliance (e.g., adhering to the recommended mental health and addiction treatment, not recidivating). Compliance is rewarded and noncompliance is punished with jail time, reprimand by the judge, or other sanctions [45]. Court participants are most often monitored within the community by probation officers and mental health professionals who confirm attendance of appointments, while maintaining confidentiality of topics discussed within the mental health setting [45]. The mental health court protocol, though variable based on location, allows for a collaborative effort between the court and mental health professionals to create a treatment plan for offenders.

Mental health courts have been moderately effective in reducing recidivism rates and sentence lengths for offenders [46, 47]. There is some evidence that the mental health treatment through the courts is successful in symptom reduction and improvement of quality of life [46, 48, 49]. Graduation from mental health courts (i.e., receiving the full intervention) leads to more successful results (i.e., lower recidivism) compared to individuals who drop out early [46]. Overall, mental health courts have been successful in reducing symptoms and reducing recidivism rates for offenders who participate.

Mental health courts can at times be ineffective dependent on various offender characteristics and choices. Failure to reduce symptoms, choosing not to participate, negative termination, and sanctions indicate non-fulfillment of the mental health court goals. History of drug crimes and racial minority status is associated with choosing not to participate in mental health courts [50]. Negative termination through failure to complete treatment is associated with multiple diagnoses and stealing crimes, while lack of negative termination is associated with offenders with drug crimes choosing to participate, as well as increased number of scheduled court appearances; however, some evidence suggests offenders with recent drug history or drug crimes are more likely to be sanctioned by mental health courts [50, 51]. Lack of successful treatment outcomes may also result from viewing the mental health courts as coercive in nature [52]. Overall, various factors impact the success of mental health courts including demographic factors, crimes committed, and how the court is viewed by offenders.

4. Therapeutic methods

There are multiple evidence-based therapeutic methods utilized in treating individuals in corrections populations (whether incarcerated or in community corrections). Due to the high levels of variability between individual TASC programs, drug courts, and mental health courts, there is no single therapeutic method which is consistently implemented across all treatment delivery systems. Further, the difficulty in assessing community corrections populations (lack of control group availability, barriers to data collection, concerns regarding treatment fidelity, etc.) limits the body of evidence supporting the use of evidence-based treatments for use specifically in community corrections. For these reasons, this section will focus on evidence-based treatments which are commonly utilized in corrections populations more broadly, and which address presenting problems believed to be relevant to community corrections populations. These include cognitive behavioral therapies, mindfulness therapies, integrative therapies, social skills training, psychopharmacology, and smoking cessation treatments.

4.1 Cognitive behavioral therapies

Cognitive Behavioral Therapy (CBT) is an umbrella term for diverse psychological treatments which share some common elements. CBT treatments have shown to be effective for treating a range of psychological disorders and presenting problems. At their core, treatments typically included under the term CBT operate under a theoretical model with roots in behaviorism (focusing on external behaviors), cognitive theory (emphasizing the importance of internal behaviors/thoughts), or both. Many CBT approaches acknowledge that thinking and behavior are interconnected and both play a role in the development of psychological problems. While there are various manualized treatments for different presenting problems, treatment packages rooted in CBT usually address learned patterns of maladaptive behavior as well as unhelpful or distorted thinking. Patients receiving CBT typically learn more adaptive ways of thinking and behaving, thereby improving their coping skills and resilience, which contributes to symptom reduction and improving the effectiveness of their behavior.

In settings where both criminological and psychological outcomes are targets of CBT treatment, this model has been adapted to address the patterns of thinking and behavior which are believed to contribute to criminal justice involvement. CBT treatments adapted for this purpose have shown to be highly effective in a variety of contexts. Barnes, Hyatt, and Sherman's [53] evaluation of a 14-week CBT intervention called "*Choosing to Think, Thinking to Choose*", designed specifically for individuals in community corrections settings at high risk of recidivism, demonstrated that participants with a history of nonviolent offending were significantly less likely to re-offend. A 16-week CBT program treating community corrections offenders with a repeated history of driving while intoxicated (DWI) was demonstrated to be significantly more effective than treatment-as-usual when recidivism was assessed during a three-year follow-up, thus providing evidence that CBT can be effective in reducing recidivism related to presenting problems which have historically been extremely challenging to treat [54].

A review of CBT's use in corrections populations, written by Milkman and Wanberg [55], identifies six treatments as being the most prominent for use with individuals in "correctional institutions, community corrections centers, and outpatient programs serving probation and parole clients" (p. xi): Aggression Replacement Training (ART), Criminal Conduct and Substance Abuse Treatment: Strategies for Self-Improvement and Change (SSC), Moral Reconation Therapy (MRT), Reasoning and Rehabilitation (R&R), Relapse Prevention Therapy (RPT), and Thinking for a Change (T4C). Milkman and Wanberg identify four primary goals that all of these therapies have in common: each attempts to assist individuals in (1) identifying the problems which contributed to their conflict with authorities, (2) identifying life goals, (3) identifying prosocial solutions to the problems conflicting with goals, and (4) putting these solutions into practice. **Table 1** provides a summary of these approaches:

CBT has accumulated significant empirical support for its effectiveness in criminal justice populations and is indicated for use with both juvenile and adult offenders. A meta-analysis of 69 research studies on the impact of CBT in a variety of criminal justice settings, including prison, jail, probation, and parole settings, from 1968 through 1996 found CBT treatment to be significantly more effective in reducing recidivism than solely behavioral treatments [61]. Another meta-analysis of 58 studies conducted between 1980 and 2004 found, on average, participants who received CBT treatment were over one and a half times as likely to remain rearrest and reincarceration free at 12-month follow-up than control participants [62]. Wilson, Bouffard, and MacKenzie [63] analyzed 20 studies conducted between

Intervention	Description
Aggression Replacement Therapy (ART)	ART was originally designed for use in juvenile justice but has since been expanded for use with adults. It is provided in three one-hour sessions per week (for 10 weeks) focusing on anger and violence reduction. ART has three components (social skills training, anger control training, and moral reasoning), alternating between components each week. It is designed to teach interpersonal skills, promote self-control competencies, and improve the moral reasoning and empathy of participants [56].
Criminal Conduct and Substance Abuse Treatment: Strategies for Self-Improvement and Change (SSC)	SSC is a long-term treatment, taking 9-12 months, for adult offenders with a history of substance-abuse. Participants progress through 12 modules separated equally into 3 phases of treatment: challenge to change, commitment to change, and ownership of change. The program is intended to assist offenders in finding the motivation to change, strengthen the basic skills they will need to make necessary changes in their life, and provide reinforcement during the stabilization and maintenance of their sobriety [55].
Moral Reconation Therapy (MRT)	MRT is highly variable in its delivery, ranging from 1 to 20 sessions per month. Originally developed for criminal justice-based drug treatment, it has since expanded to include a variety of presenting problems where client resistance likely interferes in treatment (e.g., driving while intoxicated, domestic violence, sex offenses, antisocial behavior, etc.). It attempts to gradually assist patients in transitioning patterns of selfishness, dishonesty, and victimizing toward more prosocial patterns characterized by social consideration, ethical principles, and personal fulfillment [57].
Reasoning and Rehabilitation (R&R)	R&R consists of 35 sessions, conducted in groups of 6 to 8, over the course of 8 to 12 weeks. The program was developed for use in a diverse range of settings, including both institutional settings and community corrections. R&R focuses on promoting prosocial thinking and social perspective taking, as well as helping clients develop their interpersonal problem-solving and self-regulation skills [58].
Relapse Prevention Therapy (RPT)	RPT emerged from a maintenance program designed for use following the successful treatment of addictive behavior, gradually becoming a stand-alone treatment. Throughout treatment, emphasis is placed on promoting self-management. RPT focuses on traditional cognitive therapy, cognitive-behavioral coping skills training, and teaching lifestyle modification strategies to promote overall coping capacity [59].
Thinking for a Change (T4C)	T4C is a group intervention delivered across 22 lessons, ranging from 1-2 hours each, typically 2 lessons per week. The treatment is provided in sequential lessons, emphasizing maintaining treatment integrity and continuity of care between providers and patients. T4C aims to integrate social skills and problem-solving training with cognitive restructuring to increase offenders' awareness of their own thoughts and emotions, as well as those of others [60].

Table 1.
This table provides a summary of the most wildly used and emphatically supported Cognitive Behavioral Therapies used in corrections.

1988 and 1999 and found that CBT treatment groups experienced significantly less recidivism than control groups, resulting in an overall decrease in recidivism by 8-16 percentage points. In addition to the broad support for the effectiveness of CBT treatments, meta-analyses have also provided support for the following claims: (1) CBT treatment appears to be more effective at reducing rearrest and reincarceration for moderate to high-risk offenders than for low risk offenders [62, 64]; (2) both CBT treatments emphasizing cognitive skills/cognitive restructuring and approaches emphasizing moral teachings and reasoning significantly decreased recidivism [63]; (3) CBT programming quality and dosage (measured in hours of treatment delivered rather than amount of time between first and last session) increase the effect size of treatment [62, 65].

Multiple studies have reinforced the importance of increased treatment dosage when utilizing CBT in criminal justice populations. A meta-analysis of 200 studies conducted between 1950 and 1995 with criminal justice samples found that a minimum of 100 hours of treatment was needed to reduce recidivism for juvenile offenders and suggested many programs may utilize effective treatments and technology but fail to reduce recidivism due to a lack of resources needed to provide necessary treatment dosages [66]. Based upon this earlier work, Sperber et al. [67] conducted a study of 689 adult male offenders successfully discharged from a Community-Based Correctional Facility to investigate the impact of dosage on recidivism. The results of this study further support the importance of providing a higher level of treatment dosage to high-risk offenders: the difference in recidivism for high-risk offenders was 24 percentage points between medium dosage (100-199 hours of treatment) and high dosage (200+ hours of treatment). In a replication of the Sperber [67] study, Markarios et al. [68] found the observed relationship between dosage and recidivism to be moderated by risk. This re-emphasized the importance of providing high doses of treatment to high-risk offenders, but also introduced the first evidence that high doses of treatment may increase rates of recidivism for low-risk offenders [68]. This suggests that limited resources may be allocated differently depending upon the risk level of the individual, possibly improving outcomes for both high-risk and low-risk offenders.

4.2 Mindfulness

Although mindfulness has existed within religious and spiritual traditions which long predate the study of psychology, it is only relatively recently that mindfulness practices have been integrated into clinical psychological practice and subjected to empirical tests [69]. Cognitive behavioral therapies rooted in providing patients with psychoeducation and skills training related to contemplative practices (practices which broadly fall under the umbrella of mindfulness) have been growing in influence and popularity within clinical psychology since Jon Kabat-Zinn developed Mindfulness Based Stress Reduction (MBSR) in the late 1980s and early 1990s [70]. In 1990, Kabat-Zinn published *Full Catastrophe Living*, a book introducing his landmark approach to mindfulness-based treatment, in which he defined mindfulness as "Paying attention in a particular way: on purpose, in the present moment, nonjudgmentally" [71]. In the 30 years since, growing interest in mindfulness-based therapies led to the development of multiple therapies including Mindfulness-Based Cognitive Therapy (MBCT), Mindfulness-Based Relapse Prevention (MBRP), and Metacognitive Therapy (MCT). Further evidence-based treatments have emerged which, while not exclusively mindfulness-based, integrate mindfulness-based processes into the broader cognitive behavioral therapy model to promote positive behavioral changes. Two of the most well-known of these integrative approaches are Dialectical Behavior Therapy (DBT) and Acceptance and Commitment Therapy (ACT).

Within both mindfulness-based and integrative treatments, mindfulness is utilized as a teachable skill to improve an individual's awareness of the present moment. This increased awareness of the present is purported to increase the person's ability to recognize both the salient features of their environment and how they are reacting to that environment in the moment. Mindfulness as a component of therapeutic treatment has been demonstrated to improve behavioral regulation, decrease emotional reactivity as well as psychological symptoms, and lead to increases in subjective well-being [72]. In the context of relapse prevention or emotion regulation, mindfulness skills are meant to increase the likelihood that an individual will notice and attend to internal stimuli (thoughts, emotions, cravings, physical sensations) and external stimuli (environments contributing to or worsening the problem), signaling the need to deploy behavioral regulation and coping strategies. This is a particularly salient skill for individuals in community corrections, as promoting increased self-regulation is an important component of treatment focused on rehabilitation [73].

Both mindfulness-based approaches and integrative approaches have a broad base of support for diverse presenting problems, the scope of which is beyond this chapter. However, there are specific uses for these treatments which have a more direct bearing on the treatment of presenting problems relevant to community corrections populations. Mindfulness-based treatments more broadly defined have modest evidence supporting their use in the treatment of mood disorders, chronic pain, and substance use disorders [74, 75]. MBRP in particular appears promising for the treatment of substance use disorders; early evidence comparing the outcomes of cognitively-based RPT to MBRP at 12-month follow-up suggests MBRP may be more effective in the long-term, showing reduced drug use and heavy drinking [76, 77].

Marsha Linehan [78] developed DBT, originally published under the title *Cognitive Behavioral Treatment of Borderline Personality Disorder*, as a treatment modality for chronically suicidal adults. Since its publication, DBT has accumulated strong research support for the treatment of Borderline Personality Disorder [79–81], and it is used in a variety of contexts to provide psychoeducation and skills training to address many of the same presenting problems as the CBT treatments discussed earlier; modules include mindfulness, interpersonal effectiveness training, distress tolerance, and emotion regulation [82].

In a review of transdiagnostic applications for DBT treatment, Ritschel et al. [82] describe the overall goals of DBT-based substance abuse treatment as:

1. teach emotion regulation skills that reduce the need to engage in dysfunctional emotion regulation strategies,

2. reduce behaviors and obstacles that significantly interfere with quality of life and maintain drug-seeking behavior, and

3. promote more skillful behaviors that would allow individuals to function adaptively and create a life worth living (p. 115).

There appears to be a gap in the literature specifically linking the use of DBT with community corrections populations. For example, a review of literature supporting the use of DBT in forensic settings found only 2 out of the 19 studies sampled forensic outpatient populations; of these, one was a feasibility study not reporting outcome data [83]. DBT's effectiveness, however, has been demonstrated for clients in forensic settings more generally and with mental health problems relevant to community corrections populations such as depression, substance use disorders, aggression, and violence [80, 83–85].

Although ACT was originally developed under the moniker Comprehensive Distancing, it emerged in its current form in the late 1990s [86]. ACT emphasizes identifying both a clients' values (what gives their life meaning, purpose, and vitality), as well as how their behavior is either bringing them closer to or farther from their values. As an integrative treatment, ACT also has marked similarities to the CBT treatments discussed earlier, with an emphasis on helping clients notice and identify their own thoughts and emotions, as well as promoting overall coping skills and the workability of chosen behaviors.

Since its publication, ACT has accumulated a significant body of evidence supporting its use in the treatment of a variety of disorders relevant to corrections settings. The use of ACT to improve willingness of drug and alcohol counselors to learn and apply evidence-based pharmacotherapy has been indicated; this is an important intervention given the stigmatization of pharmacotherapy in corrections settings despite its effectiveness in treating presenting problems such as substance use, stress, smoking cessation, chronic pain, and depression [87–89]. Similar to the literature surrounding the use of DBT, there is currently a gap in the literature surrounding ACT's use specifically with community corrections populations. However, an overview of the approach's applications in incarcerated populations is available in *ACT for the Incarcerated*, within the *Forensic CBT: A Handbook for Clinical Practice* [90].

4.3 Social skills training

Social skills training is a form of behavioral training and is defined as improving social relationships by building both verbal and nonverbal interpersonal skills. Originally created in the 1970s, social skills training was designed to increase socially acceptable skills, improve interpersonal skills (e.g., cooperation, empathy), and decrease socially unacceptable and harmful behaviors (e.g., aggression, exploitation) [91]. Social skills training has been used for a wide variety of psychological disorders in the general population: it has been used with children, people with schizophrenia, people with social anxiety disorder, and people with autism (e.g., [91–94]). Overall, social skills training has been used widely to increase social competence across many populations. Presentation of this therapy does not differ substantially in correctional populations; however, in community corrections, the major targets of treatment include assertiveness training, active listening, and learning to read non-verbal communication cues. These skills are taught because deficits in these areas have been shown to be precursors to aggression and conflict in this population.

Due to the high rates of comorbidity in community corrections, social skills training is often used as a supplement to other therapies, such as cognitive-behavioral therapy, and is rarely used in isolation. Social skills training begins by identifying an individual's social skills deficits and working with the individual based on their personal goals and needs [95, 96]. After goals are set, people are given psychoeducation about the social skill that is being targeted, including why it is important to learn [95, 96]. The social skills are then modelled by the therapist and practiced though role-playing within sessions [95, 96]. Use and practice of the behavior is then reinforced and given corrective feedback by the therapist. Homework assignments are also used to help generalize the skills to the clients' other relationships. In summary, social skills training is a multi-step process to create effective social skills based off an individual's needs and is adjusted based off an individual's social growth.

Social skills training has been successfully used in corrections populations as a part of treatment protocols when working with offenders. Studies indicate there are deficiencies in offenders' social skills and competence, including a lack of empathy for others, poor interpretation of social cues, and deficits in interpersonal intimacy (particularly with sex offenders) [97–99]. These social skills deficits increase the likelihood of participation in antisocial behavior. Social skills training in offender populations often focuses on how to give positive feedback and negative feedback, as well as accepting negative feedback [100, 101]. Skills addressed also include social problem-solving, recognizing non-verbal cues in order to avoid misattribution of hostile intent, and improving one's ability to reject pressure from peers to use illicit drugs or commit crimes [100–102]. Overall, social skills training with offenders can have multiple learning goals dependent upon offender-specific needs.

Social skills deficits are especially notable in sex offenders, juvenile offenders, and offenders with severe mental illness or comorbid mental illnesses [97, 102]. These populations have been popular targets for social skills training due to empathetic deficits and low functioning upon re-entry from prison. It is important to target these low functioning offenders in order achieve adequate social support upon reentry into the community [102]. Targeting of these populations in research allows for therapists to understand what populations are most important to target with supplemental social skills training.

Research on the effectiveness of social skills training has provided mixed results for corrections populations. There are concerns as to whether social skills training, when presented in isolation, has any notable impact on recidivism levels and other criminogenic outcomes, with most studies finding social skills training to have similar recidivism levels to treatment as usual or control groups [61, 103]. Some findings indicate social skills training has been successful in improving self-esteem and social competence for both sex offenders and general population offenders [103, 104]. Participants in social skills training also indicate a self-reported reduction in social problems and improved responses on role playing measures [105, 106]. Overall, it appears social skills training alone has little impact upon criminogenic outcomes but likely creates personal successes for offenders.

4.4 Pharmacotherapy

When substance abuse interventions are supplemented by pharmacotherapy, it is typically referred to in the literature as medication assisted treatment (MAT). Many of the studies conducted on the effectiveness and utilization of MAT in criminal justice populations have focused on the treatment of opioid and alcohol use disorders, given the high prevalence of these disorders in the U.S. corrections and community corrections populations [107]. Typical pharmacological treatment of alcohol use disorder involves the use of drugs disulfiram and naltrexone, while opioid use disorder involves use of methadone, buprenorphine, and naltrexone [108, 109].

Disulfiram has been FDA approved for the treatment of alcohol dependence for nearly 70 years, although clinical trials examining its effectiveness have shown mixed results. When taking disulfiram, patients typically experience strong negative physical reactions to consuming alcohol, reducing alcohol consumption and prolonging remission, but the drug is easily discontinued and difficulties in maintaining medication adherence have historically limited its effectiveness [110, 111]. In 1994, naltrexone, an opioid antagonist, was approved by the FDA for treating patients with alcohol dependency. A review of 50 randomized clinical trials found that naltrexone treatment's effect on heavy drinking was moderate, on average reducing treatment groups' risk of continued heavy drinking to 83% of the risk observed in placebo groups [112]. Overall, naltrexone has been found to be a safe and effective treatment for promoting controlled drinking behavior and reducing the risk of heavy drinking, but its effectiveness is also limited by low treatment adherence [113, 114]. Although treatment adherence is low with both of these medications, it appears the effectiveness of their treatment can be significantly increased by integrating patient monitoring strategies and compliance measurements into the treatment process, especially in combination with CBT [110, 115].

Pharmacotherapy for opioid use disorder is an effective adjunct treatment which reduces the likelihood of continued substance use, overdose, and recidivism in both incarcerated and community corrections participants [116, 117]. Naltrexone for opioid use is more commonly delivered in an injectable delayed release form, which has been demonstrated to significantly decrease opioid use, relapse, and overdose at

6-month follow-up [118]. Methadone and buprenorphine maintenance treatments are both methods of treating opioid withdrawal and are used in MAT. Methadone appears to be more effective in MAT when introduced while incarcerated and continued on an outpatient basis in community corrections settings [119, 120]. Both medications appear to be roughly equally effective in their ability to significantly lower risk of continued use, relapse, re-arrest, or re-incarceration; however, buprenorphine patients were significantly less likely than methadone patients to voluntarily withdraw from treatment [121].

In spite of the evidence suggesting MAT's effectiveness in serving offenders with substance use disorders, it appears to be underutilized nationally. Robinson and Adinoff [122] point out that both patients and providers experience confusion surrounding the efficacy and effectiveness of pharmacotherapy for the treatment of people with substance use disorders. In the United States, in both adult and pediatric populations, it appears that misinformation and stigma contribute to underutilization by limiting the likelihood that providers will even prescribe pharmacotherapy for patients with substance use disorder [122–124]. A survey of 170 providers, working in diverse contexts, found that approximately 20% of providers never prescribed these medications [125].

A study reviewing policies and practices of 50 criminal justice agencies in the United States (across 14 states) found that 83% of prisons and jails surveyed reported offering MAT on a limited basis only (e.g., detoxification during withdrawal only, or for the maintenance of pregnant women experiencing withdrawal but not for offenders more broadly; [107]). A national survey of 103 drug courts found that approximately half of all drug courts responding to the survey had policies and procedures explicitly banning MAT [126]. Opposition to MAT (political, judicial, and administrative) for treating offenders with substance use disorders appears to play a significant role in the inconsistent use of MAT in corrections and community corrections settings, due to stigmatization and general lack of understanding [107, 127]. Traditional training has been found to be minimally effective in changing the attitudes of corrections staff and treatment providers opposed to MAT, and the development and deployment of targeted interventions addressing this issue is a recent focus of community corrections research [128, 129].

4.5 Smoking cessation

Although tobacco is not an illicit substance and its use is not typically associated with committing serious or violent criminal offenses, there is substantial evidence suggesting smoking cessation treatment may positively impact treatment outcomes for other addictions by reducing overall substance use and increasing the likelihood of maintaining sobriety [130]. For example, individuals who quit smoking report reduced cravings for other stimulant drugs [131] and are less likely to experience future incidence of substance use disorders [132]. Further, smoking cessation treatment completed in conjunction with treatment for other addictions has shown to increase the likelihood of maintaining long-term abstinence from illicit drugs by 25% [133]. It has been hypothesized that successfully quitting smoking may facilitate changing other addiction-related habits. Unfortunately, despite widespread evidence of positive effects and virtually no reliable evidence of negative effects [130], smoking cessation treatment for substance addicted individuals has largely been neglected.

Over the past several decades, the proportion of cigarette smokers in the United States has steadily decreased to less than 16% [134]. However, smoking prevalence among individuals involved with the criminal justice system has remained consistently high (70-80%) constituting roughly 12% of all smokers in the U.S. [135].

Even individuals in the juvenile justice system smoke at a rate 40% greater than their peers in the general population [136]. Smoking remains a leading cause of preventable death and disability in the U.S., and individuals in the criminal justice system are at much greater risk for experiencing severe health conditions associated with smoking, including cardiovascular disease, cancer, circulatory and respiratory problems, kidney and liver problems, and diabetes, all of which may lead to premature death. Although the average age of individuals in the criminal justice system is in the mid-30's, many already report experiencing smoking-related illnesses and diseases. Further, individuals in community corrections are less likely to receive consistent medical attention to address such illnesses due to poverty and limited healthcare access encountered upon release.

The majority of prisons and jails across the country have banned smoking; however, almost all inmates released into community correctional supervision from smoke-free facilities resume smoking [137]. Widespread smoking bans in jails and prisons also limit the availability of smoking cessation treatment. Even when some forms of treatment are available, such as nicotine replacement, they are often priced so high that many inmates do not have access. Although smoking bans in correctional facilities may be a legitimate effort to aid in smoking cessation, being forced to stop smoking is not synonymous with quitting smoking, which may explain the high number of individuals released to community corrections who return to the habit.

Consequently, efforts to reduce smoking in criminal justice populations are primarily focused on community corrections, although the efforts have not been vast. Generally, smoking cessation treatment does not target criminal justice populations despite the high prevalence and associated health issues which are of great cost to the individuals and their communities. The few studies that have explored smoking cessation in criminal justice individuals have determined that more research is needed to understand the nuances associated with tailoring smoking cessation treatment to this population and its subgroups [135]. There is also an increased likelihood that those in the criminal justice system experience comorbid substance abuse issues, mental health issues, and poverty, all of which must be considered in determining the appropriateness and accessibility of treatment.

The interventions that have been studied in this population have, in some cases, been modified from traditional smoking cessation treatments, which vary widely. Some such interventions have shown to work well in certain subsets of the general population and poorly in others [138], which may further complicate the process of tailoring these treatments to individuals in community corrections. A common smoking cessation pharmacotherapy is Nicotine Replacement Therapy (NRT), which is intended to be used in place of tobacco products to relieve withdrawal symptoms and craving. When used in criminal justice populations, NRT has been successful in initiating smoking reduction even for individuals who were initially unmotivated to quit [139]. Varenicline is another leading pharmacological treatment that interferes with nicotine receptor stimulation and reduces craving. However, the cost is high and there is not presently a generic form, so it is likely not an easily accessible option for individuals in community corrections. Antidepressants such as nortriptyline and bupropion have also been utilized as smoking cessation pharmacotherapies and may be valuable for criminal justice involved individuals, as this population is at higher risk for experiencing mental illness, including mood disorders. Bupropion specifically has been shown to improve smoking cessation rates in community corrections individuals who take the medication reliably [140].

Some of the behavioral interventions utilized in smoking cessation treatment are adapted from broader therapies, such as Cognitive Behavioral Therapy (CBT), whereby individuals are taught to recognize specific circumstances that precede or trigger smoking and learn cognitive and behavioral strategies to effectively cope with those triggers. The WISE intervention (Working Inside for Smoking Elimination), which utilizes techniques from CBT and other empirically supported therapies, specifically targets inmates who are approaching discharge and has shown to reduce smoking relapse upon release from smoke-free prisons [141]. Mood Management (MM) Training was designed to prevent smoking relapse, and like CBT, it aims to identify triggers associated with smoking and to develop coping strategies. One study that adapted MM for a correctional population found it to be an effective smoking cessation treatment when combined with NRT [142]. One of the only known interventions that specifically targets smoking cessation in community corrections populations is DIMENSIONS: Tobacco Free Program, which was developed by Arkansas Community Correction (ACC) along with the University of Colorado's Behavioral Health & Wellness Program. The DIMENSIONS program is based on techniques and philosophy derived from tobacco cessation programs that target mental health populations and aims to provide holistic community-based support for individuals in community corrections. Results of the program are promising with the majority of individuals having exhibited decreased tobacco use after completing half the program, and those who completed the full program decreased tobacco use by at least 50% [143].

Along with a dearth of specifically targeted behavioral interventions, poverty and generally inadequate healthcare make even basic pharmacotherapies inaccessible for many individuals in community corrections. Unfortunately, lack of access to healthcare and negative attitudes about healthcare may contribute to exhibiting poor medication adherence, creating even more challenges in treatment. Medication adherence has shown to be the most powerful predictor of successful smoking cessation, and it is also a common issue in the community corrections population. However, individuals who have utilized pharmacological treatments in the past are more likely to succeed in subsequent cessation attempts [140]. Even short-term exposure to smoking cessation medication may be beneficial in increasing the likelihood of adherence in the future. Individuals who utilize smoking cessation medication in the presence of a treatment provider are also more likely to adhere to treatment even if the provider is minimally trained [144]. This is promising for individuals in community corrections, as they may not have consistent access to more highly trained professionals.

Smoking cessation treatment for individuals in community corrections is rife with challenges that impede success. Despite high rates of smoking in this population, as well as high interest in quitting, accessible interventions are sparse. Further research examining the effectiveness of certain interventions for individuals in community corrections, as well as methods of increasing accessibility, are certainly necessary. Future studies should also explore means of improving medication adherence to increase successful cessation. Regardless of differences in treatment effectiveness in certain subgroups, it is suspected that increasing adherence to medication will improve treatment effectiveness for the entire community corrections population.

5. Conclusions

Historically, the treatment of substance use disorders in U.S. correctional populations has been slow to take hold. Traditional models of incarceration focused almost entirely on punitive sentencing with little afterthought devoted to rehabilitation efforts. These approaches failed to reduce recidivism. Diversion rehabilitation models, particularly the Risk-Need-Responsivity model [12], which divert offenders from incarceration and provide tailored treatment in the community, have been shown to reduce recidivism rates both in research and practice. Popular implementations include TASC, Drug Court, and Mental Health Court, among others. Due to the high rates of substance abuse in these populations, most programs offer some form of substance abuse treatment. Different forms of Cognitive Behavioral Therapy (i.e., ART, SSC, MRT, R&R, RPT, and T4C) are the most commonly employed and likely have the most empirical support as well. Furthermore, substance abuse treatment in community corrections is typically complicated by high rates of comorbidity, as well as other factors such as poverty, unemployment, and inconsistent housing, which only serve to further complicate treatment [9]. As a result, these versions of therapy are often longer and more intensive than traditional forms of CBT. The cumulative product is an increased dosage and specificity of psychotherapy that had never been seen in U.S. corrections previously.

While increased substance abuse and mental health treatment are worthy of praise, especially considering the history of treatment in corrections, this same level of treatment would not be heralded as progress in a hospital or more controlled medical setting. There are multiple targets of treatment, such as traumatic brain injury and other organic issues that occur at a high base rate in both correctional and CC populations, and these diseases go almost wholly unaddressed [8, 145]. Furthermore, while the therapies employed in correction and CC specifically are comprehensive and span a multitude of presenting problems, there is a complete absence of dismantling studies to identify meaningful mechanisms of action. Furthermore, CBT based therapies are often supplemented by other forms of therapy, such as Mindfulness, social skills training, pharmacotherapy, or smoking cessation. The literature provides less support for using these other forms of therapy without some form of CBT. Therapies could likely be streamlined to focus more on the most meaningful components. Additionally, pharmacotherapy and smoking cessation can both have a positive impact on recovery but are highly underutilized in CC programs. The incorporation of treatment and therapy into the legal system has yielded very promising results, but these approaches are still in development and many have only come into existence over the past two decades. Future work needs to identify additional targets of treatment within this population, as well as streamline therapies to better emphasize the more important components.

A final component in need of change is continuity of care. The constitutional mandate to provide healthcare to prisoners does not extend to those supervised in the community. Transition from confinement back into the community is an extremely sensitive period with elevated homicide, relapse, and suicide rates [146, 147]. Furthermore, transitions from jail to CC and back to jail are often common for individuals who commit minor drug offenses, and this is especially true for individuals with limited criminal justice involvement. This period represents a window of opportunity for intervention, but coordination of treatment will require the cooperation of the treatment community and the legal system. Coordination at the national and/or state levels would likely be needed to standardize treatment and communication between jail and prison and CC providers as well as to provide consistent funding. This would likely come at considerable cost, yet the legal system in its current form was estimated to cost 182 billion in 2017 [148]. A more effective system better able to promote rehabilitation would certainly be better for offenders and may be more cost effective in the long run.

Author details

Jacob D. Armstrong, Amy Bauman, Krystal J. Moroney and C. Brendan Clark*
Wichita State University, Wichita, United States

*Address all correspondence to: c.brendan.clark@wichita.edu

References

[1] Walmsley, R. (2003). Global incarceration and prison trends. *Forum on Crime and Society, 3*(1), 65-78.

[2] U.S. Department of Justice; Bureau of Justice Statistics. (2018). Correctional Populations in the United States, 2016 (NJC Publication No. 251211). Retrieved from ttps://www.bjs.gov/content/pub/pdf/cpus16.pdf

[3] Bureau of Justice Statistics (2021). *Terms & Definitions: Community Corrections (Probation and Parole)*. Retrieved from https://www.bjs.gov/index.cfm?ty=tdtp&tid=15

[4] National Institute of Justice (2021). *Community Corrections*. Retrieved from https://nij.ojp.gov/topics/corrections/community-corrections

[5] Mumola, C. J., & Karberg, J. C. (2007). *Drug use and dependence, state and federal prisoners, 2004.* Retrieved from Bureau of Justice Statistics https://www.bjs.gov/content/pub/pdf/dudsfp04.pdf (Original work published 2006).

[6] Bronson, J., Stroop, J., Zimmer, S., & Berzofsky, M. (2017). Drug use, dependence, and abuse among state prisoners and jail inmates, 2007-2009. Washington, DC: United States Department of Justice, Office of Juvenile Justice and Delinquency Prevention.

[7] James, D. J., & Glaze, L. E. (2006, December). Mental health problems of prison and jail inmates. Retrieved fromhttp://bjs.ojp.usdoj.gov/index.cfm?ty=pbdetail&iid=789

[8] Kaba, F., Diamond, P., Haque, A., MacDonald, R., & Venters, H. (2014). Traumatic brain injury among newly admitted adolescents in the New York City jail system. Journal of Adolescent Health, 54(5), 615-617.

[9] Clark, C. B., McCullumsmith, C. B., Redmond, N., Hardy, S., Waesche, M. C., Osula, G., & Cropsey, K. L. (2013). Factors associated with rapid failure in a Treatment Alternatives for Safer Communities (TASC) program. *Journal of substance abuse treatment*, *45*(4), 376-380.

[10] Bureau of Justice Statistics. (2013). Recidivism. Retrieved from: http://www.bjs.gov/index.cfm?ty=tp&tid=17

[11] United States Sentencing Commission, (2016). Recidivism Among Federal Offenders: A Comprehensive Overview. Retrieved from: https://www.ussc.gov/sites/default/files/pdf/research-and-publications/research-publications/2016/recidivism_overview.pdf

[12] Andrews, D. A., & Bonta, J. (2010). Rehabilitating criminal justice policy and practice. Psychology, Public Policy, and Law, 16(1), 39.

[13] Anglin, M. D., Longshore, D., & Turner, S. (1999). Treatment alternatives to street crime: An evaluation of five programs. *Criminal Justice and Behavior, 26*(2), 168-195. doi:10.1177/0093854899026002002

[14] Roque, L., & Lurigio, A. J. (2009). An outcome evaluation of a treatment readiness group program for probationers with substance use problems. *Journal of Offender Rehabilitation, 48*(8), 744-757. https://doi.org/10.1080/10509670903288046

[15] Inciardi, J. A. (2008). The war on drugs IV: *The continuing saga of the mysteries and miseries of intoxication, addiction, crime, and public policy*. Boston, MA: Pearson/Allyn and Bacon.

[16] Pinker, S. (2011). The better angels of our nature: Why violence has declined. New York, NY: Viking.

[17] Weidner, R. R., & Schultz, J. (2019). Examining the relationship between U.S. incarceration rates and population health at the county level. SSM – Population Health, 9. https://doi.org/10.1016/j.ssmph.2019.100466

[18] Martinson, R. (1974). What works? — Questions and answers about prison reform. *The Public Interest, 35,* 22-54.

[19] Sarre, R. (2001). Beyond 'what works?'A 25-year jubilee retrospective of Robert Martinsons famous article. Australian & New Zealand Journal of Criminology, 34(1), 38-46.

[20] Andrews, D. A., & Bonta, J. (1995). *The Level of Service Inventory–Revised*. Toronto, Ontario, Canada: Multi-Health Systems.

[21] Mecca, A. (1978). TASC (treatment alternatives to street crime): Historical perspective and future implications. *Journal of Offender Rehabilitation, 2*(3), 279-294. doi:10.1080/10509674.19 78.9963563

[22] Ventura, L. A., & Lambert, E. G. (2004). Recidivism 12 months after TASC. *Journal of Offender Rehabilitation, 39*(1), 63-82. doi:10.1300/J076v39n01_04

[23] Marlowe, D. B. (2003). Integrating substance abuse treatment and criminal justice supervision. *Science & Practice Perspectives, 2*(1), 4-14. doi:10.1151/spp03214

[24] Mauser, E., Van Stelle, K. R., & Moberg, D. P. (2016;1994;). The economic impact of diverting substance-abusing offenders into treatment. *Crime and Delinquency, 40*(4), 568-588. doi:10.1177/0011128794040004006

[25] ***Nissen, L. B., & Kraft, M. K. (2007). The evolution of substance abuse treatment in juvenile justice. *Journal of Social Work Practice in the Addictions, 7*(3), 51-71.

[26] Maume, M. O., Lanier, C., & DeVall, K. (2018). The effect of treatment completion on recidivism among TASC program clients. *International Journal of Offender Therapy and Comparative Criminology, 62*(15), 4776-4795. doi:10.1177/0306624X18780421

[27] Drake, R. E., O'Neal, E. L., & Wallach, M. A. (2008). A systematic review of psychosocial research on psychosocial interventions for people with co-occurring severe mental and substance use disorders. *Journal of Substance Abuse Treatment, 34*(1), 123-138. https://doi.org/10.1016/j.jsat.2007.01.011

[28] Cooper, C. (1997). *1997 Drug Court Survey Report: Executive Summary*. Washington, D.C.: Drug Court Clearinghouse and Technical Assistance Project, American University.

[29] Belenko, S. (1998). Research on drug courts: A critical review. *National Drug Court Institute Review, 1*(1), 1-26.

[30] Belenko, S. (2001). Research on drug courts: A critical review, 2001 update. *National Drug Court Institute Review, 1*(1), 1-63.

[31] Shaw, M., & Robinson, K. (1999). Reports on recent drug court research. *National Drug Court Institute Review, 2*(1), 107-119.

[32] U.S. General Accounting Office. (1997). *Drug Courts: Overview of Growth, Characteristics, and Results*. Washington, D.C.: U.S. General Accounting Office

[33] Hora, P. F., Schma, W. G., & Rosenthal, J. T. A. (1998-1999). Therapeutic jurisprudence and the drug treatment court movement: Revolutionizing the criminal justice system's response to drug abuse and crime in America. *Notre Dame Law Review, 74,* 439-538. doi:10.1300/J160v07n03_04

[34] Goldkamp, J. S. (1999-2000). The drug court response: Issues and implications for justice. *Albany Law Review, 63,* 923-962.

[35] U.S. Department of Justice. Drug Courts. Retrieved from Office of Justice Programs https://www.ojp.gov/pdffiles1/nij/238527.pdf

[36] Carey, S. M., Finigan, M. W., & Pukstas, K. (2008). Exploring the Key Components of Drug Courts: A Comparative Study of 18 Adult Drug Courts on Practices, Outcomes and Costs: Executive Summary. Retrieved from U.S. Department of Justice https://citeseerx.ist.psu.edu/viewdoc/download?doi=10.1.1.160.2316&rep=rep1&type=pdf

[37] Marlowe, D. B., Festinger, D. S., Lee, P. A., Dugosh, K. L., & Benasutti, K. M. (2006). Matching judicial supervision to clients' risk status in drug court. Crime & Delinquency, 52(1), 52-76. https://doi.org/10.1177/0011128705281746

[38] National Association of Drug Court Professionals; Drug Court Standards Committee. (2004). *Defining drug courts: The key components.* (Drug Courts Program Office Grant No. 96–DC–MX–K001).

[39] Zweig, J. M., Rossman, S. B., & Roman, J. K. (2011). *The Multi-Site Adult Drug Court Evaluation Volume 2: What's Happening with Drug Courts? A Portrait of Adult Drug Courts in 2004.* Washington DC, United States: Urban Institute Justice Policy Center.

[40] Mitchell, O., Wilson, D. B., Eggers, A., MacKenzie, D. L. (2012). Assessing the effectiveness of drug courts on recidivism: A meta-analytic review of traditional and non-traditional drug courts. *Journal of Criminal Justice, 40*(1), 60-71. doi: 10.1016/j.jcrimjus.2011.11.009

[41] Wilson, D. B., Mitchell, O., & Mackenzie, D. L. (2006). A systematic review of drug court effects on recidivism. *Journal of Experimental Criminology, 2,* 459-487. doi: 10.1007/s11292-006-9019-4

[42] Fulkerson, A., Keena, L. D., & O'Brien, E. (2012). Understanding success and nonsuccess in the drug court. *International Journal of Offender Therapy and Comparative Criminology, 57*(10), 1297-1316. doi: 10.1177/0306624X12447774

[43] SAMHSA (2020). Treatment Court Locators. https://www.samhsa.gov/gains-center/treatment-court-locators

[44] Wolff, N. (2002). Courts as therapeutic agents: Thinking past the novelty of mental health courts. *Journal of the American Academy of Psychiatry and the Law Online*, *30*(3), 431.

[45] Redlich, A. D., Steadman, H. J., Monahan, J., Robbins, P. C., & Petrila, J. (2006). Patterns of practice in mental health courts: A national survey. *Law and Human Behavior*, *30*(3), 347-362.

[46] Sarteschi, C. M., Vaughn, M. G., & Kim, K. (2011). Assessing the effectiveness of mental health courts: A quantitative review. Journal of Criminal Justice, 39(1), 12-20.

[47] Steadman, H. J., Redlich, A., Callahan, L., Robbins, P. C., & Vesselinov, R. (2011). Effect of mental health courts on arrests and jail days: A multisite study. Archives of general psychiatry, 68(2), 167-172.

[48] Honegger, L. N. (2015). Does the evidence support the case for mental health courts? A review of the literature. *Law and Human Behavior, 39*(5), 478-488. https://doi.org/10.1037/lhb0000141

[49] Lowder, E. M., Desmarais, S. L., & Baucom, D. J. (2016). Recidivism following mental health court exit: Between and within-group

comparisons. Law and Human Behavior, 40(2), 118-127. https://doi.org/10.1037/lhb0000168

[50] Dirks-Linhorst, P. A., Kondrat, D., Linhorst, D. M., & Morani, N. (2013). Factors associated with mental health court nonparticipation and negative termination. *Justice Quarterly*, *30*(4), 681-710.

[51] Callahan, L., Steadman, H. J., Tillman, S., & Vesselinov, R. (2013). A multi-site study of the use of sanctions and incentives in mental health courts. *Law and Human Behavior, 37*(1), 1-9. https://doi.org/10.1037/h0093989

[52] Pratt, C., Koerner, J., Alexander, M. J., Yanos, P. T., & Kopelovich, S. L. (2013). Predictors of criminal justice outcomes among mental health courts participants: The role of perceived coercion and subjective mental health recovery. *International journal of forensic mental health*, *12*(2), 116-125.

[53] Barnes, G., Hyatt, J., & Sherman, L. (2017). Even a little bit helps. An implementation and experimental evaluation of cognitive-behavioral therapy for high risk probationers. Criminal Justice and Behavior, 44, 611-630. DOI: 10.1177/0093854816673862

[54] Quinn, T. & Quinn, E. (2015). The effect of cognitive-behavioral therapy on driving while intoxicated recidivism. Journal of Drug Issue, 45(4), 431-446. DOI: 10.1177/00220426 15603390

[55] Milkman, H. & Wanberg, K., (2007) Cognitive Behavioral Treatment: A review and discussion for corrections professionals. US Department of Justice, National Institute of Corrections., May 2007. NIC Accession Number 021657

[56] Goldstein, A.P., & Glick. B. (1987). Aggression Replacement Training: A comprehensive intervention for aggressive youth. Champaign, IL: Research Press.

[57] Little, G. L., & Robinson, K. D. (1988). Moral Reconation Therapy: A systematic step-by-step treatment system for treatment resistant clients. Psychological Reports, 62(1), 135-151. https://doi.org/10.2466/pr0.1988.62.1.135

[58] Ross, R. R., & Fabiano, E. A. (1985). *Time to Think: A Cognitive Model of Delinquency Prevention and Offender Rehabiliation.* Johnson City, Tennessee: Institute of Social Sciences and Arts.

[59] Parks, G. A., & Marlatt, G. A. (1999a). Relapse prevention therapy for substance-abusing offenders: A cognitive-behavioral approach in what works. Strategic solutions: The international community corrections association examines substance abuse, 161-233.

[60] Bush, J., Glick, B., & Taymans, J. (1997). Thinking for a change: Integrated cognitive behavior change program. National Institute of Corrections. Washington, DC: U.S. Department of Justice.

[61] Pearson, F. S., Lipton, D. S., Cleland, C. M., & Yee, D. S. (2002). The effects of behavioral/cognitive-behavioral programs on recidivism. *Crime & Delinquency*, *48*(3), 476-496.

[62] Lipsey, M.W., Landenberger, N. L., & Wilson, S. J. (2007). Effects of cognitive behavioral programs for criminal offenders. Campbell Systematic Reviews, 6, 1-27. 10.4073/csr.2007.6

[63] Wilson, D. B., Bouffard, L. A., & MacKenzie, D. L. (2005). A quantitative review of structured, group-oriented, cognitive-behavioral programs for offenders. Criminal Justice and Behavior, 32(2), 172-204.

[64] Lowenkamp, C. T., Latessa, E. J., & Holsinger, A. M. (2006). The risk principle in action: What have we

learned from 13,676 offenders and 97 correctional programs? Crime & Delinquency, 52 (1), 77-93.

[65] Kroner, D. G., & Takahashi, M. (2012). Every session counts: The differential impact of previous programmes and current programme dosage on offender recidivism. Legal and Criminological Psychology, 17, 136-150.

[66] Lipsey, M. W. (1999). Can intervention rehabilitate serious delinquents? The ANNALS of the American Academy of Political and Social Science, 564, 142-166.

[67] Sperber, K., Latessa, E., & Makarios, M. (2013). Examining the interaction between level of risk and dosage of treatment. Criminal Justice and Behavior, 40 (3), 338-348.

[68] Makarios, M., Sperber, K., & Latessa, E. (2014). Treatment dosage and the risk principle: A refinement and extension. Journal of Offender Rehabilitation, 53, 334-350.

[69] Hayes, S. C. (2002). Acceptance, mindfulness, and science. Clinical Psychology: Science and Practice, 9(1), 101-106. https://doi.org/10.1093/clipsy.9.1.101

[70] Hayes, S. C., Villatte, M., Levin, M., & Hildebrandt, M. (2011). Open, aware, and active: Contextual approaches as emerging trend in the behavioral and cognitive therapies. *The Annual Review of Clinical Psychology, 7,* 141-168. https://doi.org/10.1146/annurev-clinpsy-032210-104449

[71] Kabat-Zinn, J. (2013). *Full Catastrophe Living.* New York, United States: Bantam.

[72] Keng, S-L., Smoski, M. J., & Robins, C. J. (2011). Effects of mindfulness on psychological health: A review of empirical studies. *Clinical Psychology Review, 31*(6), 1041-1056. https://doi.org/10.1016/j.cpr.2011.04.006.

[73] Dafe, T., & Stermac, L., (2013). Mindfulness meditation as an adjunct approach to treatment within the correctional system. *Journal of Offender Rehabilitation, 52,* 198-216. https://doi.org/10.1080/10509674.2012.752774

[74] Grossman, P., Niemann, L., Schmidt, S., & Walach, H. 2004. Mindfulness-based stress reduction and health benefits: A meta-analysis. *Journal of Psychosomatic Research, 57*(1), 35-43. https://doi.org/10.1016/S0022-3999(03)00573-7

[75] Zgierska, A., Rabago, D., Chawla, N., Kushner, L., Koehler, R., & Marlatt, A. (2009). Mindfulness meditation for substance use disorders: a systematic review. *Substance Abuse, 30*(4), 266-294. https://doi.org/10.1080/08897070903250019

[76] Bowen, S., Witkiewitz, K., Clifasefi, S. L., Grow, J., Chawla, N., Hsu, S. H., . . . & Larimer, M. E. (2014). Relative efficacy of mindfulness-based relapse prevention, standard relapse prevention, and treatment as usual for substance use disorders. *JAMA Psychiatry, 71*(5), 547-556. https://doi.org/10.1001/jamapsychiatry.2013.4546

[77] Witkiewitz, K., & Bowen, S. (2010). Depression, cravin, and substance use following a randomized trial of mindfulness-based relapse prevention. *Journal of Consulting and Clinical Psychology, 78*(3), 362-374. https://doi.org/10.1037/a0019172

[78] Linehan, M. M. (1993). *Cognitive Behavioral Treatment of Borderline Personality Disorder.* New York: Guilford.

[79] Kliem, S., Kröger, C., & Kosfelder, J. (2010). Dialectical behavior therapy for borderline personality disorder: A meta-analysis using mixed-effects modeling. *Journal of Consulting and*

Clinical Psychology, 78(6), 936-951. https://doi.org/10.1037/a0021015

[80] Linehan, M. M., Schmidt III, H., Dimeff, L. A., Craft, J. C., Kanter, J., & Comtois, K. A. (1999). Dialectical behavior therapy for patients with borderline personality disorder and drug dependence. *The American Journal on Addictions, 8,* 279-292. http://dx.doi.org/10.1080/105504999305686.

[81] Stoffers-Winterling, J. M., Völlm, B. A., Rücker, G., Timmer, A., Huband, N., & Lieb, K. (2012). Psychological therapies for people with borderline personality disorder. *Cochrane Database of Systematic Reviews.* https://doi.org/10.1002/14651858.CD005652.pub2

[82] Ritschell, L. A., Lim, L. E., & Stewart, L. M. (2015). Transdiagnostic applications of DBT for adolescents and adults. *American Journal of Psychotherapy, 69*(2), 111-128. https://doi.org/10.1176/appi.psychotherapy.2015.69.2.111

[83] Ivanoff, A., & Marotta, P. L. (2018). DBT in forensic settings. In M. A. Swales (Ed.), *The Oxford Handbook of Dialectical Behaviour Therapy.* Oxford University Press. https://doi.org/10.1093/oxfordhb/9780198758723.013.14

[84] Linehan, M. M., Dimeff, L. A., Reynolds, S. K., Comtois, K. A., Welch, S. S., Heagerty, P., & Kivlahan, D. R. (2002). Dialectical behavior therapy versus comprehensive validation plus 12-step for the treatment of opioid dependent women meeting criteria for borderline personality disorder. *Drug and Alcohol Dependence, 67,* 13-26. http://dx.doi.org/10.1016/S0376-8716(02)00011-X.

[85] Lynch, T. R., Cheavens, J. S., Cukrowicz, K. C., Thorp, S. R., Bronner, L., & Beyer, J. (2007). Treatment of older adults with co-morbid personality disorder and depression: a dialectical behavior therapy approach. *International Journal of Geriatric Psychiatry, 22,* 131-143. https://doi.org/10.1002/gps.1703

[86] Hayes, S. C., Strosahl, K. D., & Wilson, K. G. (1999). *Acceptance and commitment therapy: An experiential approach to behavior change.* New York: Guilford.

[87] Powers, M. B., Vörding, M. B. Z. V. S., Emmelkamp, P. M. G. (2009). Acceptance and Commitment Therapy: a meta-analytic review. *Psychotherapy and Psychosomatics, 78,* 73-80. https://doi.org/10.1159/000190790

[88] Ruiz, F. J., (2010). A review of Acceptance and Commitment Therapy (ACT) empirical evidence: correlational, experimental psychopathology, component and outcome studies. *International Journal of Psychology and Psychological Therapy, 10*(1), 125-162. Retrieved from https://www.redalyc.org/pdf/560/56017066008.pdf

[89] Varra, A. A., Hayes, S. C., Roget, N., & Fisher, G. (2008). A randomized control trial examining the effect of Acceptance and Commitment Training on clinician willingness to use evidence-based pharmacotherapy. Journal of Consulting and Clinical Psychology, 76(3), 449-458. https://doi.org/10.1037/0022-006X.76.3.449

[90] Amrod, J., & Hayes, S. C. (2014). ACT for the incarcerated. In R. C. Tafrate & D. Mitchell (Eds.), *Forensic CBT: A Handbook for Clinical Practice,* First Edition (pp. 43-65). John Wiley & Sons.

[91] Combs, M. L., & Slaby, D. A. (1977). Social-skills training with children. In *Advances in clinical child psychology* (pp. 161-201). Springer, Boston, MA.

[92] Herbert, J. D., Gaudiano, B. A., Rheingold, A. A., Myers, V. H.,

Dalrymple, K., & Nolan, E. M. (2005). Social skills training augments the effectiveness of cognitive behavioral group therapy for social anxiety disorder. *Behavior Therapy*, *36*(2), 125-138.

[93] Kurtz, M. M., & Mueser, K. T. (2008). A meta-analysis of controlled research on social skills training for schizophrenia. *Journal of consulting and clinical psychology*, *76*(3), 491.

[94] Ozonoff, S., & Miller, J. N. (1995). Teaching theory of mind: A new approach to social skills training for individuals with autism. *Journal of Autism and developmental Disorders*, *25*(4), 415-433.

[95] Gresham, F. M. (1981). Social Skills Training with Handicapped Children: A Review. *Review of Educational Research*, 51(1), 139-176. https://doi.org/10.3102/00346543051001139

[96] Spence, S. H. (2003). Social skills training with children and young people: Theory, evidence and practice. *Child and adolescent mental health*, *8*(2), 84-96.

[97] Covell, C. N., & Scalora, M. J. (2002). Empathic deficits in sexual offenders: An integration of affective, social, and cognitive constructs. *Aggression and violent behavior*, *7*(3), 251-270.

[98] Freedman, B. J., Rosenthal, L., Donahoe Jr, C. P., Schlundt, D. G., & McFall, R. M. (1978). A social-behavioral analysis of skill deficits in delinquent and nondelinquent adolescent boys. *Journal of consulting and clinical psychology*, *46*(6), 1448.

[99] Larson, J. J., Whitton, S. W., Hauser, S. T., & Allen, J. P. (2007). Being close and being social: Peer ratings of distinct aspects of young adult social competence. *Journal of Personality Assessment*, *89*(2), 136-148.

[100] Hazel, J. S., Schumaker, J. B., Sherman, J. A., & Sheldon-Wildgen, J. (1982). Group training for social skills: A program for court-adjudicated, probationary youths. *Criminal Justice and Behavior*, *9*(1), 35-53.

[101] Hollin, C. R., & Palmer, E. J. (2004). Chapter 8: Skills Training. In C. Hollin (Eds.), *The Essential Handbook of Offender Assessment and Treatment* (pp. 117-127). West Sussex, England: John Wiley.

[102] Steadman, J.H., Peters, R.H., Carpenter, C., Mueser, K.T., Jaeger, N.D., Gordon, R.B., Fisler, C., Goss, S., Olson, E., Osher, F.C., Noether, C.D., & Hardin, C. (2013). *Six steps to improve your drug court outcomes for adults with co-occurring disorders*. National Drug Court Institute and SAMHSA's GAINS Center for Behavioral Health and Justice Transformation. Drug Court Practitioner Fact Sheet, 8(1), 1-28. Alexandria VA: National Drug Court Institute.

[103] Hollin, C. R. (1999). Treatment programs for offenders: Meta-analysis,"what works," and beyond. *International Journal of Law and Psychiatry*, *22*, 361-372.

[104] Valliant, P. M., & Antonowicz, D. H. (1991). Cognitive behaviour therapy and social skills training improves personality and cognition in incarcerated offenders. *Psychological Reports*, *68*(1), 27-33.

[105] Rice, M. E. (1983). Improving the social skills of males in a maximum security psychiatric setting. *Canadian Journal of Behavioural Science / Revue canadienne des sciences du comportement*, *15*(1), 1-13. https://doi.org/10.1037/h0080683

[106] Spence, S. H., & Marzillier, J. S. (1981). Social skills training with adolescent male offenders—II.

Short-term, long-term and generalized effects. *Behaviour Research and Therapy, 19*(4), 349-368.

[107] Friedmann, P.D., Hoskinson, R., Gordon, M., Schwartz, R., Kinlock, T., Knight, K., Flynn, P. M., . . .Frisman, L. K. (2012). Medication-assisted treatment in criminal justice agencies affiliated with the criminal justice-drug abuse treatment studies (CJ-DATS): Availability, barriers, and intentions. *Substance Abuse, 33*(1), 9-18. https://doi.org/10.1080/08897077.2011.611460

[108] Roman, P. M., Abraham, A. J., Knudsen, H. K. (2011). Using medication-assisted treatment for substance use disorders: Evidence of barriers and facilitators of implementation. Addictive Behaviors, 36(6), 584-589. https://doi.org/10.1016/j.addbeh.2011.01.032

[109] Amato, L., Davoli, M., Perucci, C. A., Ferriq, M., Faggiano, F., & Mattick, R.P. (2005). An overview of systematic reviews of the effectiveness of opiate maintenance therapies: Available evidence to inform clinical practice and research. *Journal of Substance Abuse Treatment, 28*(4), 321-329. https://doi.org/10.1016/j.jsat.2005.02.007

[110] Brewer, C., Meyers, R. J., & Johnsen, J. (2000). Does disulfiram help to prevent relapse in alcohol abuse? *CNS Drugs, 24*(5), 329-341.

[111] Fuller, R. K., & Gordis, E. (2004). Does disulfiram have a role in alcoholism treatment today? *Addiction, 99*(1), 21-24. https://doi.org/10.1111/j.1360-0443.2004.00597.x.

[112] Rösner, S., Hackl-Herrwerth, A., Leucht, S., Vecchi, S., Srisurapanont, M., & Soyka, M. (2010). Opioid antagonists for alcohol dependence. *The Cochrane Database of Systematic Reviews, 12*. https://doi.org/10.1002/14651858.CD001867.pub3

[113] Bouza, C., Angeles, M., Muñoz, A., Amate, J. M. (2004). Efficacy and safety of naltrexone and acamprosate in the treatment of alcohol dependence: a systematic review. *Addiction, 99*(7): 811-828. https://doi.org/10.1111/j.1360-0443.2004.00763.x

[114] Feeney, G. F., Connor, J. P. (2005). Review: acamprosate and naltrexone are safe and effective but have low compliance rates for people with alcohol dependence. *Evidence Based Mental Health, 8*(1): 14. https://doi.org/10.1136/ebmh.8.1.14.

[115] Baros, A. M., Latham, P. K., Moak, D. H., Voronin, K., & Anton, R. F. (2007). What role does measuring medication compliance play in evaluating the efficacy of naltrexone? *Alcoholism: Clinical and Experimental Research, 31*(4), 596-603. https://doi.org/10.1111/j.1530-0277.2007.00343.x

[116] Digiusto, E., Shakeshaft, A. P., Ritter, A., Mattick, J. W., Lintzeris, N., Bell, J., & Saunders, J. B. (2006). Effects of pharmacotherapies for opioid dependence on participants' criminal behaviour and expenditure on illicit drugs: An Australian national evaluation (NEPOD). *Australia and New Zealand Journal of Criminology, 39*(2), 171-189. https://doi.org/10.1375/acri.39.2.171

[117] Gryczynski, J., Kinlock, T. W., Kelly, S. M., O'Grady, K. E., Gordon, M. S., & Schwartz R. P. (2012). Opioid agonist maintenance for probationers: Patient-level predictors of treatment retention, drug use, and crime. *Substance Abuse, 33*(1), 30-39. https://doi.org/10.1080/08897077.2011.616816

[118] Lee, J. D., Friedmann, P. D., Boney, T. Y., Hoskinson, R. A., McDonald, R., Gordon, M., Fishman, M., . . . O'Brien, C. P. (2015). Extended-release naltrexone for opioid relapse prevention among opioid-dependent, criminal justice-involved adults. *Contemporary*

Clinical Trials, 41, 110-117. https://doi.org/10.1016/j.cct.2015.01.005

[119] Dolan, K., Shearer, J., White, B., Zhou, J., Kaldor, J., & Wodak, A. (2005). Four-year follow-up of imprisoned male heroin users and methadone treatment: Mortality, re-incarceration and hepatitis C infection. *Addiction, 100,* 820-828.

[120] Larney, S., Toson, B., Burns, L., & Dolan, K. (2012). Effect of prison-based opioid substitution treatment and post-release retention in treatment on risk of re-incarceration. *Addiction, 107,* 372-380. https://doi.org/10.1111/j.1360-0443.2011.03618.x

[121] Magura, S., Lee, J. D., Hershberger, J., Herman, J., Marsch, L., Shropshire, & Rosenblum, A. (2009). Buprenorphine and methadone maintenance in jail and post-release: A randomized clinical trial. *Drug and Alcohol Dependence, 99*(1-3), 222-230. https://doi.org/10.1016/j.drugalcdep.2008.08.006

[122] Robinson, S. M., & Adinoff, B. (2018). The mixed message behind "Medication-Assisted Treatment" for substance use disorder. *The American Journal of Drug and Alcohol Abuse, 44*(2), 147-150. https://doi.org/10.1080/00952990.2017.1362419

[123] Saloner, B., Feder, K. A., Krawczyk, N. (2017). Closing the medication-assisted treatment gap for youth with opioid use disorder. *JAMA Pediatrics, 171*(8), 729-731. https://doi.org/10.1001/jamapediatrics.2017.1269

[124] Valenstein-Mah, H., Hagedorn, H., Kay, C. L., Christopher, M. L., & Gordon, A. J. (2018). Underutilization of the current clinical capacity to provide buprenorphine treatment for opioid use disorders within the Veterans Health Administration. *Substance Abuse, 39*(3), 286-288. https://doi.org/10.1080/08897077.2018.1509251

[125] Stanciu, C. N., Penders, T. M., Wuensch, K. L., Davis, J., & Elnagar, K. (2017). Underutilization of pharmacotherapy for treatment of alcohol use disorders part II-Results from a survey of practices among North Carolina mental health providers and brief review of efficacy of available pharmacotherapies. *Journal of Alcoholism & Drug Dependence, 5*(5), 285-293. https://doi.org/10.4172/2329-6488.1000285

[126] Matusow, H., Dickman, S., Rish, J., Fong, C., Dumont, D., Hardin, C., Marlowe, J. D., Rosenblum, A. (2013). Medication-assisted treatment in US drug courts: Results from a nationwide survey of availability, barriers, and attitudes. *Journal of Substance Abuse Treatment, 44*(5), 473-480. https://doi.org/10.1016/j.jsat.2012.10.004

[127] Lee, J. D., & Rich. J. D. (2012). Opioid pharmacotherapy in criminal justice settings: Now is the time. *Substance Abuse, 33*(1). https://doi.org/10.1080/08897077.2011.616797

[128] Bonta, J., Bourgon, G., Rugge, T., Scott, T., Yessine, A. K., Gutierrez, L., & Li, J. (2011). An experimental demonstration of training probation officers in evidence-based community supervision. *Criminal Justice and Behavior, 38*(11), 1127-1148. https://doi.org/10.1177/0093854811420678

[129] Friedmann, P.D., Ducharme, L.J., Welsh, W., Frisman, L., Knight, K., Kinlock, T., Mitchell S. G., . . . Pankow, J. (2013). A cluster randomized trial of an organizational linkage intervention for offenders with substance use disorders: Study protocol. *Health & Justice, 1,* 6. https://doi.org/10.1186/2194-7899-1-6

[130] McKelvey, K., Thrul, J., & Ramo, D. (2017). Impact of quitting smoking and smoking cessation treatment on substance use outcomes: An updated and narrative review. Addictive

behaviors, 65, 161-170. https://doi.org/10.1016/j.addbeh.2016.10.012

[131] Magee, J. C., & Winhusen, T. (2016). The coupling of nicotine and stimulant craving during treatment for stimulant dependence. *Journal of consulting and clinical psychology*, *84*(3), 230.

[132] Thurgood, S. L., McNeill, A., Clark-Carter, D., & Brose, L. S. (2016). A systematic review of smoking cessation interventions for adults in substance abuse treatment or recovery. *Nicotine & Tobacco Research*, *18*(5), 993-1001.

[133] Prochaska, J. J., Delucchi, K., & Hall, S. M. (2004). A Meta-Analysis of Smoking Cessation Interventions With Individuals in Substance Abuse Treatment or Recovery. *Journal of Consulting and Clinical Psychology, 72*(6), 1144-1156. https://doi.org/10.1037/0022-006X.72.6.1144

[134] Jamal, A., Phillips, E., Gentzke, A. S., Homa, D. M., Babb, S. D., King, B. A., & Neff, L. J. (2018). Current Cigarette Smoking Among Adults - United States, 2016. *MMWR. Morbidity and mortality weekly report*, *67*(2), 53-59.

[135] Cropsey, K. L., Jones-Whaley, S., Jackson, D. O., & Hale, G. J. (2010). Smoking characteristicsof community corrections clients. *Nicotine & Tobacco Research*, *12*(1), 53-58.

[136] Cropsey, K. L., Linker, J. A., & Waite, D. E. (2008b). An analysis of racial and sex differences for smoking among adolescents in a juvenile correctional center. *Drug and Alcohol Dependence*, *92*(1-3), 156-163.

[137] Lincoln, T., Tuthill, R. W., Roberts, C. A., Kennedy, S., Hammett, T. M., Langmore-Avila, E., & Conklin, T. J. (2009). Resumption of smoking after release from a tobacco-free correctional facility. *Journal of Correctional Health Care*, *15*(3), 190-196.

[138] Ingersoll, K. S., Cropsey, K. L., & Heckman, C. J. (2009). A test of motivational plus nicotine replacement interventions for HIV positive smokers. *AIDS and Behavior*, *13*(3), 545-554.

[139] Jardin, B. F., Cropsey, K. L., Wahlquist, A. E., Gray, K. M., Silvestri, G. A., Cummings, K. M., & Carpenter, M. J. (2014). Evaluating the effect of access to free medication to quit smoking: a clinical trial testing the role of motivation. *nicotine & tobacco research*, *16*(7), 992-999.

[140] Cropsey, K. L., Clark, C. B., Stevens, E. N., Schiavon, S., Lahti, A. C., & Hendricks, P. S (2017a). Predictors of medication adherence and smoking cessation among smokers under community corrections supervision. *Addictive behaviors*, *65*, 111-117.

[141] Clarke, J. G., Stein, L., Martin, R. A., Martin, S. A., Parker, D., Lopes, C. E., ... Bock, B. (2013). Forced smoking abstinence: Not enough for smoking cessation. Journal of the American Medical Association, 173, 789-794.

[142] Cropsey, K., Eldridge, G., Weaver, M., Villalobos, G., Stitzer, M., & Best, A. (2008a). Smoking cessation intervention for female prisoners: addressing an urgent public health need. *American journal of public health*, *98F*(10), 1894-1901.

[143] Garver-Apgar, C., Young, S., Howard, B., Udochi, B., & Morris, C. (2017). Effects of a statewide tobacco cessation program among individuals involved with arkansas community correction. *Journal of Correctional Health Care, 23*(3), 259-270. doi:10.1177/1078345817709017

[144] Cropsey, K. L., Hendricks, P. S., Schiavon, S., Sellers, A., Froelich, M., Shelton, R. C., & Carpenter, M. J.

(2017b). A pilot trial of In vivo NRT sampling to increase medication adherence in community corrections smokers. *Addictive behaviors*, *67*, 92-99.

[145] Shiroma, E. J., Ferguson, P. L., Pickelsimer, E. E. (2010). Prevalence of traumatic brain injury in an offender population: A meta-analysis. Journal of Head Trauma Rehabilitation 27, E1–E10.

[146] Binswanger IA, Stern MF, Deyo RA, Heagerty PJ, et al. Release from prison-a high risk of death for former inmates. N Engl J Med. 2007; 356;157-165.

[147] Lim, S., Seligson, A. L., Parvez, F. M., Luther, C. W., Mavinkurve, M. P., Binswanger, I. A., & Kerker, B. D. (2012). Risks of drug-related death, suicide, and homicide during the immediate post-release period among people released from New York City jails, 2001-2005. American journal of epidemiology, 175(6), 519-526.

[148] Equal Justice Initiative (2017). *Mass Incarceration Costs $182 Billion Every Year, Without Adding Much to Public Safety*. Retrieved from: https://eji.org/news/mass-incarceration-costs-182-billion-annually/

Chapter 7

Conceptualizing Drug Addiction and Chronic Pain through a Biopsychosocial Framework to Improve Therapeutic Strategies

Zachary S. Harmon, Emily N. Welch and Christina L. Ruby

Abstract

The recent surge in opioid-related deaths has brought poor pain management practices to the forefront of our nation's collective consciousness. However, improving treatments for chronic pain, substance use disorders (SUD), and comorbid expression of both requires a better understanding of the pathophysiology involved in their development. In this chapter, the authors present the argument that chronic pain and SUD can be conceptualized similarly from a biopsychosocial perspective to inform a better approach to treatment. The authors describe the common neurobehavioral mechanisms of SUD and chronic pain, then discuss the efficacy of several psychotherapeutic methods employed to combat chronic pain, addiction, and related disorders. Such methods may contribute to positive health outcomes in managing chronic pain and curbing drug addiction by reducing the role of opioid analgesics for long-term pain management.

Keywords: addiction, substance use disorders, chronic pain, opioids, psychotherapy, cognitive behavioral therapy, mindfulness-based stress reduction, solution-focused brief psychotherapy, motivational interviewing

1. Introduction

Over the past two decades, the rate of prescription drug misuse has been rapidly increasing worldwide, leading to a growing number of emergency department visits, hospitalizations, and overdose deaths. The National Safety Council reported that in 2017, it was more common to die of opioid overdose than in a car crash, and by 2018, drug overdose became the number 1 cause of unintentional death in the United States. The coronavirus pandemic has only exacerbated this situation [1]. Opioid analgesics have become the most commonly prescribed class of drugs in the United States [2] in part because approximately 100 million American adults suffer from chronic pain, more than those affected by heart disease, diabetes, and cancer combined [3]. The other major piece of this puzzle is that prescription opioids were misrepresented by pharmaceutical manufacturers as non-addictive, which led to widespread over-prescription of opioids for long-term chronic pain management. Although the addictive potential of oxycodone was recognized very early [4], very few studies have been conducted on this or other opioid painkillers. Recently, the growing recognition that prescription opioids can be addictive has also led some doctors to over-correct the problem by not prescribing sufficient opioids to manage pain when it is appropriate, leaving patients to seek illegal sources or substances (e.g. heroin) to manage pain and physical withdrawal symptoms. These opposing but equally ill-informed prescription practices have culminated into a single outcome: an epidemic of opioid addiction and death in the United States.

From many different perspectives, chronic pain and substance use disorders (SUD) share a plethora of similarities and thus it is not surprising that they frequently occur in tandem, with either one preceding the other. Overall, the prevalence of chronic pain in individuals with SUD is estimated to be 27–87%, with individuals suffering from chronic pain 2-3X more likely to experience a SUD, and individuals that have a SUD 1.5 times more likely to experience chronic pain [5]. In people receiving an opioid prescription for long-term chronic pain treatment, 21–29% misuse the opioid medication and 8–12% develop an opioid use disorder (OUD) [6, 7], though some estimates are as high as 43%, with elevated risk for other substance-related disorders as well [5]. Some hypothesize that individuals self-medicate with drugs to manage the psychological aspects of pain [8, 9], while others suggest pre-existing physiological and psychological characteristics associated with OUD/SUD can be stimulated by a chronic pain condition [9, 10]. These hypotheses are not mutually exclusive, and draw attention to the fact that the relationship between chronic pain and SUD is difficult to disentangle, making it complicated to establish effective treatments.

As with many societal weaknesses exposed by the pandemic, SUD, particularly OUD, are flourishing and overdose deaths continue to rise [1]. This does not appear to be due solely to the disease itself, but rather the significant increase in life stress (e.g. job loss, social isolation, etc.) combined with lack of access to proper mental and physical health care. This illustrates well the central hypothesis we aim to present: that a biopsychosocial perspective of addiction and chronic pain, which incorporates factors from the societal to molecular levels, allows for a more thorough understanding of these disorders. We suggest that incorporating alternative therapeutic methods and reducing the role of opioid analgesics for long-term pain management may contribute to positive health outcomes in managing chronic pain, addiction, and comorbid expression of both.

2. Biopsychosocial approach to understanding health and disease

As the name suggests, the biopsychosocial (BPS) model proposes that healthcare professionals use biological, psychological, behavioral, and social lenses to understand health and disease. Psychiatrist George Engel has been credited with the formulation, and call for action, that propelled the understanding of disease and illness past that of basic Renaissance philosophy and into an understanding not solely based in biological factors [11]. Engel introduced the BPS model as a contrast to the biomedical model of health and disease, which had long reigned supreme (and still predominates clinical practice in many fields). His model also contrasts with a purely environmental/ecological model, which holds a more holistic view of health, but may neglect the importance of biological influences. The BPS model incorporates the best of both worlds, recognizing that both nature and nurture are vitally important to health and disease. This new ideal formed the foundation for behavioral and psychological conceptualizations of health and medicine [12].

The BPS model has now become the leading one in conceptualizing many forms of illness, including chronic pain, although it continues to be underutilized in practice, particularly in acute medical and surgical fields of study that prioritize biomedical views of disease and illness [13]. A large part of the problem in translating concept to practice is that the BPS model has minimal influence over provisional healthcare funding [13]. Critics of the BPS model claim that the diagnostic front would be marginalized by utilizing a threefold framework (although this had already been addressed by functional and practical analysis) [14, 15]. Biomedical model proponents suggest that the BPS model may promote a lack of focus, or that practitioners may misjudge other significant factors related to treatment, and therefore cause unintended harm to patients due to the complexity of the biopsychosocial approach and the negligence that may occur [14]. However, it is important to consider that harm can be associated with any models or frameworks, and that harm primarily results from misuse of models and failures to recognize limitations of those models [13].

The opioid epidemic is a profound and tragic illustration of the problems associated with the persistence of the biomedical model in many fields and countries (including the U.S.). This model has seen healthcare costs soar, while patient outcomes have fallen. A major cause of these failings is the lack of consideration of psychosocial factors in patients' lives, which can contribute greatly to overall health. Two recent Nature articles have drawn attention to the importance of social context - and the shortcomings of a biomedical-only approach - in relation to substance use. Hart (2017) argues that even conceptualizing addiction as a disease or disorder is not only inaccurate, but harmful, contributing to social injustice in the form of racism and socioeconomic marginalization [16]. He further takes issue with the exaggerated value placed upon neuroscientific evidence. Relatedly, Heilig et al. (2016) attributes the relative lack of addiction treatment advancements to the glaring omission of social context in neuroscience, and calls on the field to elucidate the impacts of social exclusion and marginalization on the development of drug-seeking and consumption [17]. Although these articles focus on addiction, the principles apply to chronic pain as well.

While solving the socioeconomic disparities that contribute to illness will be a formidable task that lies outside the scope of the current chapter, the authors argue that a biopsychosocial approach to addiction and chronic pain is superior to a strictly biomedical one, and that it has the potential to counteract the problems of a biomedical-only view. As noted above, the biomedical paradigm is struggling to confront rising healthcare costs and poor, patient-reported outcomes [13]. The BPS model, prided on person-centered care, can alleviate this financial and diagnostic burden, particularly as it relates to chronic pain, mental illness, and other functional disorders [13, 18]. The BPS model has the ability to yield more positive patient-reported outcomes of treatment, especially within the context of cognitive behavioral therapy, due to the person-centered approach and use of goal-setting, which has recognized utility in treating both chronic pain and SUD [19–21]. Family involvement in treatment can heavily reduce stigma related to SUD and chronic pain, and this social engagement is correlated with lasting, positive treatment outcomes [22]. If this model becomes more ingrained within the cultural sphere of Western clinical medicine and the general populace, it is predicted to drastically reduce societal stigma related to both chronic pain and SUD, thus altering perceived treatment outcomes and making non-pharmacological treatment more acceptable and accessible to those suffering [23]. Considerations of the social aspects of the BPS model would greatly advance future research, particularly that relating to psychological and behavioral functioning.

3. Neurobiological overlap between addiction and chronic pain

Epidemiological and functional imaging studies suggest a bidirectional relationship between chronic pain and many psychiatric disorders, including SUD, and that significant neurological overlap exists between them [5, 24, 25]. As described below, these similarities in affect, cognition, and behavior between addiction and chronic pain are reflected by similar changes in neural circuitry. These conditions also share many genetic and epigenetic mechanisms, but a detailed discussion is outside the focus of this chapter.

3.1 Neurobiology of substance use disorders

SUD are undeniably biopsychosocial in nature and expression, with hallmark features of impaired daily functioning in cognitive, physiological, psychological, and social domains as a result of substance use and continued use despite these negative consequences. Diagnostic criteria for SUD include impaired cognitive and behavioral control over drug use, social impairment, such as job or relationship loss, use of drugs in risky or inappropriate situations that pose physical or psychological harm, and pharmacological criteria such as tolerance and withdrawal [26]. Neuroscientists conceptualize the addicted brain in a framework that encompasses key elements of two theories of motivated behavior: incentive-sensitization theory, wherein the motivation to consume drugs is said to result from conditioned reinforcement and over-attribution of salience to drugs and drug cues [27], and opponent-processes theory [28], which holds that the motivation to consume drugs is initially driven by positive reinforcement (addition of pleasurable feelings or euphoria, e.g. reward/process A), but repeated drug use is driven by negative reinforcement (subtraction of aversive feelings or state associated with drug deprivation, e.g. antireward/process B). These theories have given rise to the concept of the addiction cycle, which is supported by abundant neuroscientific evidence (reviewed extensively in [29] and summarized below).

The addiction cycle is composed of three stages, each underlain by neuroplastic changes in the function of discrete brain circuits resulting from chronic drug exposure, with variability modulated by an individual's genetics, life experiences, and their drug(s) of choice. The binge/intoxication stage is characterized by drug-induced positive reinforcement and loss of control over the amount and duration of drug-taking. The main circuit involved in acute drug reinforcement is the dopaminergic projection from the ventral tegmental area (VTA) to the nucleus accumbens (NAc), supported by the central nucleus of the amygdala (CeA) and ventral pallidum (VP), while compulsivity in drug-taking involves the caudate/putamen (CPu). Repeated drug use reduces baseline activity of these circuits, partly setting the stage for withdrawal/negative affect to drive drug-taking. The withdrawal/negative affect stage is marked by negative reinforcement (removal of unpleasant stimulus or emotional state) driven by the recruitment of the hypothalamic–pituitary–adrenal (HPA) stress axis and circuitry connecting the basolateral amygdala (BLA) and hippocampus to the extended amygdala, CeA, basal nucleus of the stria terminalis (BNST), and a subregion of the NAc shell, which in turn project to the VP and lateral hypothalamus (LH). Acute withdrawal from several drugs, including opioids, involves hyperactive corticotropin-releasing factor (CRF) and norepinephrine (NE) neurotransmitter systems, the endogenous antireward opioid dynorphin, substance P, neuropeptide Y, vasopressin, and nociceptin. The preoccupation/anticipation stage is marked by drug craving, key to the relapsing nature of the addiction cycle. The impetus of relapse determines the neurocircuitry involved, with drug-induced relapse regulated by glutamatergic projections from the medial PFC (mPFC) to the NAc and VP, cue-induced relapse regulated by BLA-PFC-NAc glutamate signaling and VTA-PFC dopamine signaling, and stress-induced relapse activating the extended amygdalar CRF and NE systems. Compromised cognition, memory, and inhibitory control involve the hippocampus, mPFC and orbitofrontal cortex (OFC; [29]. As the authors discuss below, many of the structures, circuits, and neurochemical mediators that drive SUD are also involved in chronic pain.

3.2 Neurobiology of chronic pain

Nociception is a physiological response to a noxious stimulus wherein normally silent sensory neurons called nociceptors deliver information to the brain to elicit protective actions [30]. When stimulated, nociceptors transduce signals along spinal cord primary afferent Aδ and C fibers and converge at the dorsal horn, where afferent neurons in laminae I and V provide input to the brain [31]. Pain results from the activation of a distributed group of brain structures within the brainstem reticular formation and the limbic system, collectively referred to as the pain neuromatrix [32], a three-tiered hierarchy of experiential pain processing [33]. First order processing occurs when the spinothalamic and spinoreticulothalamic tracts carry signals from the dorsal horn into the brainstem and posterior thalamus (pTHAL), which encodes localization of pain and identification of specialized pain characteristics [31, 33]. The second tier involves perceptive and attentional internalization of pain, including cognitive structuring and modulation, attenuation, and proposition of somatic reactions to the painful stimuli, and is regulated by the posterior parietal cortex (pPAR), anterior cingulate cortex (ACC), PFC, and insula [33]. The third tier is characterized by emotional reappraisal of the nociceptive stimuli, in which emotional context is applied to the experience to modulate its psychological and social consequences. The brain regions associated with this tier are the pPAR, OFC, and anterolateral PFC [33]. These cortical structures are responsible for determining the behavioral response to nociceptive stimulation [31, 34].

Chronic pain is defined as persisting past the normal time of healing, generally for six months or more [35]. Unlike acute pain, which is protective in nature, chronic pain has negative effects on psychological and social well-being. As with SUD, chronic pain is the result of the plastic nature of molecules and circuits within the nervous system [31]. When activated persistently, the pain neuromatrix and other regions of the brain and spinal cord involved in nociceptive and cognitive-evaluative processing undergo neuroplastic changes that amplify activity, called central sensitization [36–38]. These changes result in exaggerated responses to noxious stimuli (hyperalgesia) and pain responses being triggered by normally innocuous stimuli (allodynia). The transition from acute to chronic pain is underlain by greater engagement of emotional and motivational circuitry [39], paralleling the progression through the addiction cycle.

Not surprisingly, research suggests that there is significant overlap in the neurological mechanisms involved in chronic pain with those involved in drug addiction [29, 40, 41]. Neuroplastic changes in corticolimbic structures comparable to those seen in SUD also contribute to pain chronification [42]. Specifically, chronic pain, like SUD, involves neuroadaptations that dampen reward, recruit stress-related circuitry, and promote aberrant learning that converge to negatively affect physiology and behavior [39, 42–45]. Chronic pain can disrupt the reward/antireward balance through persistent sensitization of nociceptive circuitry within the NAc, and attenuation of behavioral inhibitory signaling from the habenula [46, 47] to produce an overall shift in reward level or hedonic tone [48]. NAc functional connectivity changes have also been associated with risk-taking behavior in chronic pain patients, with high gain sensitivity in sufferers of chronic back pain correlated to greater connectivity between NAc and subcortical areas, compared to controls with strong NAc-frontal cortex connectivity [49]. These changes can promote the use of alcohol and drugs, particularly opioids, for negative reinforcement (alleviating physical and psychological pain) and ultimately predispose chronic pain sufferers to develop drug addiction [39, 43].

As discussed above, both repeated exposure to addictive drugs and chronic pain lead to changes in brain function that promote continued drug use. Conversely, recurring drug use can also promote the development of chronic pain, illustrating the logical fallacy in treating chronic pain with prescription opioids. As with other addictive drugs, repeated opioid administration can shift the balance between reward and antireward processes, affecting the ability to experience positive emotions from natural rewards over time [47]. This shift in balance is accompanied by amplification of the antireward state, effectively establishing a reward deficit state, which drives further opioid use to compensate [47, 50]. Allostatic changes from pain stimuli are amplified when opioids are misused [51–53], resulting in neural adaptations that promote hyperalgesia, drug tolerance, and difficulty regulating emotion, which can in turn amplify anhedonia, producing a downward spiral of chronic pain and further prescription opioid misuse [53].

4. Shared psychosocial factors in addiction and chronic pain

As is evident from the sections above summarizing neural circuitry involved in addiction and chronic pain, the boundary between the neurobiological and psychological aspects of these conditions is somewhat arbitrary. Likewise, the boundary between the psychological and social components is poorly defined, reflecting the central concept of the BPS model, that health and disease involve biological, psychological, and social factors that influence one another in a reciprocal, highly dynamic manner [54]. Meints and Edwards (2018) divide psychosocial variables involved in chronic pain into two main categories. General psychosocial factors include affect, trauma, social/interpersonal disposition, sex- and race-related disparities, and pain-specific psychosocial factors include catastrophizing, coping, expectations, and self-efficacy [54]. Another way of conceptualizing the division is factors that predispose an individual to develop chronic pain and those that emerge as a consequence of pain. As discussed below, there is a high degree of overlap between the psychosocial aspects of chronic pain and addiction, and it is not always easy to make the distinction between cause and consequence in SUD.

Psychosocial factors influencing reward, stress, and motivation can contribute to a downward spiral of chronic pain and comorbid conditions [46]. It is well-known that negative affect promotes drug use, while conversely, repeated drug use increases risk for depression and anxiety. Similarly, anhedonic depressive symptoms often exceed 50% comorbidity in individuals suffering from fibromyalgia, temporomandibular joint disorder, chronic spinal pain, and chronic abdominal pain [5]. Symptoms of depression and anxiety are prominent in both episodic and chronic cluster headaches, with those in the chronic subset being less likely to cognitively reframe their pain sensations and more likely to ruminate [55]. In contrast to the bidirectional nature of negative affect and SUD, depression and anxiety are strong predictors of pain and related disability, but neither pain nor related disability appear to be good predictors of depression and anxiety [54]. Affective factors are a strong predictors of opioid misuse, with mood disorders, anxiety disorders, and chronic pain conditions either preceding or overlapping with OUD [9, 56–60]. Furthermore, negative affect and cognitions increase risk of developing an OUD in surgical patients, as their pre-operative presence were major predictors of prolonged opioid cessation following the operation [61]. Childhood physical, psychological, and sexual abuse have been implicated in later-life development of several chronic pain conditions [54], as well as alcohol and drug abuse [62]. Post-traumatic stress disorder (PTSD) in adult veterans (which can be related to combat exposure and/or injuries such as traumatic brain injury) and in victims of childhood abuse are highly associated with development of chronic pain [54] and substance use [63].

Deficits in executive function can contribute to and result from repeated drug use. Likewise, chronic pain is associated with impairments in memory, attention, and cognitive flexibility, although the relationship is a complex one, owing to a lack of standard tests and poor control of confounding variables such as sleep and medication in existing studies [64]. Working memory and emotional control were shown to be impaired in chronic pain patients, but neither the intensity nor the duration of pain itself predicted executive dysfunction [65]. As with negative affect, poor executive function may predispose the development of chronic pain, a notion supported by a recent study wherein poor cognitive performance before surgery on Trail-Making Test B and Rey-Osterrieth Complex Figure copy and recall predicted the persistence of pain up to 12 months after surgery [66]. Relatedly, while impulsivity is not generally prominent in chronic pain patients [67], this trait is quite pronounced in SUD [29] and may play a key role in determining the likelihood of opioid misuse in pain patients. Specifically, urgency and attentional impulsivity have been implicated in current and future misuse of opioids by chronic pain patients, while sensation-seeking seems to have little to no influence [67, 68]. High baseline impulsivity in rats was also correlated with high impulsivity in the variable delay-to-signal test after spared nerve injury [69]. Additionally, a recent study showed that decision-making in the Iowa Gambling Task by chronic pain patients was robustly modeled mathematically by over-valuation of gains and under-valuation of losses, typical of risk-taking [70]. Risky decision-making and lifestyle is also highly prevalent with long-term substance use [9], which may, in turn, increase risk for developing a chronic pain condition. For example, prescription opioid use was associated with a 47% increased risk of car crash initiation, and thus, injury [6]. Other drug-associated behavior, such as injecting and high-risk or illegal activity to obtain drugs could also contribute to chronic pain and vice versa.

Much research underscores the importance of social support in ameliorating pain and improving function in chronic pain [12, 54], as well as preventing relapse in SUD [71]. However, negative social interactions can have the opposite effect. For example, the "sick role" of individuals experiencing chronic pain is a social context accompanied by attention, pity, and permitted exemption from daily routines [40]. Although moderately pleasurable for the individual experiencing pain, socio-emotional pain relief is stressful for family and friends, and may promote aversion and distaste of the individual that has assumed it. This can cause isolation, communication deficits, emotional setbacks, and may amplify the original chronic pain state without the presence of a nociceptive stimulus [72]. Similarly, psychosocial stressors such as aversion, isolation, and other emotional setbacks are also heavily apparent in addiction and other mood disorders [8, 10]. Relatedly, family members and peers attitudes and behaviors also influence individuals with chronic pain and SUD. Parental catastrophizing, spousal/partner depression or avoidant, anxious attachment styles, lack of social support at work, and negative interactions with co-workers and workmans compensation programs can all promote chronic pain and disability [54]. Similar interpersonal factors are at play with SUD [73], and they can be particularly important for adolescents, whose peers and parents exert heavy influences over substance use by affecting availability of drugs and the child's perception of approval/disapproval of drug use [74]. Therapies targeting positive behavioral change in the social context may be essential in combating both chronic pain and SUD.

In addition to interpersonal factors, gender and race are other aspects of the social milieu that can have profound positive or negative effects on physical and mental health. While there can clearly be biological influences in both cases, such as chromosomal and hormonal influences in gender, and genetic variability in race, it is worth considering the social features, which may be even more important in determining risk for mental health-related functioning (as appears to be the case for schizophrenia; [75]). Females have a higher prevalence of pain, decreased pain threshold, more severe, recurrent, and longer duration of pain compared to males, differences explained at least in part by social factors, such as gender roles and differences in coping strategies [54]. Compared to men, women also show greater propensity for addiction to many drugs, including opioids, but research seems to have focused primarily on potential biological explanations for such differences [76, 77]. The negative impacts of alcohol and drug use are greater on Black and Hispanic Americans, although consumption patterns between Blacks, Hispanics, and Whites do not explain this difference (at least in relation to alcohol; [78]). Data are lacking for many ethnic groups regarding chronic pain, but Blacks and Asian Americans report higher levels of pain and lower pain tolerance compared to Caucasians, differences which may stem from racism, socioeconomic strain, and ineffective pain coping strategies [54]. Other structural vulnerability factors such as poor access to health care are likely to contribute to the unequal impacts of SUD and chronic pain on minority groups [79]. Further research is needed to gain a better understanding of how complex social and structural factors shape risk for chronic pain and SUD. The field of epigenetics, which has begun to address the neurobiological effects of well-known social context-related risk factors for schizophrenia - early life adversity, growing up in an urban environment, minority group position, and cannabis use [75] - holds great promise in advancing science, therapeutics, and social change, and underscores the strengths of the biopsychosocial perspective.

5. Non-pharmacological treatments for addiction and chronic pain

The focus of biomedical interventions to manage chronic pain is primarily pharmacological, using opioid analgesics or surgical procedures [80]. However, surgery inherently subjects patients to risks associated with the surgical procedures, including more pain [80]. Likewise, opioids do not show substantial evidence for beneficial long-term pain management [80–82] and as discussed above, may even exacerbate it. For example, in a study of 26,014 individuals experiencing chronic back pain, psychological distress (depression, anxiety, posttraumatic stress disorder, and SUD), unhealthy lifestyle (obesity and smoking), and health care utilization increased incrementally with duration of opioid use [83]. As chronic pain and long-term opioid use may cross-sensitize across multiple biopsychosocial domains, it is essential to identify alternative treatment options.

A large body of clinical evidence suggests that treatments such as cognitive behavioral therapy (CBT) and mindfulness-based stress reduction (MBSR) alleviate symptoms of depression, anxiety, SUD, and chronic pain [84] and that the core mesocorticolimbic structures impacted by SUD and chronic pain can be effectively targeted by innovative therapies [85]. The CDC has also recommended treatments like exercise therapy and CBT to reduce pain and improve function in patients with chronic pain [86]. These alternative treatments aim to directly dismantle the negative biofeedback created by drug- or pain-induced maladaptive changes within reward and stress circuitry. Although more research is needed, the authors suggest that a more integrated approach for managing chronic pain and addiction should include clinical mental health therapeutic techniques, discussed below.

5.1 Cognitive behavioral therapy (CBT)

The goal of cognitive behavioral therapy (CBT) is to educate the client in the realm of positive coping strategies utilizing cognitive, respondent, and behavioral techniques [87]. CBT is designed to manage individual patient characteristics through a collaborative reframing of negative prediction, selective abstraction, and depersonalization to help the patient assume responsibility for their cognitions and behaviors. Cognitive behavioral therapists highlight the direct link between negative emotional states, sedentary cognitions, and resulting behaviors and seek to alter them in a holistic fashion that allows patients to grow through therapeutic change. This patient-therapist collaboration shakes sedentary perspectives and faulty core beliefs surrounding their ailment and allows the patient to reframe their thoughts and learn from new experiences.

Many individuals with SUD present to treatment unwillingly and approximately 45–50% will continue to use one or more drugs while in treatment [88]. In one study, CBT-treated individuals with SUD showed a 31% rate of abstinence compared to 13% abstinence rate in controls [89]. Compared to other psychosocial treatments, such as insight-oriented therapies involving psychoeducation, CBT appears more durable [90]. In the context of OUD, studies have shown that CBT alone does not lead to consistent therapeutic outcomes in patients, although it does seem to enhance the effects of methadone maintenance treatments (MMT) [91–93]. Combined treatment outcomes include greater attendance and treatment adherence and an increase in abstinence as evidenced by urine toxicology [88, 94]. Although reductions in substance use are often modest, sleeper effects, the notion that positive responses to CBT will increase over time, have been historically documented [95]. Relatedly, compared to MMT-only groups, or MMT and another independent counseling strategy, CBT has been associated with latent positive effects on psychosocial functioning. For example, employment consistency was shown to increase in parallel to daily functioning, and stress was shown to decrease with increased cognitive coping skills, reduced opioid use, and less depressive symptomology [91, 92]. Contingency management utilized within the context of CBT has been found to increase the likelihood of abstinence, and therefore may further enhance effectiveness of SUD treatment [89, 96]. A study in rats also supports the use of contingency management to enhance the relative value of nondrug reinforcers (in this case, delayed food reward) versus immediate opioid delivery, suggesting that people may similarly develop delay-discounting (a behavioral component of impulsivity) because of contingencies in their environment [97]. Combining pharmacological treatment with CBT to increase coping skills appears to be a promising strategy for SUD and its effectiveness may lie in addressing the individual's biopsychosocial functioning rather than simply treating withdrawal symptoms.

Recent international guidelines prescribe psychological interventions, rather than strictly pharmacological interventions, for the treatment of chronic nociceptive pain [98]. In chronic pain, CBT aims to help the patient channel their pain-related negative affect pain into a new cognitive interpretation of their sensations to increase their quality of life. Evidence has shown that outcomes from CBT-based interventions for chronic pain are moderate and comparable in efficacy to those for SUD. While CBT does not have a direct impact on the disability causing chronic pain [99], it has positive effects on patients' cognitions and appears to increase quality of life. For example, participants were 3X as likely to report no pain interference after CBT techniques to target and reframe negative cognitive patterns associated with the perceptions of pain [100]. Likewise, unrelenting chronic pain from terminal illness can increase desire for hastened death, but CBT-based activities like education, targeting of negative appraisal states, and relaxation association have been shown to allow management and attenuation of pain [101]. Experimental, graded *in vivo* exposure therapy, a broad-spectrum CBT technique, has been shown to have some success in targeting the fear-avoidance model of chronic pain. Here, exposure to fearful movements gradually reduces classically conditioned fear/anxiety to reduce avoidance of these movements over the long-term [102]. Although more research is necessary, CBT appears promising as an adjunctive treatment in chronic pain. It may also be effective in augmenting treatment for patients with comorbid chronic pain and OUD by targeting patients' ability to cope with pain- and stress-related opioid craving.

5.2 Mindfulness-based stress reduction (MBSR)

Mindfulness is a novel treatment strategy with roots in Eastern religions and philosophies that aims to enhance the experience and understanding of positive emotions and dismantle aberrant learning underlying pathological thoughts and behaviors. At the core of mindful therapeutic practice is acceptance that the stressors that trigger drug use or exacerbate chronic pain cannot be eliminated from one's life, but that their responses to those stressors can be modified. Relatedly, MBSR teaches a non-judgmental approach to affective, cognitive, and behavioral states; whether a particular stimulus is positive or aversive makes no difference. Invocation of the present moment is also key, allowing the patient to moderate their awareness and attention by attending to themselves in the here-and-now. The idea is that this systematic awareness of the present state coupled with a non-judgmental, accepting attitude ameliorates stress by weakening the negative emotional states attached to stressors, and thereby interrupting the cycle of addiction/chronic pain and eliminating the need to self-medicate.

Mindfulness programs are particularly efficacious for SUD because they address aberrant learning related to distressing stimuli and promote an openness to experience that leads to a reduction in future distress from those stimuli [103], rather than promoting avoidance of stressors or triggers, which does not address the underlying pathology. Mindfulness strategies also lead to pro-adaptive changes in intrapersonal thought patterns and ingrained belief systems, such as cues and cravings [104], while momentary awareness enhances an individual's ability to accept and cope with negative experiences, such as relapse and risky behavior [105]. This momentary acceptance of unpleasant stimuli leads to neurobiological alterations related to new learning, and consequently protects against relapse [103]. MBSR has been found to alter neurostructural changes in the mesocorticolimbic system and reduce autonomic arousal, physiological correlates to individual perceptual shifts, value and priority clarification, increased self-awareness, urge and craving shifts, and the ability to "let go" [106]. This sensory- and perception-focused strategy system has also been found to positively impact hedonic processing in the context of chronic pain and opioid management that interferes with habit-forming behaviors associated with addiction [107].

MBSR and similar strategies that target aberrant learning have been shown to interrupt the progression of addiction to opioids [107]. Mindfulness trainings reduce the intense neural reactivity to drug-cues, reduce cravings, and uncouple negative affective states from the previously induced, self-medicated state [108]. Functional MRI studies have revealed that MBSR can enhance top-down limbic-striatal connections by strengthening associations between the PFC and the parietal regions of the brain [109, 110], suppressing the influences of craving and autonomic responses, and enhancing cognitive control and flexibility related to attention [109]. Furthermore, by promoting gratitude for positive experiences and acceptance of negative physical and affective states, MBSR has been shown to reduce craving, downregulate sympathetic arousal, and heighten natural reward [111], essentially breaking the cycle of addiction. Compared to typical treatments for OUD that focus patient attention on suppression of craving, which can actually increase self-medication and relapse, mindfulness strategies that focus the attention of the patient on acceptance of substance use uncouples opioid craving and opioid use to promote long-term relapse prevention [109, 112, 113].

Utilizing mindfulness in the context of treating chronic pain is new to Western society. Eastern practices, such as Zen Buddhism and Hatha yoga, have been applied to a plethora of physical ailments for centuries, but now these are combined with traditional psychotherapies such as CBT and acceptance and commitment therapy [114]. As in addiction treatment, a non-judgmental stance is vitally important to MBSR-based treatment of chronic pain. The patient focuses their attention on uncomfortable physical sensations with no attempt to alter them, instead developing compassion toward both positive and aversive bodily experiences [114, 115]. Neuroimaging studies support the notion that MBSR strategies have allowed patients to adopt a new perception of their chronic pain. The chronic pain experience involves the interplay of nociceptive cues, cognitive distortions, and negative emotional appraisal. Compared to controls, subjects receiving mindfulness instruction showed reduced activity in the right amygdala, parahippocampus, and insula, and increased activation in the dorsomedial and other PFC subregions during the presentation of unpleasant visual stimuli, consistent with attenuated emotional activation [116]. Mindfulness training has also been shown to reduce pain severity and uncouple pain from opioid use by helping the patient attenuate negative appraisals, reduce fixation and hypervigilance from chronic pain, and reduce pain catastrophizing [86, 107, 117–120]. As in SUD, MBSR interventions help to disengage the cycle of maladaptive pain coping strategies and prevent related behaviors, such as opiate stockpiling and other habits [107]. Together, these lines of evidence suggest that mindfulness-based therapeutic interventions hold great promise for treating and preventing OUDs, chronic pain, and co-expression of both, and the authors hypothesize that the biopsychosocial nature of the approach is key to its effectiveness.

5.3 Solution-focused brief psychotherapy (SFBP)

Solution-focused brief psychotherapy (SFBP) applies a postmodern constructivist approach to counseling, meaning that an individual's experience of their substance use acts as the "objective truth" [121]. In this way, the therapist will collaborate with the client in order to develop a working, clinical understanding of the client's problem situation in terms of experience, perception, and meaning related to ambiguous stimuli and events [122]. Like CBT and MBSR, SFBP hinges on the development of a personalized construction of the problem behaviors or experiences and reframing of meaning that perpetuates maladaptive cycles of thought and behavior. Some researchers believe that it is not the specific interventions, but the demeanor and actions of the therapist that promote the therapeutic effects of solution-focused therapy. The collaborative relationship extended by the therapist, use of core facilitative conditions of the counseling process, mindfulness of the stages of change, and a focus on solutions instead of problems provides moderate empirical backing [123–125]. SFBP practitioners believe that therapy relies on the therapist's ability to engage the client in examining their negative *status quo* and that they become aware of exceptions to problem situations so as to direct insight toward future change [126]. SFBP allows the client to determine their own goals related to recovery, which includes harm-reduction strategies, and does not rely upon all-or-nothing measures such as complete abstinence from drugs.

Many reports support the notion that solution-focused brief psychotherapy (SFBP) has worked well for individuals with SUD, and more modern group-based SFBP approaches have continued to be successful [121, 122, 127]. Although research has stagnated somewhat, SFBP group therapy appears to be effective for treating SUD, sometimes outperforming traditional programs [127]. This success may lie in allowing patients to choose their own goal structures and giving them more responsibility, which generally increases the likelihood of a positive therapeutic alliance between clinician and patient and typically yields better treatment outcomes [127]. Because depression and anxiety, like chronic pain, are highly comorbid with SUD, clinicians have had more success in targeting these disorders in order to address the other habitual drug-seeking behaviors [122, 127] and solution-focused techniques have been found to outperform traditional therapies in this regard [127]. Specifically, interpersonal functioning, symptom severity, and social roles pre- and post- treatment, have shown improvements in those receiving solution-focused interventions [127–129]. Meta-analyses have also shown that 23% of systematic reviews have reported positive trends in depression-related outcomes [130, 131]. Applying a solution-focused mindset to other psychotherapies, including CBT and MBSR, has also led to positive outcomes in the treatment of SUD and depression [127, 132]. Another advantage of SFBP is its cost effectiveness, due to its brief duration yet surprisingly long-term positive outcomes for many. Although no studies to date have examined the efficacy of SFBP specifically for the treatment of OUD, application of this approach to OUD seems promising.

In the context of chronic pain, the emphasis of solution-searching in SFBP may be advantageous, as individuals living with chronic pain typically react passively to their pain sensations, or develop coping strategies that can be misguided or unhelpful [133]. The idea of a "preferred future," a concept at the core of SFBP wherein the therapist assists the patient in identifying exceptions to their painful *status quo*, has elicited unique responses from patients often lacking in hope [126, 133]. Research on the therapeutic effects of SFBP for chronic pain is quite limited. However, SFBP has been helpful when coupled with physical rehabilitative practices. Two studies have shown improvement of individuals undergoing orthopedic rehabilitation while on sick leave, with over 60% of participants returning to homeostatic daily functioning levels as a result of solution-focused practices, as opposed to a 13% return rate from the waitlisted control groups [134, 135]. A case study also supports the efficacy of combined biofeedback (galvanic skin response) and SFBP in order to manage chronic pain associated with gastro-esophageal reflux disease, with the patient showing a significant decrease in chest pain and increase in personal life satisfaction lasting two months post-treatment [136]. Further research on biopsychological interventions such as combining biofeedback with SFBP for chronic pain could be illuminating.

5.4 Motivational interviewing (MI)

Originally developed by Dr. William Miller for alcohol use disorders in 1983, motivational interviewing (MI) can be described as a therapeutic conversation, held by the therapist and client, about aspects of change [137]. Therapists use specific communication strategies that allow the client to explore their arguments for why change is not possible, seeking to elicit "change talk" from the client by developing discrepancies in the way the client thinks and speaks about their issues. These discrepancies arise from a collaborative exploration of the client's story pertaining to how substance use, for example, has impacted their lives. The therapist's role is to highlight ambivalence that has arisen from the storytelling and provide space for the client to think about what changes they are capable of making [138]. Eventually, by weighing personalized positive and negative aspects related to change outcomes, the client breaks down the lines of logic sustaining pathological behaviors [139, 140]. MI addresses four processes: engaging, focusing, evoking, and planning [141]. Engaging the client in a person-centered style develops the therapeutic bond that will facilitate change [141]. Focus revolves around the change target of the client, which is developed collaboratively to avoid negative power dynamics, polarization, or fractures to the therapeutic relationship [142]. Evocation involves intentional change talk wherein the client must identify their own personal reasons for change and therapist feedback aims to prevent potential losses in motivation related to these reasons. Planning involves collaboration and commitment as the primary method for enforcing the desired change. The ability for the client to elicit their own motivations for change rather than the therapist imposing their own advice is the driving force of this therapy.

MI has become one of the leading theoretical interventions for treating individuals with SUD. Some early explanations of its popularity are its cost effectiveness, theoretical fluidity, usefulness for non-treatment-seeking populations, and motivational enhancement of the client, which is highly important in addiction treatment [143, 144]. Although there have only been a handful of studies, MI has shown clinical efficacy in the treatment of a variety of SUD [143, 145]. For example, the ability to resolve ambivalence related to drug use and to reframe one's perspective of change ultimately reduced active drug use to a larger extent in an MI group compared to a more confrontational counseling style focused on the consequences of risky drug use [138, 139, 146]. Change talk has been shown to play a vital role in treatment outcomes and researchers have hypothesized that it promotes a neurocognitive shift negatively correlated with substance use [147, 148]. For example, an fMRI study showed that positive change talk inhibited activation of reward circuitry by alcohol-associated cues, suggesting that change talk can nullify reward activation under high-risk circumstances and thereby prevent cue-induced relapse [147, 149]. A single-blinded, randomly controlled trial found that bimonthly MI treatment significantly reduced the number of opioid overdose events and promoted a lower attrition rate amongst participants [150] compared to psychoeducation and tertiary prevention strategies [150, 151]. Educational programs did reduce other risk factors, such as viral infections as a result of needle misuse and enhanced protective factors including how to detect overdose, promotion of needle exchanges, and safe injection habits [151]. Future studies examining potential benefits of combined pharmacological and MI methods on treatment outcomes for patients with OUD will be important.

Although controlled studies have been limited by the fluidity of motivational strategies and their implementation, researchers have found that MI can augment treatment of chronic pain, and is moderately effective for lower-back pain, asthma, hypertension, cardiac and respiratory issues, and fibromyalgia [152]. In this context, the focus of MI is on resolving ambivalence through change talk and enhancing the ability to cope with chronic pain by incorporating mindfulness and cognitive restructuring techniques [153–155]. In addition, MI interventions used in conjunction with physiotherapy enhance the therapeutic relationship between the physician and patient, which correlates to more positive outcome expectancies of the patient that ultimately decrease subjective pain intensity and increase range in physical functioning [156]. Another study found that infusing a biopsychosocial assessment of chronic pain with MI also had more favorable outcomes, including marital satisfaction, reductions in pain intensity, stability in positive mood, lower ratings of personal distress, and higher ratings of empathy [155]. Future studies examining the efficacy of MI in treating comorbid SUD and chronic pain would be informative.

6. Conclusions

Chronic pain and addiction are widespread, pervasive, and significant public health burdens that demonstrate a need for more effective management strategies. The known effectiveness of opioids for managing acute pain combined with the limited therapeutic alternatives for chronic pain, have led to an overreliance on opioids for long-term pain management and the current opioid crisis in the United States [2]. In this chapter, the authors have discussed conceptualizing chronic pain and SUD using a similar biopsychosocial framework and suggest that both can be more effectively managed by including clinical mental health therapeutic techniques as opposed to a purely biomedical approach. While psychotherapy has long been used in treating SUD, applying these techniques to chronic pain is fairly novel. Evidence of the effectiveness of these nonpharmacological treatments for chronic pain, particularly for long-term management, is still sparse [157]. However, the techniques highlighted in this review, CBT, MBSR, SFBP, and MI are promising in managing mental illnesses that are frequently comorbid with chronic pain, suggesting further research into their efficacy for chronic pain is warranted. Moreover, the biopsychosocial parallels between chronic pain and SUD represent potential areas of translational research to further improve these nonpharmacological pain management practices and foment social change. By addressing these areas of biopsychosocial overlap, nonpharmacological approaches may hold great promise in reducing the negative impacts of chronic pain and the opioid epidemic simultaneously.

Author details

Zachary S. Harmon[1], Emily N. Welch[2] and Christina L. Ruby[3*]

1 Department of Counseling, Indiana University of Pennsylvania, Indiana, PA 15705, USA

2 Department of Biological Sciences, Kent State University, Kent, OH 44242, USA

3 Department of Biology, Indiana University of Pennsylvania, Indiana, PA 15705, USA

*Address all correspondence to: cruby@iup.edu

References

[1] Haley, D.F. and R. Saitz, The Opioid Epidemic During the COVID-19 Pandemic. JAMA, 2020.

[2] Volkow, N.D. and A.T. McLellan, Opioid Abuse in Chronic Pain--Misconceptions and Mitigation Strategies. N Engl J Med, 2016. 374(13): p. 1253-63.

[3] (IOM), I.o.M., Relieving pain in America: A blueprint for transforming prevention, care, education, and research. 2011, Washington, DC: The National Academic Press.

[4] Bloomquist, E.R., The addiction potential of oxycodone (Percodan). Calif Med, 1963. 99: p. 127-30.

[5] Hooten, W.M., Chronic Pain and Mental Health Disorders: Shared Neural Mechanisms, Epidemiology, and Treatment. Mayo Clin Proc, 2016. 91(7): p. 955-70.

[6] Chihuri, S. and G. Li, Use of Prescription Opioids and Initiation of Fatal 2-Vehicle Crashes. JAMA Netw Open, 2019. 2(2): p. e188081.

[7] Hedlund, J. and K. Macek Drug-impaired driving: Marijuana and opioids raise critical issues for states. 2018.

[8] Cho, J., M.D. Stone, and A.M. Leventhal, Anhedonia as a phenotypic marker of familial transmission of polysubstance use trajectories across midadolescence. Psychol Addict Behav, 2019. 33(1): p. 15-25.

[9] Ilgen, M.A., et al., The timing of onset of pain and substance use disorders. Am J Addict, 2010. 19(5): p. 409-15.

[10] Gatchel, R.J. and D.C. Turk, Psychological approaches to pain management: A practicioner's handbook. 2002, New York, NY: Guilford Press.

[11] Engel, G.L., The need for a new medical model: a challenge for biomedicine. Science, 1977. 196(4286): p. 129-36.

[12] Gatchel, R.J., et al., The biopsychosocial approach to chronic pain: scientific advances and future directions. Psychol Bull, 2007. 133(4): p. 581-624.

[13] Wade, D.T. and P.W. Halligan, The biopsychosocial model of illness: a model whose time has come. Clin Rehabil, 2017. 31(8): p. 995-1004.

[14] Weiner, B.K., Spine update: the biopsychosocial model and spine care. Spine (Phila Pa 1976), 2008. 33(2): p. 219-23.

[15] Gatchel, R.J. and D.C. Turk, Criticisms of the biopsychosocial model in spine care: creating and then attacking a straw person. Spine (Phila Pa 1976), 2008. 33(25): p. 2831-6.

[16] Hart, C.L., Reply to 'Addiction as a brain disease does not promote injustice'. Nat Hum Behav, 2017. 1(9): p. 611.

[17] Heilig, M., et al., Time to connect: bringing social context into addiction neuroscience. Nat Rev Neurosci, 2016. 17(9): p. 592-9.

[18] Alvarez, A.S., M. Pagani, and P. Meucci, The clinical application of the biopsychosocial model in mental health: a research critique. Am J Phys Med Rehabil, 2012. 91(13 Suppl 1): p. S173-80.

[19] Smith, R.C., et al., An evidence-based patient-centered method makes the biopsychosocial model scientific. Patient Educ Couns, 2013. 91(3): p. 265-70.

[20] Wade, C.L., et al., Compulsive-like responding for opioid analgesics in rats with extended access. Neuropsychopharmacology, 2015. 40(2): p. 421-8.

[21] Weiner, S.J., et al., Patient-centered decision making and health care outcomes: an observational study. Ann Intern Med, 2013. 158(8): p. 573-9.

[22] Daley, D.C. and A.B. Douaihy, Relapse Prevention Counseling: Clinical Strategies to Guide Addiction Recovery and Reduce Relapse. 2015, Eau Claire, WI: PESI Publishing & Media.

[23] Buchbinder, R., D. Jolley, and M. Wyatt, 2001 Volvo Award Winner in Clinical Studies: Effects of a media campaign on back pain beliefs and its potential influence on management of low back pain in general practice. Spine (Phila Pa 1976), 2001. 26(23): p. 2535-42.

[24] Ballantyne, J.C. and K.S. LaForge, Opioid dependence and addiction during opioid treatment of chronic pain. Pain, 2007. 129(3): p. 235-55.

[25] Tegethoff, M., et al., Comorbidity of Mental Disorders and Chronic Pain: Chronology of Onset in Adolescents of a National Representative Cohort. J Pain, 2015. 16(10): p. 1054-64.

[26] (APA), A.P.A., Dianostic and statistical manual of mental disorders. 5th ed. 2013, Arlington, VA: American Psychiatric Publishing.

[27] Robinson, T.E. and K.C. Berridge, The neural basis of drug craving: an incentive-sensitization theory of addiction. Brain Res Brain Res Rev, 1993. 18(3): p. 247-91.

[28] Solomon, R.L. and J.D. Corbit, An opponent-process theory of motivation. I. Temporal dynamics of affect. Psychol Rev, 1974. 81(2): p. 119-45.

[29] Koob, G.F. and N.D. Volkow, Neurocircuitry of addiction. Neuropsychopharmacology, 2010. 35(1): p. 217-38.

[30] Dubin, A.E. and A. Patapoutian, Nociceptors: the sensors of the pain pathway. J Clin Invest, 2010. 120(11): p. 3760-72.

[31] Basbaum, A.I., et al., Cellular and molecular mechanisms of pain. Cell, 2009. 139(2): p. 267-84.

[32] Fuchs, P.N., et al., The anterior cingulate cortex and pain processing. Front Integr Neurosci, 2014. 8: p. 35.

[33] Garcia-Larrea, L. and R. Peyron, Pain matrices and neuropathic pain matrices: a review. Pain, 2013. 154 Suppl 1: p. S29-43.

[34] (SAMHSA), C.f.S.A.T., Managing chronic pain in adults with or in recovery from substance use disorders. Treatment Improvement Protocol (TIP). 2012, Rockville, MD: Substance Abuse and Mental Health Services Administration.

[35] (IASP), I.A.f.t.S.o.P., Classification of chronic pain. 2012.

[36] Latremoliere, A. and C.J. Woolf, Central sensitization: a generator of pain hypersensitivity by central neural plasticity. J Pain, 2009. 10(9): p. 895-926.

[37] Luo, C., T. Kuner, and R. Kuner, Synaptic plasticity in pathological pain. Trends Neurosci, 2014. 37(6): p. 343-55.

[38] Moseley, G.L., A pain neuromatrix approach to patients with chronic pain. Man Ther, 2003. 8(3): p. 130-40.

[39] Taylor, A.M.W., Corticolimbic circuitry in the modulation of chronic pain and substance abuse. Prog Neuropsychopharmacol Biol Psychiatry, 2018. 87(Pt B): p. 263-268.

[40] Elman, I. and D. Borsook, Common Brain Mechanisms of Chronic Pain and Addiction. Neuron, 2016. 89(1): p. 11-36.

[41] Leknes, S. and I. Tracey, A common neurobiology for pain and pleasure. Nat Rev Neurosci, 2008. 9(4): p. 314-20.

[42] Thompson, J.M. and V. Neugebauer, Cortico-limbic pain mechanisms. Neurosci Lett, 2019. 702: p. 15-23.

[43] LeBlanc, D.M., et al., The affective dimension of pain as a risk factor for drug and alcohol addiction. Alcohol, 2015. 49(8): p. 803-9.

[44] Mansour, A.R., et al., Chronic pain: the role of learning and brain plasticity. Restor Neurol Neurosci, 2014. 32(1): p. 129-39.

[45] McCarberg, B. and J. Peppin, Pain Pathways and Nervous System Plasticity: Learning and Memory in Pain. Pain Med, 2019. 20(12): p. 2421-2437.

[46] Borsook, D., et al., Reward deficiency and anti-reward in pain chronification. Neurosci Biobehav Rev, 2016. 68: p. 282-297.

[47] Finan, P.H., B. Remeniuk, and K.E. Dunn, The risk for problematic opioid use in chronic pain: What can we learn from studies of pain and reward? Prog Neuropsychopharmacol Biol Psychiatry, 2018. 87(Pt B): p. 255-262.

[48] Gardner, E.L., Addiction and brain reward and antireward pathways. Adv Psychosom Med, 2011. 30: p. 22-60.

[49] Berger, S.E., et al., Risky monetary behavior in chronic back pain is associated with altered modular connectivity of the nucleus accumbens. BMC Res Notes, 2014. 7: p. 739.

[50] Koob, G.F. and M. Le Moal, Plasticity of reward neurocircuitry and the 'dark side' of drug addiction. Nat Neurosci, 2005. 8(11): p. 1442-4.

[51] Cahill, C.M., et al., Allostatic Mechanisms of Opioid Tolerance Beyond Desensitization and Downregulation. Trends Pharmacol Sci, 2016. 37(11): p. 963-976.

[52] Garland, E.L., B. Froeliger, and M.O. Howard, Allostatic dysregulation of natural reward processing in prescription opioid misuse: autonomic and attentional evidence. Biol Psychol, 2015. 105: p. 124-9.

[53] Garland, E.L., et al., Anhedonia in chronic pain and prescription opioid misuse. Psychol Med, 2019: p. 1-12.

[54] Meints, S.M. and R.R. Edwards, Evaluating psychosocial contributions to chronic pain outcomes. Prog Neuropsychopharmacol Biol Psychiatry, 2018. 87(Pt B): p. 168-182.

[55] Valade, D., et al., Emotional status, perceived control of pain, and pain coping strategies in episodic and chronic cluster headache. Eur J Psychology, 2012. 8: p. 461-74.

[56] Degenhardt, L., et al., Global burden of disease attributable to illicit drug use and dependence: findings from the Global Burden of Disease Study 2010. Lancet, 2013. 382(9904): p. 1564-74.

[57] Hser, Y.I., et al., Long-term course of opioid addiction. Harv Rev Psychiatry, 2015. 23(2): p. 76-89.

[58] Hser, Y.I., et al., Chronic pain among patients with opioid use disorder: Results from electronic health records data. J Subst Abuse Treat, 2017. 77: p. 26-30.

[59] Larson, M.J., et al., Persistent pain is associated with substance use after detoxification: a prospective cohort

analysis. Addiction, 2007. 102(5): p. 752-60.

[60] Rosenblum, A., et al., Prevalence and characteristics of chronic pain among chemically dependent patients in methadone maintenance and residential treatment facilities. JAMA, 2003. 289(18): p. 2370-8.

[61] Hah, J.M., et al., Self-loathing aspects of depression reduce postoperative opioid cessation rate. Pain Med, 2014. 15(6): p. 954-64.

[62] Moustafa, A.A., et al., The relationship between childhood trauma, early-life stress, and alcohol and drug use, abuse, and addiction: An integrative review. Current Psychology, 2018.

[63] Stewart, S.H., et al., Functional associations among trauma, PTSD, and substance-related disorders. Addict Behav, 1998. 23(6): p. 797-812.

[64] Berryman, C., et al., Do people with chronic pain have impaired executive function? A meta-analytical review. Clin Psychol Rev, 2014. 34(7): p. 563-79.

[65] Baker, K.S., et al., Everyday Executive Functioning in Chronic Pain: Specific Deficits in Working Memory and Emotion Control, Predicted by Mood, Medications, and Pain Interference. Clin J Pain, 2016. 32(8): p. 673-80.

[66] Attal, N., et al., Does cognitive functioning predict chronic pain? Results from a prospective surgical cohort. Brain, 2014. 137(Pt 3): p. 904-17.

[67] Marino, E.N., et al., Impulsivity but not sensation seeking is associated with opioid analgesic misuse risk in patients with chronic pain. Addict Behav, 2013. 38(5): p. 2154-7.

[68] Vest, N., C.J. Reynolds, and S.L. Tragesser, Impulsivity and risk for prescription opioid misuse in a chronic pain patient sample. Addict Behav, 2016. 60: p. 184-90.

[69] Cunha, A.M., et al., High trait impulsivity potentiates the effects of chronic pain on impulsive behavior. Neurobiol Pain, 2020. 7: p. 100042.

[70] Hess, L.E., et al., Beyond pain: modeling decision-making deficits in chronic pain. Front Behav Neurosci, 2014. 8: p. 263.

[71] Havassy, B.E., S.M. Hall, and D.A. Wasserman, Social support and relapse: commonalities among alcoholics, opiate users, and cigarette smokers. Addict Behav, 1991. 16(5): p. 235-46.

[72] Navratilova, E. and F. Porreca, Reward and motivation in pain and pain relief. Nat Neurosci, 2014. 17(10): p. 1304-12.

[73] Leach, D. and H.R. Kranzler, An Interpersonal Model of Addiction Relapse. Addict Disord Their Treat, 2013. 12(4): p. 183-192.

[74] Trucco, E.M., A review of psychosocial factors linked to adolescent substance use. Pharmacol Biochem Behav, 2020. 196: p. 172969.

[75] van Os, J., G. Kenis, and B.P. Rutten, The environment and schizophrenia. Nature, 2010. 468(7321): p. 203-12.

[76] Fattore, L., S. Altea, and W. Fratta, Sex differences in drug addiction: a review of animal and human studies. Womens Health (Lond), 2008. 4: p. 51-65.

[77] Zlebnik, N.E., Females pay a higher price for addiction. Neuropsychopharmacology, 2019. 44(7): p. 1179-1181.

[78] Wallace, J.M., Jr., The social ecology of addiction: race, risk, and resilience. Pediatrics, 1999. 103(5 Pt 2): p. 1122-7.

[79] Jegede, O., Addiction, Race, and the Structurally Vulnerable. Am J Addict, 2020. 29(5): p. 428-429.

[80] Gatchel, R.J., et al., Interdisciplinary chronic pain management: past, present, and future. Am Psychol, 2014. 69(2): p. 119-30.

[81] Chou, R., et al., The effectiveness and risks of long-term opioid therapy for chronic pain: a systematic review for a National Institutes of Health Pathways to Prevention Workshop. Ann Intern Med, 2015. 162(4): p. 276-86.

[82] Frank, J.W., et al., Patient Outcomes in Dose Reduction or Discontinuation of Long-Term Opioid Therapy: A Systematic Review. Ann Intern Med, 2017. 167(3): p. 181-191.

[83] Deyo, R.A., et al., Opioids for back pain patients: primary care prescribing patterns and use of services. J Am Board Fam Med, 2011. 24(6): p. 717-27.

[84] Zwart, J.A., et al., Depression and anxiety disorders associated with headache frequency. The Nord-Trondelag Health Study. Eur J Neurol, 2003. 10(2): p. 147-52.

[85] Brewer, J.A., H.M. Elwafi, and J.H. Davis, Craving to quit: psychological models and neurobiological mechanisms of mindfulness training as treatment for addictions. Psychol Addict Behav, 2013. 27(2): p. 366-79.

[86] Dowell, D., T.M. Haegerich, and R. Chou, CDC Guideline for Prescribing Opioids for Chronic Pain--United States, 2016. JAMA, 2016. 315(15): p. 1624-45.

[87] Turk, D.C., Cognitive-behavioral approach to the treatment of chronic pain patients. Reg Anesth Pain Med, 2003. 28(6): p. 573-9.

[88] Copenhaver, M.M., R.D. Bruce, and F.L. Altice, Behavioral counseling content for optimizing the use of buprenorphine for treatment of opioid dependence in community-based settings: a review of the empirical evidence. Am J Drug Alcohol Abuse, 2007. 33(5): p. 643-54.

[89] Dutra, L., et al., A meta-analytic review of psychosocial interventions for substance use disorders. Am J Psychiatry, 2008. 165(2): p. 179-87.

[90] Hides, L., et al., Quik Fix: a randomized controlled trial of an enhanced brief motivational interviewing intervention for alcohol/ cannabis and psychological distress in young people. Psychother Psychosom, 2013. 82(2): p. 122-4.

[91] Otto, M.W., et al., A randomized, controlled trial of the efficacy of an interoceptive exposure-based CBT for treatment-refractory outpatients with opioid dependence. J Psychoactive Drugs, 2014. 46(5): p. 402-11.

[92] Pan, S., et al., Efficacy of Cognitive Behavioral Therapy on Opiate Use and Retention in Methadone Maintenance Treatment in China: A Randomised Trial. PLoS One, 2015. 10(6): p. e0127598.

[93] Weiss, R.D., et al., Adjunctive counseling during brief and extended buprenorphine-naloxone treatment for prescription opioid dependence: a 2-phase randomized controlled trial. Arch Gen Psychiatry, 2011. 68(12): p. 1238-46.

[94] Montoya, I.D., et al., Randomized trial of buprenorphine for treatment of concurrent opiate and cocaine dependence. Clin Pharmacol Ther, 2004. 75(1): p. 34-48.

[95] Hides, L., S. Samet, and D.I. Lubman, Cognitive behaviour therapy (CBT) for the treatment of co-occurring depression and substance use: current evidence and directions for future

research. Drug Alcohol Rev, 2010. 29(5): p. 508-17.

[96] Prendergast, M., et al., Contingency management for treatment of substance use disorders: a meta-analysis. Addiction, 2006. 101(11): p. 1546-60.

[97] Panlilio, L.V., et al., Choice between delayed food and immediate opioids in rats: treatment effects and individual differences. Psychopharmacology (Berl), 2017. 234(22): p. 3361-3373.

[98] Glombiewski, J.A., et al., Exposure and CBT for chronic back pain: An RCT on differential efficacy and optimal length of treatment. J Consult Clin Psychol, 2018. 86(6): p. 533-545.

[99] Chou, R., et al., Nonpharmacologic Therapies for Low Back Pain: A Systematic Review for an American College of Physicians Clinical Practice Guideline. Ann Intern Med, 2017. 166(7): p. 493-505.

[100] Deol, H.S. and E. Gondles, Strategies in managing chronic pain. Corrections Today, 2018. 80: p. 76-85.

[101] Morley, S., A. Williams, and S. Hussain, Estimating the clinical effectiveness of cognitive behavioural therapy in the clinic: evaluation of a CBT informed pain management programme. Pain, 2008. 137(3): p. 670-80.

[102] Boersma, K., et al., Lowering fear-avoidance and enhancing function through exposure in vivo. A multiple baseline study across six patients with back pain. Pain, 2004. 108(1-2): p. 8-16.

[103] Chiesa, A. and A. Serretti, Are mindfulness-based interventions effective for substance use disorders? A systematic review of the evidence. Subst Use Misuse, 2014. 49(5): p. 492-512.

[104] Teasdale, J.D., Z. Segal, and J.M. Williams, How does cognitive therapy prevent depressive relapse and why should attentional control (mindfulness) training help? Behav Res Ther, 1995. 33(1): p. 25-39.

[105] Linehan, M.M., Dialectical behavior therapy for treatment of borderline personality disorder: implications for the treatment of substance abuse. NIDA Res Monogr, 1993. 137: p. 201-16.

[106] Shonin, E. and W. Van Gordon, The Mechanisms of Mindfulness in the Treatment of Mental Illness and Addiction. Int J Ment Health Addict, 2016. 14(5): p. 844-849.

[107] Garland, E.L., et al., The downward spiral of chronic pain, prescription opioid misuse, and addiction: cognitive, affective, and neuropsychopharmacologic pathways. Neurosci Biobehav Rev, 2013. 37(10 Pt 2): p. 2597-607.

[108] Westbrook, C., et al., Mindful attention reduces neural and self-reported cue-induced craving in smokers. Soc Cogn Affect Neurosci, 2013. 8(1): p. 73-84.

[109] Garland, E.L., B. Froeliger, and M.O. Howard, Mindfulness training targets neurocognitive mechanisms of addiction at the attention-appraisal-emotion interface. Front Psychiatry, 2014. 4: p. 173.

[110] Smallwood, R.F., J.S. Potter, and D.A. Robin, Neurophysiological mechanisms in acceptance and commitment therapy in opioid-addicted patients with chronic pain. Psychiatry Res Neuroimaging, 2016. 250: p. 12-4.

[111] Quoidbach, J., et al., Positive emotion regulation and well-being: Comparing the impact of eight savoring and dampening strategies. Personality and Individual Differences, 2010. 49(5): p. 368-373.

[112] Imani, S., et al., Comparing Mindfulness-Based Group Therapy With Treatment as Usual for Opioid Dependents: A Pilot Randomized Clinical Trial Study Protocol. Iran J Psychiatry Behav Sci, 2015. 9(1): p. e216.

[113] Imani, S., et al., Effectiveness of Mindfulness-Based Group Therapy Compared to the Usual Opioid Dependence Treatment. Iran J Psychiatry, 2015. 10(3): p. 175-84.

[114] Davenport, J., L.C. Koch, and P.D. Rumrill, Mindfulness-based approaches for managing chronic pain: Applications to vocational rehabilitation and employment. Journal of Vocational Rehabilitation, 2017. 47(2): p. 247-258.

[115] Marchand, W.R., Mindfulness-based stress reduction, mindfulness-based cognitive therapy, and Zen meditation for depression, anxiety, pain, and psychological distress. J Psychiatr Pract, 2012. 18(4): p. 233-52.

[116] Opialla, S., et al., Neural circuits of emotion regulation: a comparison of mindfulness-based and cognitive reappraisal strategies. Eur Arch Psychiatry Clin Neurosci, 2015. 265(1): p. 45-55.

[117] Chiesa, A. and A. Serretti, Mindfulness-based interventions for chronic pain: a systematic review of the evidence. J Altern Complement Med, 2011. 17(1): p. 83-93.

[118] Froeliger, B.E., et al., Neurocognitive correlates of the effects of yoga meditation practice on emotion and cognition: a pilot study. Front Integr Neurosci, 2012. 6: p. 48.

[119] Vago, D.R. and Y. Nakamura, Selective Attentional Bias Towards Pain-Related Threat in Fibromyalgia: Preliminary Evidence for Effects of Mindfulness Meditation Training. Cognitive Therapy and Research, 2011. 35(6): p. 581-594.

[120] Zeidan, F., et al., Mindfulness meditation-related pain relief: evidence for unique brain mechanisms in the regulation of pain. Neurosci Lett, 2012. 520(2): p. 165-73.

[121] O'Hanlon, B. and M. Weiner-Davis, In search of solutions: A new direction in psychotherapy. 2003, New York, NY: WW Norton & Company.

[122] Linton, J., Mental health counselors and substance abuse treatment: Advantages, difficulties, and practical issues to solution-focused interventions. J Mental Health Counseling, 2005. 27: p. 297-310.

[123] de Shazer, S., Clues: Investigating solutions in brief therapy. 1988, New York, NY: WW Norton & Company.

[124] Gingerich, W.J. and S. Eisengart, Solution-focused brief therapy: a review of the outcome research. Fam Process, 2000. 39(4): p. 477-98.

[125] Rogers, C.R., The interpersonal relationship: The core of guidance. Harvard Educational Review, 1962. 32: p. 176.

[126] Simon, J.K. and I.K. Berg, Solution-focused brief therapy with long-term problems. 1999.

[127] Smock, S.A., et al., Solution-focused group therapy for level 1 substance abusers. J Marital Fam Ther, 2008. 34(1): p. 107-20.

[128] McCollum, E.E., T.S. Trepper, and S.A. Smock, Solution-focused group therapy for substance abuse: Extending competency-based models. J Family Psychotherapy, 2004. 14: p. 27-42.

[129] Sundstrom, S.M., Single-session psychotherapy for depression: Is it better to focus on problems or solutions?, in Psychology. 1993, Iowa State University: Ann Arbor, MI.

[130] Dargan, P.J., R. Simm, and C. Murray, New approaches towards chronic pain: patient experiences of a solution-focused pain management programme. Br J Pain, 2014. 8(1): p. 34-42.

[131] Gingerich, W.J. and L.T. Peterson, Effectiveness of Solution-Focused Brief Therapy: A Systematic Qualitative Review of Controlled Outcome Studies. Research on Social Work Practice, 2013. 23(3): p. 266-283.

[132] Berg, I.K. and N.H. Reuss, Solutions step by step: A substance abuse treatment manual. 1998, New York, NY: WW Norton & Company.

[133] Eccleston, C. and G. Crombez, Worry and chronic pain: a misdirected problem solving model. Pain, 2007. 132(3): p. 233-6.

[134] Cockburn, J.T., F.N. Thomas, and O.J. Cockburn, Solution-focused therapy and psychosocial adjustment to orthopedic rehabilitation in a work hardening program. Journal of Occupational Rehabilitation, 1997. 7(2): p. 97-106.

[135] Thorslund, K.W., Solution-focused group therapy for patients on long-term sick leave: A comparative outcome study. J Family Psychotherapy, 2007. 18: p. 11-24.

[136] Brooks, P., et al., Biofeedback and solution-focused therapy: Case study of chronic pain, in Applied Psychopathology and Biofeedback. 2005, Springer/Plenum New York, NY. p. 417-8.

[137] Miller, W.R., Motivational Interviewing with Problem Drinkers. Behavioural Psychotherapy, 1983. 11(2): p. 147-172.

[138] Littrell, J., How addiction happens, how change happens, and what social workers need to know to be effective facilitators of change. J Evidence-Based Social Work, 2011. 8: p. 469-86.

[139] Miller, W.R. and G.S. Rose, Toward a Theory of Motivational Interviewing. American Psychologist, 2009. 64(6): p. 527-537.

[140] Wagner, C. and K. Ingersoll, Motivational interviewing in groups. 2013, New York, NY: Guilford Press.

[141] Miller, W.R. and S. Rollnick, Applications of motivational interviewing. Motivational interviewing: Helping people change. 3rd ed. 2013, New York, NY: Guilford Press.

[142] Madson, M.B., et al., Measuring Client Experiences of Motivational Interviewing During a Lifestyle Intervention. Measurement and Evaluation in Counseling and Development, 2015. 48(2): p. 140-151.

[143] Bjork, A., Stabilizing a fluid intervention: The development of Motivational Interviewing, 1983-2013. Addiction Research & Theory, 2014. 22(4): p. 313-324.

[144] Heather, N., Motivational interviewing: Is it all our clients need? Addiction Research & Theory, 2005. 13(1): p. 1-18.

[145] Burke, B.L., H. Arkowitz, and M. Menchola, The efficacy of motivational interviewing: A meta-analysis of controlled clinical trials. Journal of Consulting and Clinical Psychology, 2003. 71(5): p. 843-861.

[146] Karno, M.P. and R. Longabaugh, Does matching matter? Examining matches and mismatches between patient attributes and therapy techniques in alcoholism treatment. Addiction, 2007. 102(4): p. 587-96.

[147] Feldstein Ewing, S.W., et al., Proposed model of the neurobiological

mechanisms underlying psychosocial alcohol interventions: the example of motivational interviewing. J Stud Alcohol Drugs, 2011. 72(6): p. 903-16.

[148] Moyers, T.B., et al., Can Specialized Training Teach Clinicians to Recognize, Reinforce, and Elicit Client Language in Motivational Interviewing? Alcoholism-Clinical and Experimental Research, 2011. 35(6): p. 84a-84a.

[149] Kalivas, P.W., N. Volkow, and J. Seamans, Unmanageable motivation in addiction: a pathology in prefrontal-accumbens glutamate transmission. Neuron, 2005. 45(5): p. 647-50.

[150] Coffin, P.O., et al., Behavioral intervention to reduce opioid overdose among high-risk persons with opioid use disorder: A pilot randomized controlled trial. PLoS One, 2017. 12(10): p. e0183354.

[151] Walley, A.Y., et al., Opioid overdose rates and implementation of overdose education and nasal naloxone distribution in Massachusetts: interrupted time series analysis. BMJ, 2013. 346: p. f174.

[152] Chilton, R., R. Pires-Yfantouda, and M. Wylie, A systematic review of motivational interviewing within musculoskeletal health. Psychol Health Med, 2012. 17(4): p. 392-407.

[153] Cano, A. and M. Leonard, Integrative behavioral couple therapy for chronic pain: promoting behavior change and emotional acceptance. J Clin Psychol, 2006. 62(11): p. 1409-18.

[154] Goubert, L., et al., Facing others in pain: the effects of empathy. Pain, 2005. 118(3): p. 285-8.

[155] Miller-Matero, L.R. and A. Cano, Encouraging couples to change: a motivational assessment to promote well-being in people with chronic pain and their partners. Pain Med, 2015. 16(2): p. 348-55.

[156] Cheing, G., et al., Testing a path-analytic mediation model of how motivational enhancement physiotherapy improves physical functioning in pain patients. J Occup Rehabil, 2014. 24(4): p. 798-805.

[157] Skelly, A.C., et al., in Noninvasive Nonpharmacological Treatment for Chronic Pain: A Systematic Review. 2018: Rockville (MD).

Chapter 8

Supervision of Substance Abuse Therapeutics Emphasizing the Discrimination Model of Supervision and Motivational Interview Practices

John A. Mills and Maren Krizner

Abstract

There is considerable pressure from varied sources to provide effective supervision to professionals who deliver therapeutic services to persons being treated for substance use disorders. The literature of supervision continues to evolve as the utility of supervision models and their applicability with substance abuse therapeutics are explored. Among the many models of supervision, Bernard's Discrimination Model of supervision is experiencing on-going development in the context of a variety of clinical services. The current chapter will describe how Bernard's model can be used effectively to enhance the supervision of substance abuse professionals as well as how further development of the model would enhance the approach. The Discrimination Model will be combined with existing literature of Motivational Interviewing approaches to describe key elements of effective clinical supervision with professionals delivering services in a complex and challenging industry.

Keywords: Discrimination model, motivational interviewing, supervision of substance use therapeutics

1. Introduction

Clinical supervision is indispensable to the professional development and well-being of therapists in all areas of mental health intervention.[1] Supervision is unavoidably a process that involves at least three participants: a Supervisor, a therapist, and at least one client. In most supervision cases, the supervisory activity attends to the work of the therapist with more than one client and each client then becomes part of this relationship triad (one triad for each client). Therapists must contend with challenges associated with patient difficulties and possess a great range of skills and knowledge to be successful. Besides the extensive array of personal and professional attributes necessary to promote therapeutic effectiveness in general, therapists must understand particular and unique patient concerns in the context in

[1] "Therapist" will be used interchangeably with comparable professional titles such as "counselor" and "service provider." No substantive difference is intended or implied.

which the therapist works. Intervention with patients with substance use disorder (SUD) requires a uniquely broad and complex body of knowledge as well as the ability to thrive under an emotionally charged set of stressors that are intrinsic to the treatment industry [1]. SUDs are serious and commonly long-term disorders that requires systematic and vigorous interdisciplinary intervention, education, and support [2]. As a result, successful work as a therapist with clients with SUDs requires skills associated with all types of psychological intervention as well as issues that are uniquely relevant to intervention with SUD patients [2].

In addition to the challenges of work with persons with SUDs, the treatment setting is further complicated by the fact that the professional background of SUD treatment providers is quite heterogeneous. While it may not be obvious to people outside the industry, SUD treatment professionals function in their roles on the basis of many different specific forms of professional training [2–5]. In fact, SUD treatment programs are unique within the spectrum of mental health services in that professionals within these programs are qualified to provide services even if they do not have a master's degree (e.g. [6]). While many jurisdictions have established certifications for SUD professionals, the variety of therapist backgrounds and characteristics is a reality that heightens the need for effective and persistent mentorship. Tatarsky [7] described the main components of intervention with SUDs. The author asserted that any supervision of SUD intervention must include how the therapist works with the therapeutic alliance, fosters corrective emotional experiences with the client, and how to teach of self-regulation. These challenges are considerable.

There are more than sufficient rational arguments for attending to the nature and quality of the supervision of SUD therapists. First, there is great variability in therapist training, so initial preparation to provide SUD treatment is critical. The range of issues that are essential to even beginning SUD treatment include skill with addiction processes, diagnostic concepts and practices, and methods of intervention. Next, these aforementioned basics that may be considered internal to treatment can be made more complicated by political realities. For example, there have been widely shifting attitudes in both public and professional circles about the status of persons with SUDs ("junkies," "addicts") throughout history [7]. The ethical and effective clinician will be sensitive to the varieties of client backgrounds and will use supervision as a part of on-going efforts to be expand these sensibilities. Such a clinician will refrain from a narrow view of patients and strive to build a therapeutic alliance in the context of the client's cultural context. These forces have real consequences for persons with SUDs that may become a focus in treatment. In addition to the initial considerations training, SUD therapists have considerable on-going training needs as they continue working in the field. For example, legal and ethical issues are persistent challenges that must be resolved. Adding to the demands already noted, the stress of continued work in the field places real demands on therapists, rendering continued emotional support essential. One can readily see how supervision may be essential to the well-being of clinicians and the utility of treatment efforts.

As already established, therapists and supervisors are called upon to function effectively in the context of differing demands for results, significant ethical, legal, and cultural consideration, gaps in training, increasing pressure to use empirically supported practices, differences pertaining to services being provided by persons with and without prior SUDs, and differing models for intervention [4]. As a result, the demand on SUD treatment supervisors is more complex and demanding than what might be found in other contexts. The question then arises about how to think of optimal clinical supervision. The Center for Substance Abuse Treatment [8] attempted to define effectively functioning clinical supervisors as those who are knowledgeable about SUDs as well as all other areas of therapeutic practice. Much of this definition was grounded in technical skills of supervisors because of the complexities of clinical tasks for therapists. While this need for the highest quality supervision is seemingly irrefutable, there is a relative dearth of recent empirical literature to support this idea. There is some evidence to support the role of supervision in the job performance of therapists [5, 9]. Laschober and colleagues [2] reported the results of an investigation of the quality of counselor preparation as a function of supervision effectiveness. Harkening to the complexities of supervisory tasks, the authors confirmed the demands on practitioners and supervisors discussed above, and described the perceptions of SUD counselors in this regard. It is important to note that Laschober and her colleagues concluded that significant emphasis must be placed on the quality of the supervisory relationship. Their work was a survey design that lacked the elements necessary to infer causality between effective clinical supervision and the job performance of counselors, but it did support the link between supervisory skill and counselor outcomes. This remains an area in which experimental designs are still needed.

As just described, there is real importance to the development of a strong supervisory alliance. This reality has been echoed in many works in the field (e.g. [10, 11]). This connection has been discussed in the literature of both the supervision of mental health and SUD clinicians. The supervisory alliance is a medium for social influence in a critical professional area [12, 13]. The working alliance in supervision is most commonly defined as a supportive relationship that includes three components: agreement on goals, agreement on tasks to pursue the goals, and the bond that develops between the supervisor and therapist. [14–16]. There are some reports of research that suggest that the alliance and the associated mentoring are a distinct predictor of therapist proficiency relative to technical proficiency of the supervisor [2].

2. The discrimination model

There is undisputed importance to the identification, examination, and application of effective and appropriate models for clinical work. This is also true for clinical supervision for SUDs. Optimal supervision requires a keen sense for the wide range of difficulties of the therapist, and models of supervision can hasten and sharpen the processes by which supervisors identify and work with training needs. Suitable models of supervision may function as a guard against toxic fluctuations in the strategies used by supervisors [11].

2.1 Development and concept of the discrimination model

In 1979, Bernard introduced the "Discrimination Model" (DM) of supervisor training, at least partly in response to confusion in the literature about the significance of supervision, a dearth of literature regarding the training of supervisors, and a wish to promote an effective training model that addresses the processes of supervision. The majority of the following description comes directly from Bernard's 1979 seminal paper [17]. The model has been applied in a number of subsequent works that highlight its applicability [18–22]. The discrimination model is named as such because its main function is to provide the supervisor with a variety of approaches that they may apply within a given situation at their discretion without the limitations of theory. In the discrimination model, the supervisor must identify the area of skill or behavior with which the counselor most requires assistance at a particular time (process, conceptualization, or personalization), and then subsequently assume one of three roles (teacher, counselor, or consultant) by which to provide said assistance. The variety of combinations that result from this process grant the supervisor with nine possible approaches to a given situation, allowing for the maximization of effective communication between the supervisor and the counselor. It is important to explicate these approaches as prelude to the discussion of integration with other supervisory skills.

The ultimate goal of supervisor training is to provide counselors with the necessary skills for successful intervention. Bernard divides these necessary skills into three major categories: process skills, conceptualization skills, and personalization skills. At any given time, a counselor may be exhibiting behaviors that relate to these skill categories, and the discrimination model assists the supervisor in identifying the nature of the trainee behavior for supervisory intervention. "Process" behaviors are those which relate to the conduct of the session, such as effectively opening and closing the session, implementing different intervention techniques, or encouraging communication with nonverbal cues. Process behaviors indicate to the client that the counseling has begun and how it is progressing. Counselor-trainees typically learn these skills early in their training, though they may also be skill areas that evolve throughout their career. A counselor-trainee who struggles in this area may incorrectly implement a specific technique, have difficulty maintaining a robust working alliance, or fail to effectively communicate with the client. When evaluating and assisting counselors with the development of process skills within the discrimination model, the supervisor is to focus on how these skills and techniques are executed, as opposed to whether or not they are the appropriate skills to apply within the given situation. "Conceptualization" behaviors are skills which pertain to comprehension, analysis, recognizing themes or patterns, and deciding which strategies and techniques would be most effectively applied to help the client achieve their goals. Since these behaviors take place primarily as cognitive functions, they are more difficult for a supervisor to observe within the session. Conceptualization should occur both within the session and between sessions. It is possible for a counselor the struggle with, say, recognizing patterns within the client during the session, but easily do so when writing a case report of the same client. Therefore, it is important for a supervisor to differentiate between these two areas of conceptualization and determine where the counselor-trainee is struggling in order to maximize effectiveness of supervision. Lastly, "personalization" skills are the counselor's ability to maintain professionalism, take responsibility and authority within their position as counselor, use their inner experience as professional guidance, accept challenges, feedback, or criticism from the client, avoid projecting personal beliefs and values onto the client, and maintain a basic, fundamental respect for the client. Development of these skills requires a willingness for personal growth within the counselor. Because the advancement of personalization skills requires the counselor to identify personal flaws and biases that inhibit their ability to be objective toward the client, such advancement is simultaneously emotionally difficult and perpetually necessary in all counselors. It is important the supervisor treats the learning of personalization skills as not a sign of personal shortcoming in the counselor, but as being equivalent to learning any process or conceptualization skills. The ability of the counselor to possess adequate skills in each of these three areas of behavior is vital to the success of intervention. The discrimination model aims to train both the counselor and the supervisor to recognize which areas specific behaviors pertain to and better understand where issues arise.

As the supervisor is able to recognize an issue as falling into one of these three areas, the supervisor must determine the best approach with which to present instruction. Bernard identifies three possible approaches or roles the supervisor may take on in order to do so: teacher, counselor, or consultant. When taking on the "teacher" role, the supervisor's goal is to impart knowledge and information to the counselor-trainee. This might include, but not be limited to, introducing relevant professional literature or directly explaining a concept or technique. Within the "counselor" role, the supervisor works with the personal needs of the counselor, helping them to overcome personal or emotional barriers that inhibit their development as a counselor. While maintaining appropriate professional boundaries, the supervisor evokes the inner subjective experience to facility the trainee having the most fluid and adaptative access to this part of their reaction and approach to a client. Lastly, when taking the role of "consultant," the supervisor acts less authoritatively, engaging in reciprocal dialog and offering suggestions and discussions of professional and case material in order to come to solutions or more advanced understanding in the trainee. It is deeply important that the supervisor chooses their role based on the needs of the counselor within the situation. The model does not work if the supervisor chooses a role because it is most comfortable or natural to their disposition.

2.2 Application of the discrimination model

Bernard [23] saw supervision as an activity that emerged more from the training of therapists than the nature of therapy relationships despite the fact that many models of supervision closely followed models of psychotherapy. Given the above-noted significance of mentorship in supervision the skilled and purposeful application of the seemingly simple discrimination model may be critical. It is important, then, to consider how the DM is used.

The discrimination model offers an array of approaches that a supervisor can employ by first identifying the skill type within which an issue occurs, and then assuming the role which they feel is best fit for the situation. For example, a counselor-trainee may approach the supervisor expressing that they wish to use a technique that they have not learned with a client. This would be an instance of building process skills, and the supervisor may take on the role of "teacher", providing the counselor-trainee with resources and information on how to use the desired technique. In another instance, the supervisor may notice that the counselor-trainee is more hesitant to work with clients of the opposite gender, an issue which relates to the counselor-trainee's personalization skills. Here, the supervisor might choose to take on the role of counselor and attempt to help the counselor-trainee understand what aspects of their own world view may be contributing to this bias. Although it may be tempting to associate specific supervisor roles with specific skill areas, such as, for example, assuming the development of process skills always necessitates the teacher role, it is important to remember that any combination may occur. The discrimination model is most effective when the supervisor's approach is selected based solely on the circumstances of the given situation.

Use of the supervisor role from the DM is based on the real needs of the supervisee and this may not be directly evidenced by the manifest nature of the dilemma as just described. For example, when confronting ethical, legal, and professional issues in SUD treatment, the trainee may have a lack of information for which they need instruction, a need for help considering alternatives about which they are already familiar, or more personal assistance working through more subjective blocks to effective and appropriate application of relevant standards. Thus, the supervisor must develop an appreciate the dynamics of a supervisees dilemma before adopting the teacher, consultant, or counselor role with a specific dilemma.

The complex skill needs of the therapist in SUD treatment may make the simple structure of the DM a useful framework for the consideration of the areas of supervision that merit the greatest focus. Given the extent and nature of the complexities of the SUD diagnosis and treatment planning, conceptual problems are readily encountered. Between diagnostic categories, complexities of treatment planning, and implementation of a treatment program, the therapist has a significant array of ideas to consider and integrate. In addition, the SUD treatment environment can be highly evocative for the professional therapy environment, and it is natural for an inexperienced therapist could need support and counsel with the emotional components of the work. Finally, SUD treatment can be very difficult to implement, and the process tasks of a therapist can be very important to address to maximize the likelihood of proper treatment implementation.

Specific settings can further highlight the utility of the DM. Byrne and Sias [24] reported on the application of the DM model to supervision of direct care professionals in adolescent residential treatment programs. In particular, they focused on therapist intentionality, flexibility, and professionalism as target themes for supervision activities. The authors highlighted how the conceptualization role could be tailored to the exact needs of the trainees. With widely varying amounts of experience and training, the therapist would have differing needs for how to understand clinical situations. In addition, careful focus on conceptualization allows the supervisor to be responsive to the different needs while allowing for team collaboration in shared understanding of clinical dilemmas. This focus enhanced the effectiveness of the therapists. Their effectiveness was further enhanced by a suitable attention to personalization. By encouraging the therapist to employ their own personal style to interventions and being careful of their own reactions in an evocative environment, focus could remain on planned interventions without the interference of unmodulated therapist emotions.

The DM can also magnify the impact of specialized or advanced supervisory functions. The prospect of the "parallel process" in supervision is also a challenge to supervision that is such an example for the DM. The idea of a parallel process began in psychodynamic writings as a replication of the therapy relationship and supervision outside of the awareness of the participants [25]. The concept was not initially named in the seminal literature, but the parallel process concept received increasing attention and has evolved into a well-articulated principle. The parallel process notion was clarified extensively in the literature, beginning with Doehrman's [26] work. Doehrman's work was a landmark contribution in identifying issues of power, control, dependency, intimacy, and judgment as manifest in the parallel process of supervision [27]. The concept of the parallel process began to receive successful empirical examination in subsequent decades [28]. The parallel process is now clarified as a set of sometimes parallel phenomena between the supervision relationship and the treatment relationship. Many authors now recognize the phenomenon with or without the psychodynamic trappings and independent of theoretical orientations.

2.3 Limitations of the discrimination model

With any clinical approach there are limitations that may be anticipated. For now, we will consider limitations of the DM that are associated with the application of the model. Some approaches to, activities of, and contexts for supervision are inconsistent with parts of the nine "cells" in the model. The cells of the model have to be applied in a manner that is optimally targeted to the specific milieu. Therapists in such a context must learn about the significance of supervision, the responsibilities and functions of supervisors, and the responsibilities of therapists in the supervisory conditions. For example, quick application of supervision that occurs in front of clients can be corrosive to the delicate work that needs to happen within the supervision. This could easily complicate the delivery of group services in the

SUD treatment context. In addition, the model does not prescribe exact approaches for exact situations and has not been empirically investigated for doing so. As a result, the model is useful for considering possible approaches and enjoys some rich descriptions of its application, but the DM is not yet supported by well-designed empirical work.

The model does not appear to provide a locus for what may be considered "external" or "political" considerations or when disciplinary action is in the offing. There are a number of possible components that fit in this area of concern. First, if supervision needs to turn to issues of therapist accountability, it is not clear what supervisory function is invoked. That is, when there are deficiencies in practical dimensions of a therapist's work and development efforts seem to have been exhausted, the preferred cells in the DM are not clear. Perhaps obviously, the counselor would not be the preferred role. It is possible that the consultant role could be invoked, particularly in situations in which the therapist was bringing some of the issues to the table on their own. In the end, however, if discussions of objective components of performance or considerations of job action were imperative, the DM may be irrelevant or at least not instructive.

A political consideration might be the career development of the therapist. It is quite appropriate for such discussions to be some part of supervision and mentorship, but the DM might not be helpful. One might argue that the consultant role would be useful in general professional mentorship, but this has not been suggested or discussed in the literature [29].

A final limitation of note was raised by the work of Crunk and Barden [18] who began a discussion of the relative lack of research into the integration of the discrimination model with other supervisory factors. In particular, their work integrated the "common factors" of supervision that by themselves have already received such robust support [30]. Their preliminary efforts are a part of future developments that are spawned by the discrimination model but are yet to be realized.

3. Motivational interviewing

3.1 Development and concepts

This chapter is based on the notion that Motivational Interviewing (MI: [31]) is a highly useful approach to treatment *and* supervision and with SUD patients and therapists in particular. MI was originally designed to assist with persons suffering from mental health conditions whose difficulties seemed particularly challenging because of internal conflict about treatment and behavior change. The applicability of MI to SUD treatment was readily made when MI was introduced, and its widespread utility has been reflected in the literature since then [32]. After introducing and describing MI, the discussion will turn to an integration of MI concepts and methods with the DM to maximize supervisory effectiveness.

MI is a technique which focuses on working with the client to uncover motivation for change that is already posited as being present within the client. The goal of MI is to use the client's own desires and feelings in order to overcome resistance to change which would otherwise inhibit the therapeutic process [33]. MI develops many of its key goals and practices based upon Rogers' [34] necessary and sufficient conditions for constructive personality change. Rogers proposes six conditions which must be met in order for personality change to occur within the therapeutic setting.

The first and most basic of these conditions is that two people must be in psychological contact. In other words, there must be some sort of relationship between the counselor and the client of which both parties are aware. Conditions 2–6 relate to the nature of this relationship. The second condition is that the client must be in some state of incongruity. Within this state of incongruity, the client is experiencing a disconnect between their perceived self and their actual behaviors and experience. This idea relates closely with Festinger's theory of cognitive dissonance, a principle which is also frequently employed within MI [35]. Rogers' third condition for change is that the counselor is consistent and genuine within their relationship with the client. The counselor must be aware and accepting of their own feelings within the relationship, and must not attempt to act in any way that is disingenuous or performative. The fourth condition requires the counselor to experience unconditional positive regard toward the client. The counselor must aim to be accepting of all of the client's experiences or statements, without the presence of judgment or persuasion. The fifth condition proposes that the counselor must hold an empathetic understanding of the client's internal perception of their own experiences, and effectively communicate this understanding to the client. It is important not only that the counselor is able to understand the client's experiences as if they themselves were experiencing them from the client's perspective, but that the client feels understood as a result of this. Lastly, Rogers' sixth condition for change is that the client is aware of the unconditional positive regard, acceptance, and empathy which the counselor feels toward them.

Miller and Rollnick [31] described four general concepts that were important for the implementation of MI. These were 1) express empathy, 2) develop discrepancy, and 3) roll with resistance, and 4) support self-efficacy. It is important to clarify these foundational elements and recall that these factors are central to the conditions in the relationship and may underlie and/or precede a variety of other interventions. First, motivational interviewing includes the expression of reflective listening to communicate understanding of what a client is saying. The second component is the cultivation of the client experience of any inconsistency between the client's most cherished values and their recent behavior. The third element of MI is the practice of understanding and tolerating a client's resistance to change in contrast with a more confrontational stance with forces that seem to interfere with change. Finally, MI encourages clients to believe that wished-for change can happen.

3.2 Application of motivational interviewing for supervision

Clarke and Giordano [33] articulated a compelling case for the applicability of MI in supervision. This relevance is rooted in the fundamentally essential nature of the relationship in therapy *and* supervision. Bordin [14] described the working alliance in supervision in part by applying therapeutic principles to supervision. He stated that a working alliance in supervision included shared goals, mutual understanding of the work to be done, and a constructive timbre of the working bond as foundational themes. Clarke and Giordano extended Bordin's supervisory alliance notion to include a greater range of supervision complexities. A significant part of this development was to highlight the difficulties associated with conditions in which Bordin's three conditions of the alliance were awry any way. In particular, difficulties with any of the three areas of the working alliance in supervision can promote anxiety and resistance in the therapist to learning and change. The presence of such conflict, then, highlights the need for supervisory methods that address the resistance. As discussed when MI was defined above, the principles and practices of MI are well-suited to such situations. As a result, there is a call to clarify the usefulness of MI in supervision.

Because of the paucity of relevant literature, it is instructive to review Clarke and Giordano's description of supervisory components that foster anxiety and resistance in the therapist and how the key features of MI can enhance a response. As they noted, while MI has expanded rapidly in the development of therapeutic approaches, most of the work related to MI and supervision has been to clarify how to conduct supervision of therapists' MI work rather than using MI in supervision itself. This is a key distinction, and a notable exception to the relative neglect of MI as a supervisory method was Madson et al.' [4] consideration of a MI model of supervision in the context of SUD treatment.

In most supervisory contexts, it is likely that a supervisor may serve at different times as a teacher, consultant, and supporter. We will soon turn to a consideration of these roles from the DM perspective, but it is instructive to talk about the supervisory roles from an MI perspective first. As has been discussed, supervision is an intervention that is based on a relationship in which a more advanced professional provides the necessary activities to a less experienced professional for the sake of maximizing client welfare, increasing therapist competence and promoting their ongoing development [23]. In discussing the contribution of MI to the supervision of SUD treatment, Madson and his colleagues [4] stated that"a supervisor may adopt roles as educator, consultant, supporter, and evaluator" (p. 350). Here is clear groundwork for the upcoming discussion of using MI and DM jointly.

3.3 Limitation of motivational interviewing

MI is widely characterized by well specified theory and technique [36]. MI has also been afforded a wide range of training resources and increasing empirical support for the efficacy of those efforts. At the same time, there is some increasing concern about the ability to evaluate MI and transfer it among settings because of inconsistencies in practice and the ongoing changes to the underlying theory that have been articulated [37]. Scholarship of MI needs to become more transparent so that developments are better examined, replicated, and advanced [38]. Such enhanced scholarship will also solidify the impact of clinical trials and the resulting guidance for practitioners.

There is still a lack of knowledge about the exact connection between the activities of MI and the outcomes that are associated with it [39]. There are a number of hypothesized mechanisms for this connection, but the specific action is not known. The relationship is considered to be an important part of how MI in addition to the technical advantage of altering the inner dialog of clients [40]. It is also possible that the investment of a client in behavioral changes could be enhanced by reducing the client talk that reinforces the persistence of old patterns [41].

4. The discrimination model and motivational interviewing in supervision

It is argued here that these two models for different kinds of intervention contexts may be considered in an integrated fashion to enhance the supervision of the treatment of substance use disorders. As previously discussed, Bernard's Discrimination Model (DM: [17]) was developed as an atheoretical guide for supervisors in the decision to adopt different roles or approaches to issues manifest in supervision. In the context of teaching, consulting, or counseling roles, flexible and intentional approaches are available in any given situation [41]. In the DM, three possible supervisor roles are employed in conjunction with three possible areas of trainee concern. So, the supervisor may work from flexible roles to address the conduct of intervention, understanding of clinical dynamics, and optimizing the presence of the person of the therapist.

This chapter contends that the DM can be productively integrated with the principles and practices of Motivational Interviewing (MI) to even further strengthen the supervision of the treatment of SUDs. MI was developed with an emphasis on four basic principles for intervention in treatment and supervision [31]. Briefly, MI includes the expression of understanding, the cultivation of the awareness of tension between actions and values, gentleness with expressions of resistance to change, and support for the experience of what is possible. The four basic principles and practices in MI are designed to work with a therapist (in supervision) or a client (in treatment for SUDs) include attitudes about emotional, cognitive, and behavioral aspects of experience. Challenging these attitudes from different positions is essential for the effectiveness of interventions.

4.1 Joint implementation of MI and DM

The best use of DM and MI is grounded in the common factors of psychotherapy. While there is little literature that describes the common factors in supervision [23], the common factors have been suggested as an important dimension of any form of supervision. In fact, it has been suggested that DM be expanded into a "Common Factors DM" [18]. Full treatment of the Common Factors DM is beyond the scope of this chapter, but the application of common factors to DM shows the significance of the common factors when it is combined with a supervisory approach (DM) that is so widely associated with effective supervision. The *integration* of DM and MI actually depends on the common factors. First, Bernard clearly recommended that the supervisor give careful consideration of exact supervisee needs and adopting interventions that match them carefully [17]. This attention requires the supervisory conditions that are fostered through the common factors. Therefore, when examining *any* dilemma faced in supervision, it is important to consider the exact nature of the dilemma, the subjective reaction of the supervisee, the extent to which the supervisee harbors adequate knowledge, and to the extent to which the supervisee can serve as their own expert in a particular matter (tenets of the DM).

One can readily see that in the exploration of these supervisory themes, the common factors quickly rise to the surface. The exploration of supervisory dilemmas must be conducted with empathy for the conditions of treatment relationship as well as the individual experience of the supervisee. Adding MI to the work *also* begins with the reflection of empathy by the supervisor encourages the expression of the therapist and facilitates the assessment and associated of supervisory work. The accuracy of the supervisory assessment and the effectiveness of the MI interventions are also promoted by a supervisory stance that refrains from evaluating or judging the therapist as they work to express and resolve their dilemma. Finally, it is critical that the supervisor conduct the assessment and supervisory interventions in a manner that is genuine. As MI is applied to supervision in this way, one can see some ways that MI works naturally with the DM.

The integration of MI and DM may be illustrated at the abstract level by examining the 9-cell Discrimination model grid presented by Bernard in her seminal work [17] accompanied by MI concepts. **Figure 1** shows the DM grid first advanced by Bernard with three columns for the supervisor roles (teacher, counselor, consultant) and three rows for the therapy functions that may be a supervisory focus (process, conceptualization, personalization). Each cell is populated by an index number for the list sample activities that represent one of the MI basic activities as implemented in that particular cell.

DOI: http://dx.doi.org/10.5772/intechopen.97626

		Supervisor Role		
		Teacher	Counselor	Consultant
Therapeutic function	Process	1	2	3
	Conceptualization	4	5	6
	Personalization	7	8	9

Figure 1.
Integrative examples of motivational interviewing functions in the discrimination model context.

What follows are indexed examples of SUD treatment supervision activities for each of the nine cells of the DM (with a sample MI function):

1. The supervisor is concerned about the extent to which the therapist feels capable of enduring the vicissitudes of the SUD treatment relationship. The supervisor provides instruction to the therapist about the typical elements of the treatment process. (fostering therapist self-efficacy)

2. The therapist has been enduring a particularly challenging treatment relationship, so the supervisor provides time for the therapist to express some conflicted and negative therapist feelings that have accumulated and not been expressed through the SUD treatment. (rolling with the resistance)

3. The therapist has been very confused about some of the ways that their client has been behaving, particularly in relation to some of the more difficult aspects of therapy. The supervisor helps the therapist by discussing clinical data combined with knowledge of recovery processes (addressing incongruities).

4. The young therapist is not very sure about how to understand recovery processes, so the supervisor provides instruction in what is known about recovery from conditions such as those face by the client. This includes attention to stages of change and how those are resisted naturally (roll with resistance)

5. The therapist is so angry with the client's public SUD-related behavior that the supervisor feels that the therapist understanding of the client's condition has become cloudy. The supervisor knows that it is important for the therapist to feel calmer and so spends time listening to the therapist's pain for the sake of clarifying her/his thinking (being in contact)

6. The therapist has become slightly disorganized in presenting treatment activities to the client. The supervisor spends some time helping the therapist re-organize SUD treatment goals and objectives because it appears that the therapist has lost some sense of feeling able to plan treatment effectively (support self-efficacy).

7. The therapist has felt very concerned and sad for some developments with her/his SUD patient. The supervisor listens very carefully for the personal impact of this development and treatment (being in contact).

8. The patient in SUD treatment has been vigorously blaming the therapist for their problems with the probation department. This has had little emotional impact on the therapist and the therapist her/his indifference disturbing. The therapist thinks that she/he should be upset by this intense blame. The therapist evokes the experience of the therapist to help sort out feelings that might be interfering with acceptance of a natural reaction (highlighting incongruities)

9. The supervisor shows compassion and flexibility with the therapist need to discuss techniques of various types. The therapist feels that they are going through a time of professional growth and transition and are reviewing a lot of different elements of the SUD treatment that they provide. (being in contact).

The originators of MI were clear about the important principles for intervention [40]. As noted above, the MI components that are central to this discussion are well matched to the common factors and the specific techniques associated with DM. For example, genuineness in the supervisory stance is a fundamental dimension of a working alliance and a major component of the common factors approach; genuineness is also a central tenet of MI. As previously noted, the conditions of the working alliance is associated with supervision outcomes. The optimal timing of feedback is best realized when the supervisor and trainee agree that the supervisory climate reflects the mutual trust and respect that are hallmarks of a strong alliance. Feedback is also made more useful when the trainee has had an opportunity to fully discuss their perspective on the supervisory dilemma; this is a common activity that maintains the supervisory alliance. The quantity of feedback is critical in providing the optimal balance of frustration and support for a supervisee. As has often been suggested, the specificity and concreteness of observations made in the feedback can enhance the receptivity of the trainee to the information and its eventual utility. Finally, it is important to close a difficult discussion with reflections on the trainee's experience of the feedback and its discussion. This final suggestion is critical to the continued largess of the supervisory alliance. It is an opportunity review the feedback process, revise the process for future discussions, and to renew shared goals and values for the continued supervision.

4.2 Examples of supervision of SUD treatment using MI & DM

Madsen and his colleagues claimed that MI is useful in a number of situations that are unique to the supervision of SUD treatment [4]. This chapter argues that the DM *adds* to the MI approach and will now expand some of Madsen's examples to illustrate the synergy that is possible with the combined application of these two approaches. It is beyond the scope of this chapter to fully explicate all possible details of the integration of these two useful models, but the discussion of some key issues in the supervision of the treatment of SUDs can be very useful and lead to further experimentation by experienced supervisors. Some basic examples of the integration are presented in the prior section and we now turn to more extensive examples.

Madsen and colleagues [4] claimed that supervision of SUD treatment from an MI perspective is most likely to include critical functions in three particular situations that are likely to be a part of the treatment of SUDs. While the exact function of the supervision may be discussed from a variety of perspectives, these situations *are* critical in the treatment of SUDs in general. Madsen's common SUD treatment scenarios include 1) when it appears that a client has lied to a therapist, 2) when a therapist is unsure of how to properly maintain privacy with the treatment, and 3) the optimal procedures for working with recidivism. When a client has lied to a therapist in a manner that is challenging to a therapist, this can be evocative to the therapist, disrupt treatment success, and present specific dimensions which may call for different types of clinical approaches. The assessment of supervisee needs when she/he has been lied to begins in a careful understanding from the supervisor of the supervisee's description of their dilemma. In such a discussion, the supervisor will use MI concepts to develop and express understanding of conflicts in the supervisee and their experience of the dilemma. It is likely that the supervisee with have a variety of conflicting thoughts and feelings. Given the nature of this supervisory condition, the DM provides a window on the nature of the clinical dilemmas and supervisee turmoil without making assumptions about the therapeutic situation. With these complex understanding, the supervisor develops an opinion about the extent to which the supervisee needs help with the conduct of the session, how to understand the session, or how to work with their own reaction. During this process, the supervisor will cultivate an awareness of any conflict that exists within the supervisee that contributes to the expressed dilemma. This awareness contributes to the understanding of the locus of the dilemma (process, personalization, conceptualization) and the nature of any resistance experienced in the supervisee. Adopting the suitable role (DM: teacher, consultant, counselor), the supervisor can then begin to consider supervisory interventions in a strategic manner. One possible version of this scenario is that the therapist has been emotionally hurt by the betrayal by the client that is embedded in the patient's deception. However, the therapist feels restricted in their ability to fully experience and work with the nature of this reaction as well as feeling constricted in their ability to use their feelings to shape interventions. This supervisor could readily begin in the counselor role from an MI approach to assist the therapist with the richness and spontaneity of their reaction until its toxic quality has dissipated. The supervision then can shift to a consultant role regarding the therapy process and assist the therapist to consider possible interventions while instilling optimism regarding their potential success as a therapist at this juncture. As this unfolds, the supervisee is naturally encouraged to experience the optimism that characterizes the last step of MI. While this description of the process associated with deception from a client with an SUD has been necessarily brief, one can readily see how DM and MI readily work together and with the common factors to bring greater focus an optimal strategy to the supervisory encounter.

In the second common scenario, the therapist is presented with privacy in SUD treatment that be challenging to therapists at all levels. A hypothetical situation helps illustrate the use of DM an MI together in dealing with a thorny privacy matter. A loved one of a person in SUD treatment has called the therapist to advise the therapist that the patient has succeeded in eluding detection of their continued use of psychoactive substances. The loved one wants to know what the patient has really told the therapist about their current level of adaptation. The loved one suspects that the client has less than candid or potentially misleading to the therapist. On one hand, the therapist believes that the family of the patient could be very instrumental in assisting with the progress of the patient. This could be particularly true if the family knew about the nature of the patient's real struggles in treatment and could respond accordingly. Since there are legal and ethical prohibitions against the therapist disclosing such information outside the treatment relationship, the therapist is frustrated that what is perceived to be a tool for treatment is not available. This may be compounded by the reluctance of the patient to be forthcoming with loved ones because of a host of factors associated with SUD and recovery. The frustration of the therapist can interfere with the spontaneous generation and implementation of effective and appropriate viable treatment approaches because of this conflict, so the dilemma clearly merits supervisory attention. The development of the supervisory themes should progress much as described in the prior scenario. The empathic stance of the supervisor assists in the process of open communication by the therapist and allows supervisor understanding of the dilemma. This can bring to light the impediments to clear clinical thinking as well as a greater understanding of the ways in which the therapist is tempted to behave in ways that are inconsistent with prevailing professional standards. This segment of the work which is promoted by the principles of MI allows for clarification of the focus of therapeutic the supervisory attention (concerning therapy process, therapist reaction, or therapist conceptualization of the treatment dilemma). Further exploration assists the supervisor in considering the most likely supervisory role to promote the desired educational effect (teacher, consultant, counselor). It is likely in this scenario that there are a variety of alternatives in the treatment that could respond to in some fashion to the prompting of the loved one without violating professional standards regarding privacy. However, such alternatives require careful consideration of the complex factors that converge on this dilemma and the proper DM role and focus can be brought to bear through MI methods as the painful and complicated dilemmas as sorted. As a result, the supervisor might be well advised to adopt more than one of the DM rolls in order to thoroughly provide the supervisory influence needed.

A final scenario to be considered is the somewhat common but regrettable circumstance of the SUD patient relapsing to substance use during the course of treatment. Despite the fact that such an occurrence is not particularly uncommon, its occurrence can be particularly difficult for early career therapists and an occasion for which heightened supervision can be critical for therapists at any level. The relapse of a patient can suggest failure to a therapist and be discouraging in the context of the therapist's considerable investment in learning to be a therapist and believing deeply in the importance of the work. This sensation can also be enhanced by their sentiments and perceptions associated with the work with a particular patient. Therapist responses to patient relapse can also be exacerbated by the therapist's reaction to treatment approaches espoused by the facility in which they work and the therapist's knowledge of treatment approaches in general. Given the possible emotionality and professional complexity of responding to a relapse, the initial assessment conducted by the supervisor as described in the prior two scenarios may garner even more importance and sensitivity. Despite these challenges, the principles that have already been described remain relevant in this particular treatment possibility. The supervisor is advised to listen carefully to how the dilemma uniquely impacts the therapist and the nature of the clinical restriction that follows. The integration of DM and MI can be particularly noticeable in this scenario because the patient relapse is not the end of the possibilities for the patient or for the treatment. The therapist's perception of the situation may be aggravated by policies and procedures of a treating facility and relevant legal situations for the patient, but it is unlikely that the long-term considerations are determined by a single relapse. As a result of the complexity of this dilemma, the supervisor must take care at the assessment phase to interact with the therapist in a way that helps the therapist come to an understanding of the supervisory goals and methods around this specific therapeutic occurrence.

5. Discussion

This chapter has described the Discrimination Model of Supervision, the Motivational Interviewing approach to intervention, and how the two may be considered together in the context of the common factors of supervision as a way to promote the most sensitive and powerful supervision of the therapy of SUDs. MI was originally designed as a foundation for clinical work in which the service recipient was in conflict about change. After widespread and dissemination and some empirical support, MI was extended into the realm of supervision. The DM has been discussed and applied widely and appears to enjoy considerable clinical utility. Unfortunately, there is a paucity of empirical support for the structure of efficacy of the model. With the well-supported context of the common factors, this chapter has argued that MI and DM are significant contributions to the supervision of treatment of SUDs. Abstract considerations of combining the perspectives were followed by practical examples that demonstrated how these ideas could be integrated in practice.

Since this is one of the first attempts to integrate these two strong traditions, there is no empirical support for any of the intuitively plausible suggestions made in this work. As already noted, this further extends areas of clinical practice, such as the DM, for which there is a dearth of empirical support. Empirical support for these ideas will require difficult research designs with carefully delineated controls and predictions. In addition, employment of these methods will continue to evolve in parallel with any research efforts. Clearly this is an area of supervision practice in early stages. However, given the pressure on SUD treatment resources, supervision of such work should be supported through the continued promotion of clinical practice, cultivation of enhanced supervisory methods, and extensive research. The research must pursue support for the efficacy of supervision that uses DM and MI in combination in general as well as in specific conditions of SUD treatment.

Conflict of interest

The authors have no conflict of interest, financial or otherwise.

Author details

John A. Mills* and Maren Krizner
Indiana University of Pennsylvania, Indiana, PA, USA

*Address all correspondence to: jamills@iup.edu

References

[1] National Institute on Drug Abuse. Treatment approaches for drug addiction. 2018. https://www.drugabuse.gov/publications/principles-drug-addiction-treatment-research-based-guide-third-edition/evidence-based-approaches-to-drug-addiction-treatment/behavioral-therapies. Retrieved January 5, 2021.

[2] Laschober T.C., Eby L. T. de T., Sauer, J.B. Effective clinical supervision in substance use disorder treatment programs and counselor job performance. Journal of Mental Health Counseling. 2013; 35 (1): 76-94

[3] Culbreth J.R., Borders L.D. Perceptions of the supervisory relationship. Journal of Substance Abuse Treatment. 1998; 15: 345-352.

[4] Madson, M.B., Bullock, E. E., Speed, A.C., & Hodges, S. A. Supervising substance abuse treatment: Specific issues and a motivational interviewing model. 2008. In Hess, Hess, & Hess (ed.) *Psychotherapy supervision: Theory, research, and practice*. (2nd ed). pp. 340-358. Wiley.

[5] Powell D.J., Brodsky A. Clinical supervision in alcohol and drug abuse counseling: Principles, models, methods. San Francisco, CA: Jossey-Bass; 2004

[6] Knudsen, H.K., Roman, P.M., Abraham, A.J. Quality of clinical supervision and counselor emotional exhaustion: the potential mediating roles of organizational and occupational commitment. 2013; 44:528-533.

[7] Tatarsky A. The challenge of harm reduction. Psychotherapy Networker. 2019; 43: 29-35,52.

[8] Center for Substance Abuse Treatment, (CSAT). Competencies for substance abuse treatment clinical supervisors. Technical assistance publication (TAP) Series 21-A (HHS Publication No. (SMA) 07-4243. 2007. Rockville, MD: Substance Abuse and Mental Health Services Administration.

[9] Substance Abuse and Mental Health Services Administration. (2009). *Clinical supervision and professional development of the substance-abuse counselor*. Treatment improvement protocol (TIP) Series 52,

[10] Efstation J.F., Patton M.J., Kardash C.M. Measuring the work alliance in counselor supervision. Journal of Counseling Psychology. 1990; 37: 322-329.

[11] Szecsody I. Supervision: A didactic or mutative situation. Psychoanalytic Psychotherapy. 1990; 4: 245-261

[12] Culbreath J.R. Clinical Supervision of Substance Abuse Counselors: Current and Preferred Practices. Journal of Addictions & Offender Counseling. 1999; 20: 15-25.

[13] Usher C.H., Borders L.D. Practicing counselors' preferences of supervisory style and supervisory emphasis. Counselor Education and Supervision. 1993; 33: 66-79.

[14] Bordin E.S. A working alliance based model of supervision. The Counseling Psychologist. 1983; 11: 35-42. DOI: 10.1177/0011000083111007

[15] Ladany, N., & Friedlander, M. L. The relationship between the supervisory working alliance and supervisee role conflict and ambiguity. Counselor Education and Supervision. 1995; 34: 220-231

[16] Strickler, A. Valenti, M.W., & Mihalo, J.R. Mechanisms for building working alliances in clinical supervision. Clinical Social Work Journal. 2018; 46:

361-373.https://doi.org/10.1007/s10615-018-0684-3

[17] Bernard J.M. Supervisor training: A discrimination model. Counselor Education and Supervision. 1979; 19: 60-68. DOI: 10.1002/j.1556-6978.1979.tb00906.x

[18] Crunk A. E., Barden S. M. The Common Factors Discrimination Model: An integrated approach to counselor supervision. The Professional Counselor. 2017; 7 (1): 62-75.

[19] Knight, C. Trauma-informed supervision: Historical antecedents, current practice, and future directions. The Clinical Supervisor. 2018; 37 (1): 7-37. https//doi.org/10.1080/07325223.1017.1413607

[20] Koltz, R.L. Intergrating creativity into supervision using Bernard's discrimination model. Journal of Creativity in Mental Health. 2008; 3(4): 416-427. doi:10.1080/15401380802530054

[21] Rubel, D. & Okech, J. E. A. The expert work group supervision process: Apperception, actions, interactions. Journal for Specialists in Group Work. 2009; 34 (3): 227-250. doi:10.1080/01933920903032596

[22] Timm, M. Creating a preferred counselor identity in Supervision: A new application of Bernard's discrimination model. The Clinical Supervisor. 2015; 34 (1): 115-125. doi:10.1080/07325223.2015.1021499

[23] Bernard J. M., Goodyear R. K. Fundamentals of clinical supervision. 5th ed. Upper Saddle River, NJ: Pearson Education; 2014

[24] Byrne A.M., Sias S.M. Conceptual application of the Discrimination Model of clinical supervision for direct care workers in adolescent residential treatment settings. Child Youth Care Forum. 2010; 39: 201-209.

[25] Searles, H. F. The informational value of the supervisor's emotional experiences. 1955. Psychiatry, 18, 135-146 PMid: 14384968

[26] Doehrman M.J.G. Parallel processes in supervision and psychotherapy. Bulletin of the Menninger Clinic. 1976; 40: 9-104.

[27] Alpher, V. S. Interdependence and parallel processes: A case study of structural analysis of social behavior in supervision and short-term dynamic psychotherapy. Psychotherapy. 1991, 28 (2), 218-231

[28] Tracey T. J. G., Bludworth J, Glidden-Tracey C. E. Are there parallel processes in psychotherapy supervision? An empirical examination. Psychotherapy. 2012; 49 (3): 330-343.

[29] Kram K. F. Mentoring at work. Glenview, IL: Scott, Foresman & Company; 1985

[30] Watkins, C.E., Jr., Budge, S. L., & Callahan, J.L. Common and specific factors converging in psychotherapy supervision: A supervisory extrapolation of the Wampold/Budge psychotherapy relationship model. 2015; 25: 214-235. doi:10.1037/a0039561

[31] Miller W. R., & Rollnick S. Motivational interviewing: Preparing people for change. 2nd ed. New York: Guilford Press; 2002

[32] Rollnick, S., Butler, C.C., Kinnersley, P., Gregory, J. & Mash, B. Motivational interviewing. British Medical Journal. 2010; 340: 1242-1245. doi:10.1136/bmj.c1900 https://www.jstor.org/stable/40701844

[33] Clarke P.B., Giordano A.L. The motivational supervisor: Motivational Interviewing as a clinical supervision

approach. The Clinical Supervisor. 2013; 32 : 244-259. DOI: 10.1080/07325223.2013.851633.

[34] Rogers C. R. The necessary and sufficient conditions of therapeutic personality change. Journal of Consulting Psychology. 1957; 21(2): 95-103. http://doi.org/10.1037/h0045357

[35] Miller, W.R. & Rose, G.S. Toward a theory of motivational interviewing. American psychologist. 2009; 64: 527-537.

[36] Vansteenkiste, M. & Sheldon, K. There's nothing more practical than a good theory: integrating motivational interviewing and self-determination theory. British Journal of clinical psychology. 2006; 45: 63-82.

[37] Atkinson, C. & Woods, K. establishing theoretical stability and treatment integrity for motivational interviewing. Behavioral and cognitive psychotherapy. 2017; 45:337-350. doi:10.1017/S1352465817000145

[38] Dobson, K. S. Cautionary tales regarding the dissemination of motivational interviewing. Addiction. 2016; 111: 1152-1153

[39] Burke, B., Arkowitz, H., & Dunn, C. (2002). The efficacy of motivational interviewing. 2002. In W. R. Miller & S. Rollnick (Eds.), motivational interviewing: preparing people for change (2nd ed, –-. 217-250). Guilford.

[40] Rollnick, S., Miller, W. R., & Butler, C.C. Motivational interviewing in health care: Helping patients change behavior. 2007 Guilford.

[41] Amrhein, P.C., Miller, W.R., Yahne, C.E., Palmer, M & Fulcher, L. Client commitment language during motivational interviewing predicts drug use outcome. Journal of consulting in clinical psychology. 2003, 71, 862-878

Chapter 9

An Evaluation of Diverse Therapeutic Interventions for Substance Use Disorders: Serotonergic Hallucinogens, Immunotherapy, and Transcranial Magnetic Stimulation

William M. Meil, William Farrell and Reem Satti

Abstract

Substance Use Disorders are a substantial public health concern whose treatment remains challenging. High rates of relapse are in fact a hallmark of drug addiction despite the wide variety of psychotherapeutic and pharmacotherapeutic approaches. This chapter discusses three innovative and controversial therapeutic approaches for Substance Use Disorders that have received considerable attention: the use of classic serotonergic hallucinogenic drugs (LSD and psilocybin), addiction immunotherapy and anti-addiction vaccines, and the use of transcranial magnetic stimulation. These treatments are not necessarily new but are discussed because they represent a diverse set of approaches that address varied aspects of drug addiction. Furthermore, they have an accumulated body of research from which to assess their future viability. For each of these therapeutic approaches this chapter considers the theoretical basis for use, history, status of the literature supporting their use, limitations, and potential applications. While these three interventions represent highly varied approaches to the treatment of Substance Use Disorders, this diversity may be necessary given the complex nature of addictive disorders.

Keywords: Pharmacotherapy, hallucinogens, addiction vaccines, addiction immunotherapy, transcranial magnetic stimulation

1. Introduction

Substance Use Disorders (SUDs) are likely to be chronic conditions for many effected individuals [1, 2] and are associated with a variety of negative physical and psychological health outcomes [3, 4]. Among those treated for drug and alcohol dependence, 40–60% relapse within a year of treatment cessation [5, 6]. Longitudinal cohort studies have demonstrated significant relapse rates across a variety of substances and yielded insight into predictors of remission and relapse. A recent meta-analysis of 21 long-term remission studies, conducted between 2000 and 2015, examined follow-up periods with a minimum of three years or reported lifetime remission. The results showed 35–54% achieved remission after a mean follow-up of 17 years. Moreover, the pooled estimated annual remission rates suggested yearly remission was uncommon ranging between 6.8% and 9.1% [2]. The conclusion that SUDs are likely to be long-term in nature is consistent with studies likening them to other chronic diseases and highlights the need for treatment to address the chronicity of SUDs [5].

Despite the poor long-term prognosis of SUDs, research suggest treatment is often efficacious in the short-term [7] as well as able to positively affect the long-term outcomes [7, 8]. Multiple longitudinal cohort studies support the efficacy of a variety of therapeutic approaches while at the same time revealing significant heterogeneity of treatment responsivity. For example, individuals treated for Alcohol Use Disorders (AUDs) via Alcoholics Anonymous (AA), formal treatment, or a combination of the two are more likely to be abstinent after 8 years than untreated individuals, however the AA only group surpassed the formal treatment group at 1- and 3-year follow-ups [9]. Another study of adults with AUD, most of whom were entering treatment, revealed five trajectory classes distinguished by their changes in drinking patterns across three years with AA involvement predicting abstinence and/or declines in drinking over time [10]. A recent prospective longitudinal cohort study examining heroin use and treatment utilization over 10–11 years also identified five trajectory groups related to treatment utilization and continued drug use [8].

Addiction is fundamentally a brain disease in which chronic use of substances produce neuroplastic changes across multiple brain systems rendering a person more vulnerable to drug craving, escalating use, and relapse. Depending on the effected system, these changes yield increased incentive salience towards the drug and drug associated cues, attenuated reward, motivation, emotion, and altered stress responsivity. These changes are also coupled with deficits in the prefrontal

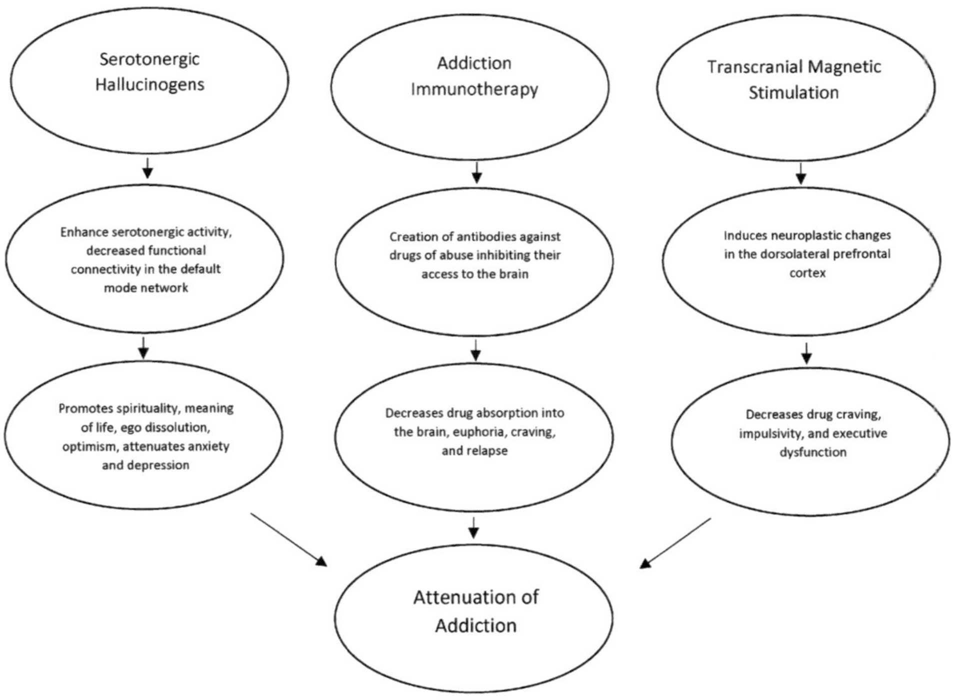

Figure 1.
Therapeutic interventions under development and their putative mechanisms of action (second row from top) and posited anti-additive effects (third row from the top).

cortex and related circuitry leaving drug addicted individuals with diminished executive function and enhanced impulsivity. Moreover, the extent to which these neural adaptions change over time appears to vary, but many have been shown to be highly durable. These neural changes must also be considered within the context of an individual's genetic and epigenetic vulnerabilities, and life circumstances [11–13]. The complexity of variables which contribute to the development of SUDs make them particularly challenging to understand and treat, but they also offer a bevy of targets to develop new treatment approaches.

The purpose of this chapter is to examine three putative treatments for SUDs: serotonergic hallucinogens, immunotherapy approaches, and transcranial magnetic stimulation [TMS]. These treatments are not necessarily new but were chosen because they represent a diverse set of approaches that address varied aspects of drug addiction (see **Figure 1**). Moreover, they have an accumulated body of research from which to assess their future viability. For each of these therapeutic approaches this chapter will address the theoretical basis for use, history, status of the literature supporting their use, limitations, and potential applications.

2. Serotonergic hallucinogens and substance use disorders

Hallucinogenic drugs represent a diverse set of naturally occurring and synthetic substances which vary based on their pharmacological actions and psychoactive effects. The term hallucinogen typically refers to a drug that produces perceptions in the absence of sensory stimuli. However, it is now recognized that hallucinogens produce a broader range of effects across cognition and mood and that hallucinations themselves are less common than the perceptual illusions and sensory distortions they produce. For this reason, the term psychedelic, or mind manifesting, is often used to describe this class of drugs [14, 15]. This section of the chapter focusses on lysergic acid diethylamide (LSD) and psilocybin, two hallucinogens typically referred to as classic serotonergic hallucinogens because they act primarily as agonists on the serotonin (5-HT) 2A receptor and share behavioral effects and proposed therapeutic mechanisms [14].

Psilocybin occurs naturally in more than 200 species of mushrooms and has long been consumed by indigenous cultures to engage with the spiritual world [16, 17]. Albert Hofmann isolated psilocybin and its active metabolite psilocin and subsequently synthesized them in 1958 [18]. LSD was first synthesized in 1938 by Hofmann from ergotamine, a compound found in ergot fungus. After preclinical administration failed to reveal many observable effects in laboratory animals its psychoactive properties were recognized following an accidental ingestion of the drug by Hofmann in 1943. Beginning in the mid-1950s LSD and psilocybin were widely distributed under the names Delysid and Indocybin for study of multiple psychological disorders resulting in more than 1000 papers, treating more than over 40,000 individuals by the mid-to-late 1960's [16, 18–20].

The main focus of research through the late 1960s on the efficacy of hallucinogens in the treatment of addiction was the ability of LSD to attenuate alcoholism [21]. Among the first studies was that of Hoffer & Osmond [22] who followed 24 treatment resistant alcoholics. After taking several weeks to establish a psychotherapeutic relationship, participants were administered a single dose of 200–400 micrograms of LSD while accompanied by a nurse and/or a psychiatrist and in many cases, efforts were made to create a therapeutic environment. The next day, participants were asked to write about their experience. Six participants were considered much improved (complete abstinence and positive lifestyle changes) and another six improved at the conclusion of the study [22].

This early research was influential in establishing a treatment model referred to as "psychedelic therapy" [22], though over time the nature of treatment sessions has varied greatly [21, 23]. Central to this therapeutic approach is the idea that patients will experience a psychedelic peak characterized by an ecstatic state, visual hallucinations, a loss of boundaries between the individual and the objective world, feelings of unity with others, nature, God and the universe [19, 21]. The result of this peak being the induction of a mystical experience that would profoundly alter the way a person views themselves and the world [20]. The dramatic nature of this experience is then interpreted with the assistance of a trained therapist who helps the patient appreciate the psychotherapeutic benefits of the experience [24].

In the following years more than 20 studies with larger sample sizes were published illustrating the effectiveness of LSD for treating alcoholism with many describing unprecedented levels of success [19, 25]. From, 1954–1960 Osmond and colleagues studied the effects of LSD on approximately 2000 alcoholics finding almost half were abstinent after a year [26]. However, by and large this body of research suffered from significant methodological flaws among them a lack of diagnostic specificity, non-random assignment of participants, lack of control and or placebo groups, inconsistent participant follow-up, participant attrition, absence of blind raters, and a lack of clarity in assessing treatment efficacy. Despite these flaws, these early findings were encouraging enough that by the late 1960s six alcoholism treatment programs in North America used LSD based therapy [19, 23, 25].

Gradually some of the methodological problems that plagued earlier studies were partially addressed and a meta-analysis was conducted of six randomized controlled studies (five of which were double-blind) between 1966 and 1970 examining the efficacy of LSD in the treatment of alcoholism [27]. Across these studies 536 adults suffering from alcoholism were compared to 211 control participants receiving a low-dose LSD, d-amphetamine, ephedrine sulphate or non-drug control. While the characteristics of LSD sessions and follow up varied considerably, the results supported the efficacy of a single dose of LSD. Decreases in alcohol misuse were observed at 2–3 and 6 months, but not 12 months post-treatment. Moreover, in three studies reporting total abstinence from alcohol, LSD showed benefits 1–3 months after discharge from treatment programs. Despite these results, research examining the utilization of LSD for alcoholism stalled by the late 1960s due to increased recreational use, its association with the drug counterculture movement, increased restrictions on human drug research, continued methodological concerns, ambiguous results, and passage of the Controlled Substances Act of 1970, which placed LSD in the most restrictive category of drugs [15, 18, 25, 28].

After a cessation of almost 30 years, controlled studies in humans using hallucinogens resumed in the late 1990s [18, 24]. However, Psilocybin, not LSD, emerged as the drug of choice to study the effects of hallucinogens on SUDs [18, 23, 24]. Multiple reasons have been put forward for psilocybin's emergence in this context. Psilocybin has a shorter duration of action compared to LSD, and psilocybin is believed to have a milder side effect profile producing less anxiety, affective disturbances, and milder vegetative side effects [16, 28]. Also, LSD may still suffer from its negative counterculture reputation of the 1960s and a litany of mass media misinformation including exaggerated claims of drug-induced insanity, chromosomal damage, and other falsehoods [14, 15]. In contrast there is growing interest in certain locales to legalize psilocybin's use in licensed facilities for mental health purposes and decriminalize it in others [29].

Among the limited number of recent studies is a small open-label trial with psilocybin for AUD [30]. Psilocybin was administered to 10 alcohol dependent individuals in context of a 12-week program of motivational enhancement therapy. Participants were initially administered 0.3 mg/kg of oral psilocybin followed by a second dose of 0.3 or 0.4 mg/kg, 4 weeks later. The two doses of psilocybin were separated by four therapy sessions and the final dose was followed by another four sessions. Following the initial psilocybin treatment self-reported alcohol use significantly decreased and remained below baseline at a 36-week follow-up. In addition, significant correlations were reported between the overall intensity and mystical quality of psilocybin sessions and reductions in the percent of drinking days, alcohol craving, and self-efficacy to abstain.

Research examining psilocybin's ability to treat nicotine addiction is also promising. An open-label study was conducted with 15 treatment-resistant, nicotine dependent participants administered 2–3 moderate and high doses of oral psilocybin integrated within a 15-week cognitive behavioral therapy program. Using biologically based verification procedures at a 6-month follow-up 80% of participants were abstinent, at 12 months 67% remained nicotine free, and at 16 months 60% were abstinent. After a long-term follow-up averaging 2.5 years, 75% of study participants were verified as nicotine free. Moreover, participants abstinent at 6-months scored higher on measures of mystical experiences following psilocybin compared to those who relapsed. Greater mystical-type experiences following psilocybin administration also correlated with reduced nicotine cravings at 6 months. At the 12-month follow-up participants rated their psilocybin experience among the 5 most personally meaningful and spiritually significant of their lives [31, 32].

A variety of additional factors speak to the potential viability of serotonergic hallucinogens for the treatment of SUDs. A single or a limited number of drug administrations during supervised treatment sessions may negate a number of liabilities associated with other pharmacotherapies such as high cost, problems with medication adherence, drug interactions and side effects [24]. LSD and psilocybin have a limited addictive liability as indicated by a lack of drug self-administration by laboratory animals [28, 33], relatively slow onset of effects after oral administration not typically characterized by pleasure or craving and has no direct effects on the brain dopamine pathways [15]. Physical withdrawal symptoms do not develop even following prolonged use of LSD and psilocybin and the rapid development of dramatic tolerance, on the order of days, does not facilitate the acquisition of addictive behavior [14, 33]. Methodological details associated with the use of psilocybin for treatment of SUDs can be found in several sources [21, 31, 33].

The general public's perception that psychedelic drugs are dangerous, contradicts the fact that from a physiological perspective they are among the safest classes of drugs [15]. Both drugs are not without their liabilities [14, 15, 28, 33], yet substantial toxicity has only been associated with a small number of users [28] In the context of clinical use, the incidence of problems is substantially mitigated as patients are typically prescreened for psychotic symptoms and cardiovascular issues, receive a single or a small number of doses, pharmacotherapies may be available to reverse untoward effects, and therapeutic sessions are supervised by a trained clinician [24, 34]. Recent trials examining the efficacy of these hallucinogens for SUDs have reported no serious adverse effects [30–34] nor have trials examining these hallucinogens in patients with anxiety, depression, or healthy volunteers [18].

A variety of mechanisms have been suggested to explain the therapeutic efficacy of LSD and psilocybin for SUDs and many overlap with proposed explanations for addressing other psychological disorders [18, 34]. Depression and anxiety are hallmarks of addiction [17]. Both negative affective states have been shown to be ameliorated following LSD and psilocybin administration [18, 19, 34] and are linked to prolonged increases in optimism and wellbeing [17]. While it cannot be ruled out that these drug's effects on mood and anxiety are part of a broader mechanism, the fact that antidepressants [35] and anxiolytics [36] alone are generally not effective treatments for managing SUDs suggest this represents at best an incomplete explanation for hallucinogens therapeutic effects for SUDs.

It has been widely suggested that LSD and psilocybin's experiential effects underly their benefits for treating SUDS [17]. Alcoholics Anonymous has long argued that addiction follows from deficits in spirituality and meaning [37]. Bill Wilson one of the co-founders of Alcoholics Anonymous, credited his experiences with hallucinogens as the reason for his own abstinence and advocated for LSD as a pathway to sobriety [38]. Spirituality has been demonstrated to play a role in the success of Alcoholics Anonymous [39] and other therapeutic approaches [40] and a sense of purpose in life decreases chronic heavy drinking [10]. The benefits of hallucinogenic-based therapeutic experiences may also lie in their intensity [17] as their effects are often described as life changing in nature [31, 32] and research has shown users who experience the most profound mystical experiences consistently undergo the greatest symptom relief [15]. Moreover, stronger mystical experiences and greater intensity of subjective effects of psilocybin are associated with alcohol and nicotine abstinence suggesting a mediating role of mystical experience in psychedelic-facilitated addiction treatment [30, 41].

Consistent with the importance of hallucinogen induced experiential effects recent research using brain imaging in healthy volunteers has shown LSD and psilocybin decrease functional connectivity in the default mode network (DMN), a pathway bilaterally spanning the medial and lateral parietal, medial prefrontal, and medial and lateral temporal cortices, and whose activity appears augmented in depressed patients [24, 42, 43]. Moreover, administration of both drugs was associated with "ego-dissolution" and "altered meaning" suggesting the importance of this circuit for the maintenance of "self" or "ego" and its processing of "meaning" [43, 44]. These results and those of other studies support the idea that classic hallucinogens may function to increase processing of positive stimuli and decrease processing of negative stimuli, elevate mood, and decrease coupling of neural networks allowing for unrestrained exploration of spirituality and meaning [21, 24]. Imaging studies of this network in those with SUD following administration of hallucinogens and after periods of abstinence are needed.

It is noteworthy that past and present research examining the efficacy of LSD and psilocybin in combination with psychotherapy for the treatment of SUD has been consistently promising [18]. Their benefits compare favorably with daily administration of naltrexone, acamprosate, and disulfiram for the treatment of AUD [27] and exceed success rates of behavioral and pharmacological interventions for nicotine dependence [31]. In addition, this approach represents a sea change in the dramatic, broad, and long-lasting nature of its effects and appears relatively safe when administered in a clinical setting. Recently a therapeutic model specifically for psilocybin-assisted treatment of AUD has been proposed [21], as have a neuroscience based mechanistic theory of explaining psilocybin's efficacy for treating SUD [28], and larger randomized studies are now being conducted on the efficacy of psilocybin for AUD, nicotine, and cocaine dependence [34, 45]. However, the above advances should be tempered with the knowledge that recent research has had small samples, this approach is demanding on both the patient and therapist, hallucinogens and hallucinogen-assisted psychotherapy have a negative reputation and are misunderstood by many [24, 45, 46].

3. Addiction immunotherapy: anti-addiction vaccines

The primary immunotherapies being developed for SUDs are vaccines that cause the generation of antibodies directed against drugs of abuse such as cocaine, nicotine, and opioid analgesics. The underlying rationale is that once drugs of abuse are bound to antibodies, the resulting complex is too large to cross the blood–brain barrier. This reduces the amount of abused substance that reaches the central nervous system (CNS) and thereby reduces the rewarding effects of the drugs. The development of vaccines for drugs of abuse is complicated by the fact that the drugs themselves are small molecules that do not inherently elicit an immune response. To overcome this obstacle, drug molecules or their derivatives (haptens) are typically attached to an immunogenic carrier molecule and administered with adjuvants to stimulate the generation of antibodies directed against the drug. Vaccine candidates have been developed against several drugs of abuse using variations on this approach [47].

Cocaine abuse represents a condition for which a vaccine could be of particular use since there are currently no approved pharmacotherapies to promote abstinence or prevent relapse. Studies in the 1990s conducted in rodents demonstrated that anti-cocaine vaccines could induce the generation of cocaine-specific antibodies and reduce cocaine levels in the brain following peripheral cocaine administration [48, 49]. Additionally, vaccination reduced the psychostimulant (locomotion and stereotopy) effects of cocaine in rats [48], and vaccination or the administration of monoclonal antibodies against cocaine reduced cocaine self-administration and the reinstatement of cocaine self-administration following extinction in rats [49, 50].

Two cocaine vaccines are currently listed on ClinicalTrials.gov. The vaccine that has been most studied is the TA-CD vaccine. This vaccine, which consists of succinylnorcocaine (SNC) attached to a recombinant cholera toxin B (rCTB) carrier administered with aluminum hydroxide adjuvant, caused the generation of cocaine-specific antibodies in rats and reduced cocaine self-administration [51]. The results of a randomized, double-blind, placebo controlled, Stage I clinical trial in which 34 former cocaine abusers in a residential treatment facility were randomized to receive three vaccine injections during the first two months of the study at doses of 13, 82 or 709 mg or an equivalent number of placebo injections (n = 6) indicated that the vaccine was well tolerated and elicited the dose-dependent production of cocaine-specific antibodies which peaked after the third injection and declined over the remainder of the year-long study [52]. A subsequent open-label, outpatient, treatment study involving 18 cocaine-dependent participants indicated that participants who received a total of 2000 mg of vaccine administered in five equal injections over 12 weeks achieved higher mean peak antibody titers and reduced cocaine use over 12 weeks relative to participants who received a total of 400 mg of vaccine administered in four equal injections over 8 weeks [53]. The majority of participants who did use cocaine during the study reported a reduction in the euphoric effects of the drug. The results of a subsequent study conducted in a laboratory setting with participants who were actively abusing cocaine indicated that participants with immune responses to the TA-CD vaccine above the 50th percentile reported reduced positive subjective effects of smoked cocaine [54].

The results from a 24-week Phase IIb clinical trial conducted with 115 cocaine- and opioid-dependent participants enrolled in an outpatient methadone program found that participants who mounted a robust antibody response (≥43 mg/ml) following five vaccine injections (360 mg each) administered over the course of 12 weeks had a higher number of cocaine free urine tests during weeks 9–16 of the study than participants who received placebo injections or who produced a smaller antibody response to the vaccine [55]. These participants were also more likely to exhibit a 50% reduction in cocaine use between weeks 8–20 of the study relative to those who mounted a less robust immune response to the vaccine. However, a subsequent randomized, double-blind, placebo-controlled, Phase III clinical trial involving 300 cocaine-dependent participants in outpatient treatment programs across six sites failed to demonstrate efficacy of the TA-CD vaccine [56]. Participants in this study received five vaccinations (400 mg each or placebo) over the course of 13 weeks, and 67% of the fully vaccinated participants displayed a robust antibody response (≥42 mg/ml). Vaccinated participants did not, however, have fewer cocaine-positive urine tests than participants receiving placebo injections, and participants with a robust antibody response did not exhibit a significant reduction in cocaine-positive urine tests relative to participants who mounted a lesser immune response. Participants who generated robust immune responses to the vaccine were, however, more likely to complete the study than those with weaker immune responses.

The second cocaine vaccine undergoing clinical trials is the dAd5GNE vaccine. One major drawback to the TA-CD vaccine was that it did not consistently elicit high titers of cocaine-specific antibodies. For example, in one study [55] only 38% of the vaccinated participants generated antibodies at the concentration projected to be required for efficacy. The dAd5GNE vaccine consists of the cocaine analog, GNE (6-(2R,3S)-3-(benzoyloxy)-8-methyl-8-azabicyclo [3.2.1] octane-2-carboxoamido-hexanoic acid) connected to disrupted adenovirus capsid proteins administered with Adjuplex (Advanced BioAdjuvants, LLC, Omaha, NB) adjuvant, and was designed to elicit a strong immune response from humans [57]. In rodents, this vaccine has been demonstrated to elicit high and persistent titers of cocaine-specific antibodies, attenuate the passage of cocaine from the peripheral circulation to the brain, reduce cocaine self-administration on a progressive-ratio schedule, and reduce cocaine-induced reinstatement of cocaine self-administration following extinction [57, 58]. The vaccine also produced high antibody titers in Rhesus macaques, reduced the penetration of cocaine to the CNS [59], and reduced reacquisition of cocaine self-administration following extinction [60]. The dAd5GNE vaccine is currently in a Phase I clinical trial, but results are not yet available.

Vaccines have also been developed against nicotine with the intention of helping users quit and remain abstinent. Vaccines that have been or are being examined in clinical trials include NicVax, Nic-002 (Nic-Qb), TA-NIC, Niccine, and SEL-068. None of these vaccines are currently approved for the treatment of tobacco use disorder, but further refinement and evaluation appears to be warranted. Because peer reviewed data related to many of these vaccines are limited, this discussion will focus on NicVax and Nic-002 (Nic-Qb). NicVax (3′-AmNic-rEPA) was one of the earliest candidate vaccines directed against nicotine. In preclinical studies, antibodies generated in response to this vaccine in rabbits and injected into rats reduced the passage of intravenously administered nicotine to the brain in a dose-dependent manner and attenuated the effects of nicotine on systolic blood pressure and locomotor activity [61]. Similarly, active immunization of rats elicited the production of nicotine-specific antibodies and also attenuated the passage of nicotine to the brain [61]. Active immunization also reduced nicotine self-administration in rats [62].

Single photon emission computed tomography (SPECT) data collected from nicotine-dependent human participants, indicates that active immunization with NicVax reduces the binding of nicotine to β2-nicotinic acetylcholine receptors in the brain [63], and the results of a study involving 68 current smokers assigned to receive four injections of vaccine (50, 100, or 200 mg) or placebo indicated that the vaccine was well tolerated and that the nicotine-specific antibodies were elicited in quantities believed to be sufficient for efficacy at the highest dose [64]. Participants receiving the highest dose of vaccine were also more likely to achieve 30 days of abstinence than participants receiving lower doses of the vaccine or placebo injections. The results of a subsequent Phase II clinical trial [65] in which 301 smokers were assigned to receive four or five doses of NicVax (200 or 400 mg/injection) or placebo over the course of 26 weeks indicated that participants who received five

400 mg doses of vaccine had higher prolonged abstinence rates through both 6 and 12 months relative to participants receiving placebo. In addition, participants with the highest antibody response (top 30% across all vaccine doses) were more likely to achieve eight weeks of abstinence between weeks 19–26 of the study, had higher rates of continuous abstinence from weeks 19–52 of the study, and had higher rates of 7-day point prevalence abstinence at weeks 26 and 52 of the study compared to participants receiving placebo. Participants in the high antibody response group were also more likely than participants receiving placebo to exhibit prolonged abstinence through 6 and 12-months. Unfortunately, while two subsequent Phase III clinical trials with NicVax confirmed that the vaccine was safe and well tolerated, six injections (400 mg each) of NicVax failed to significantly alter abstinence rates relative to placebo [66]. An additional Phase IIb study was conducted on the effectiveness of NicVax in combination with varenicline and motivational interviewing, however, this study too failed to establish a significant effect of NicVax on abstinence rates relative to participants receiving placebo [67].

Nic-002 (Nic-Qb), a vaccine consisting of a virus-like particle (VLP)-nicotine conjugate also showed both preclinical and clinical potential for reducing nicotine use. This vaccine yielded high titers of nicotine-specific antibodies in mice, rats, and rabbits, and vaccination of mice significantly reduced brain nicotine levels [68]. The report of the results from a European Phase I randomized, placebo controlled clinical trial in which 32 healthy human participants received two vaccinations separated by four weeks and 8 participants received control injections indicated that the vaccine was generally well-tolerated and produced a robust immune response with high affinity, nicotine-specific antibodies [68]. The results of a subsequent phase II study in which participants, were scheduled to receive five 100 mg vaccinations of Nic-002 with alum adjuvant (n = 229) over four months or alum alone as the placebo (n = 112) [69] indicated that, continuous abstinence rates from months 3 to 6 of the protocol, did not differ between the vaccination (30.1%) and placebo groups (26.1%), the 1/3 of participants with the highest antibody response had a significantly higher continuous abstinence rate from months 2 through 6 of the study (56.6.%) compared to participants receiving placebo (31.3%). Furthermore, this effect was maintained through month 12 of the study (41.5% vs. 21.3%). While researchers believed these results to be encouraging, Novartis announced that an interim analysis of data from a subsequent Phase II study indicated that the vaccine failed to improve continuous abstinence rates, likely due to insufficient antibody titers [70], and its development appears to have been halted.

Developing vaccines against opioid analgesics presents some unique challenges. One consideration is that unlike nicotine and cocaine the metabolites of many opioid drugs are active and can have physiological and psychological effects of their own. A second consideration is that if vaccines are to be used for the treatment of opioid use disorder, they should not bind to and inactivate opioids that are used to assist with treatment for the disorder or are used to prevent overdose. Finally, vaccines directed against one opioid analgesic will ideally not bind to other analgesics which may be needed for pain management. While no opioid vaccines have been tested in clinical trials, several candidate vaccines have emerged from preclinical investigations with promising results against heroin, oxycodone and fentanyl.

One example of a vaccine that appears promising for the treatment of heroin use consists of a heroin-tetanus toxoid (TT) combination [71]. Following administration heroin is rapidly metabolized to 6-acetyl morphine (6 AM) and subsequently to morphine, and these two metabolites act via mu-opioid receptors to generate heroin's antinociceptive and rewarding effects. Preclinical studies with this vaccine have demonstrated that it generates substantial antibody titers with high affinity for

6 AM and heroin and much lower affinity for morphine, oxycodone, and methadone in both mice and monkeys. Additional vaccines using haptens derived from morphine, have also been demonstrated to reduce the CNS-mediated behavioral effects of heroin [72].

Vaccines have also been developed that attenuate the behavioral and physiological effects of oxycodone and/or hydrocodone in rodents [72]. One of these vaccines, comprised of an oxycodone-based hapten conjugated to keyhole limpet hemocyanin (KLH), is notable, in part, for the specificity of its action [73]. Rats immunized with this vaccine generated antibodies with high affinity for oxycodone and, to a lesser extent oxymorphone, an active metabolite of oxycodone. Importantly cross-reactivity with naloxone and naltrexone was 1.2% or less and was undetectable for methadone and buprenorphine. Vaccination also reduces brain oxycodone levels by as much as 51% following intravenous administration of 0.5 mg/kg of oxycodone and significantly reduced the antinociceptive effects of oxycodone as indicated by performance on the hot-plate test. Furthermore, vaccination significantly reduced the acquisition of oxycodone self-administration and the number of infusions administered indicating a reduction in reinforcing effects of the drug.

Given the ongoing opioid crisis, a vaccine with clinical potential has also been developed against fentanyl [74]. This vaccine consists of a fentanyl-based hapten conjugated to either KLH or GMP-grade subunit KLH (sKLH). Vaccination elicited an immune response containing fentanyl-specific antibodies in mice and reduced the antinociceptive effects of fentanyl (0.05 mg/kg, s.c.) by 60% as assessed by the hotplate test. In addition, this vaccine elicited an immune response from rats and reduced the antinociceptive effects of fentanyl (0.05 mg/kg, s.c.) by 93% without significantly attenuating the antinociceptive effects of heroin or oxycodone. Fentanyl levels in the brain were also reduced by 30% following peripheral fentanyl administration (0.05 mg/kg, i.v.), and vaccination attenuated fentanyl-induced respiratory depression. Importantly, naloxone (0.1 mg/kg, s.c.) still reversed fentanyl-induced antinociception and respiratory depression following vaccination, indicating the vaccine does not render this important, life-saving drug ineffective.

While the results of clinical trials conducted thus far with vaccines against drugs of abuse have failed to yield consistent results indicating effectiveness, examination of the results obtained from participants who mounted a robust immune response has been encouraging. One hope is that advances in vaccine design improve will immune responses from participants [75]. Providing exogenous monoclonal antibodies against drugs of abuse to vaccinated participants might also provide a means of assuring that vaccine recipients have high antibody titers. This approach yielded improvements in combating the behavioral effects of nicotine in rats relative to vaccine administration alone [76]. It is also possible that modifying the route of administration could improve the efficacy of vaccines. For example, intranasal vaccine administration has been demonstrated to increase mucosal antibody levels against nicotine which could aid in the rapid immobilization of inhaled nicotine [77]. Intranasal administration of a cocaine vaccine has also recently been demonstrated to have advantages preventing cocaine-induced locomotion in mice [78].

Beyond simply attenuating the rewarding effects of drugs of abuse, vaccines may present additional advantages for SUD. Unlike available pharmacotherapies, the effects of vaccines can be long-lasting and require only periodic booster immunizations to maintain effectiveness. This may make vaccination more cost-effective than other treatments and preclude the need for daily adherence to drug regimens. Vaccines against drugs of abuse should also have a reasonably low behavioral/psychological side-effect profile as they do not have CNS effects of their own. Because of the lack of direct CNS effects, well designed vaccines should also not interfere with other pharmacotherapies for substance use and could be combined with such therapies to enhance effectiveness. For example, while antagonist medications may be able to reduce the rewarding effects of drugs of abuse, users may increase their drug use in an attempt to override the blockade. This could leave the individual vulnerable to dangerous peripheral effects of the drugs. Vaccines may aid in combating these peripheral effects by limiting drug availability in the periphery as well. Co-administrations of vaccines against multiple drugs also has potential usefulness for individuals who abuse a mixture of substances such as fentanyl-laced heroin. The effectiveness of one such vaccine mixture (heroin/fentanyl) has recently been seen in mice [79].

Despite their promise, vaccines against drugs of abuse have several limitations. For example, vaccinated individuals could potentially increase substance intake to overwhelm the antibodies generated in response to the vaccine, and evidence of increased substance use by at least some participants has been reported in some of the studies discussed above [55, 56]. Additionally, participants with insufficient motivation to remain abstinent could discontinue treatment. Current skepticism about vaccines may also reduce the attractiveness of vaccines as an SUD treatment. Despite these limitations, with improvement, vaccination against drugs of abuse may still prove to be an efficacious tool to aid motivated individuals in recovery.

4. Transcranial magnetic stimulation and substance use disorders

Transcranial Magnetic Stimulation (TMS) is a noninvasive medical procedure involving the application of fluctuating magnetic pulses generated from a coil placed over the scalp that passes through the skull and into the brain generating electrical currents which alter neural activity by electromagnetic induction. The coil design can influence intensity, localization, and depth of stimulation. Multiple TMS pulses administered consecutively are referred to as repetitive or rTMS. Low frequency rTMS (LF-rTMS; ≤ 1 Hz) typically attenuates neural excitation and cortical excitability and higher frequency rTMS (HF-rTMS; 1–20 Hz) augments neural excitation, cortical excitability, and regional cerebral blood flow. Stimulation parameters, anatomical loci, and the current cortical activity also influence its facilitative or suppressive effects. rTMS results in strong moderately localized intracranial currents in the underlying cortex but also produces long lasting complex changes, neurotransmitter release, plasticity, and connectivity in distal neural circuitry [80–83]. The present form of TMS traces its origins to Barker and Colleagues who demonstrated the effects of magnetic stimulation on human motor cortex in 1985 [84]. The therapeutic efficacy of rTMS is currently under study for many psychological disorders and has U.S. Food and Drug Administration approval for the treatment of Major Depressive Disorder in adults [80].

The methods and mechanisms associated with rTMS-induced neuroplasticity and therapeutic efficacy for SUD are complex and reviewed elsewhere [80–83], however, the majority of studies have targeted the prefrontal cortex, more specifically the dorsolateral prefrontal cortex (DLPFC) [81–83]. This structure represents a desirable target not only for its accessibility but because it has been directly linked to neuroplastic changes associated with craving, impulsivity, and executive function all of which play central roles in addiction [80, 81]. Moreover, the DLPF is highly interconnected with other cortical and subcortical circuits associated with anhedonia, escalation of use, and relapse [82]. The potential of this approach has resulted in a significant number of studies in a relatively short period across a variety of addictive substances, brain loci, and employing a wide range of rTMS methods [81–83]. Most studies on the effects of rTMS for SUD have focused on alcohol, cocaine, and nicotine and those literatures are highlighted below. Limited research has examined opiates, methamphetamine, and cannabis [85–87].

Multiple sham-controlled studies have been conducted to examine the efficacy of HF-rTMS on individuals with AUD with mixed results. One single-blind study examined rTMS (10 Hz) in 10 sessions to the right DLPFC and measured self-reported cravings at baseline following treatment and after 4 weeks. Significant decreases in craving were reported in patients who received rTMS versus sham rTMS [88]. A similar double-blind study comparing 10 sessions of right versus left DLPFC HF-rTMS (10 Hz) stimulation following treatment in those with AUD showed no difference in efficacy based on the side of treatment of administration but a significant reduction in craving scores in those administered rTMS [89]. Other studies using rTMS on the DLPC have failed to show effects of alcohol craving in those with AUD. A single session of rTMS versus sham treatment to the right DLPFC did not reduce craving immediately following treatment or when measured at home several days later [90]. Similarly, no significant differences in alcohol craving were reported after 10 days between sham rTMS and HF-rTMS of the left DLPFC, (20 Hz) [91]. Moreover, rTMS targeting the insula in alcohol-dependent participants in a double-blind, sham-controlled, randomized trial receiving 10 Hz rTMS or sham stimulation 5 days a week for 3 weeks showed no effects of rTMS on craving and alcohol consumption. A recent systematic review and meta-analysis of the effects of transcranial direct current stimulation (tDCS; 11 studies) and rTMS (23 studies), most targeting aspects of the prefrontal cortex, on alcohol craving concluded there was no evidence of positive effects on alcohol craving [92]. However, the positive results found in some studies and the variability in study quality and methodology underscore the need for further research in this area [93].

To date no medication has clearly emerged as an efficacious treatment for cocaine or methamphetamine addiction [81], making the positive results with r-TMS for psychostimulant addiction particularly noteworthy. The benefits of a single 10 Hz rTMS exposure over right, but not left, DLPFC was found to transiently attenuate cocaine craving [94] and many studies have now illustrated the ability of multiple administrations to attenuate craving and use in cocaine dependent individuals. Among these is a between-subject randomized study examining stimulation of the left DLPFC using HF-rTMS (15 Hz administered during 8 sessions) versus a control group receiving a mixture of putative medications for cocaine addiction during a 29-day period. Results showed significantly more cocaine-free urine tests and lower craving scores in the rTMS treatment group [95]. In a study examining use, craving, and other markers indicative of cocaine dependence 20 individuals with cocaine use disorder (CUD) received 2 weeks of rTMS administration (15 Hz; 5 days/week, twice daily totaling 20 sessions) of the left DLPC, followed by 2 weeks of maintenance sessions (15 Hz, 1 day/week, twice a day). Of the 16 participants who completed rTMS treatment, 56% had negative urine tests, craving scores significantly decreased as did participants depressive symptoms, anhedonia, and anxiety [96]. Other studies have reported benefits of rTMS for CUD when applied to the medial prefrontal cortex [81] and rTMS induced reductions in methamphetamine craving [85]. As with other rTMS research, study protocols vary greatly when examining rTMS for psychostimulant craving and addiction, and it is of note that investigators are now attempting to synthesize knowledge gained across studies to design and optimize a rTMS protocols for treating CUD [97].

The significant degree of support for the efficacy of rTMS for SUD comes from research on nicotine dependence [83]. Multiple studies have reported 1–2 rTMS sessions applied to the left DLPC results in reduced craving for cigarettes [83]. Repeated rTMS has also consistently yielded attenuated nicotine craving though the persistence of the effects remains unclear. For example, a randomized sham-controlled study administering 10 daily (10 Hz) rTMS to the left DLPC reduced cigarette consumption as measured by self-report and urine cotinine levels and cue-induced craving, though these effects dissipated with time [98]. The majority of studies of rTMS for SUD have focused on the efficacy of rTMS alone while some started to examine it in combination with other therapies. One study examined participants randomly assigned to receive 13 daily treatments of high-frequency, low-frequency or sham rTMS with and without cue exposure prior to treatment. Deep rTMS was bilaterally administered above the lateral prefrontal cortex and insula. High, but not low, frequency deep rTMS significantly attenuated cigarette smoking and when combined with smoking cues further facilitated reduction in cigarette use leading to an abstinence rate of 44% following the treatment and an estimated abstinence rate of 33% at 6 months [99]. A recent systematic review of the efficacy of rTMS for nicotine consumption and craving concluded that no recommendation beyond the possibility that HF-rTMS of the left DLPFC is effective for attenuating craving and consumption could be made and that while rTMS may be most effective when combined with other approaches, recent results obtained when combining approaches require replication and more rigorous evaluation [100].

Because rTMS is a neural circuit-based treatment approach rather than neurotransmitter focused and is directly administered to the brain, rather than systemically given, it is well tolerated. Adverse events are uncommon and tend to include transient headache and scalp discomfort. However, caution applying rTMS may be warranted in those with greater seizure risk such as individuals actively using psychostimulants or undergoing alcohol withdrawal [80]. rTMS may also be advantageous as it circumvents issues of medication adherence, cost, and side effects associated with most pharmacotherapies. The long-term efficacy of rTMS for decreasing drug craving in those with SUD is a potential concern given most studies assess these variables following relatively short-term administration periods (days-weeks) [81–83] or after limited follow-up periods [89]. However, one recent study suggests rTMS effects have the potential to be more protracted [85].

While initial rTMS results investigating craving and substance use among those with SUD are promising current findings still require replication in double blind studies with larger sample sizes [81–83]. Moreover, studies showing reduction in symptoms of SUD beyond craving are uncommon [82] and given long-term effects from rTMS are only achieved following weeks of stimulation sessions the approach may be time intensive and costly [86]. Several aspects of rTMS treatment are robust and reliable such as regional specificity, depth of magnetic field, dose dependent amplification of behavior, polysynaptic engagement, and frequency dependent effects. However, many treatment parameters are yet to be determined including the optimal number of daily sessions, the optimal number of total sessions, efficacy of rTMS for attenuating drug consumption when applied to regions other than the DLPFC, optimal coil orientation relative to anatomy, and an appreciation of the synergy between rTMS and other therapeutic approaches [80–82]. It is also worth highlighting that much of our understanding of addiction has moved away from purely drug-centered model which focuses on the neurochemical changes that result from drug exposure towards a more individual-centered model whereby individual differences in vulnerability to developing addiction are recognized. With this paradigm shift future application of rTMS might benefit from using individual MRIs and TMS navigator devices to individualize and maximize its physiological and therapeutic effects [82, 93].

5. Conclusion

The process of bringing a new therapeutic approach into practice in a larger population is multifaceted and hinges on regulatory procedures, safety, efficacy, need, cost, among other variables. Moreover, this process is rarely linear as new research is published and the zeitgeist for various therapies changes. Where there remains little controversy is that while SUD treatment has seen growing success, evidenced-based therapeutic options are still limited and not effective for all patients. Developing novel approaches continues to be paramount given the psychological, social, healthcare, and economic costs of drug addiction.

The reemergence of research on serotonergic hallucinogens, most notably psilocybin, is of particular significance as it appears effective and well tolerated for treating SUD in the limited research that has been conducted. This conclusion is further bolstered by research examining the efficacy of psilocybin and related drugs for the variety of psychological disorders that are also part of the milieu of addiction. The dramatic and long-lasting nature of psilocybin's effects on meaning, spirituality and drug use appears to address the chronic nature of SUD in ways not achieved by most treatment approaches. Likewise, the potential therapeutic use of rTMS for SUD and other psychological disorders is notable for its efficacy, safety, and anti-craving effects, the latter of which is both central to addiction yet remains particularly challenging to resolve. The promise of these two approaches is hard to overstate yet in the absence of findings from larger randomized, double-blind clinical trials these approaches will continue to be viewed as merely promising. Anti-addiction vaccines, while potentially beneficial, require further technical refinement and appreciation of their place among therapeutic modalities.

As research on these approaches progresses it is not too early to consider how these therapies might be scaled to treat the large number of people affected by SUD. While some of these questions have begun to be addressed, such as the optimization of treatment protocols and how to best integrate them with other treatment modalities, larger issues loom. Who will be trained to administer these therapies and where will they be administered? Overcoming the public's negative perception and misunderstanding of hallucinogenic drugs, electroshock therapy, and vaccine hesitancy are all barriers to scaling these therapeutic approaches which are unfamiliar to most and therefore susceptible to misunderstanding and misinformation. The use of newer pharmacotherapies for SUD over the past 30 years has been slow to be adopted by healthcare providers partially due to their lack of awareness and comfort with these new approaches. The inclusion of these interventions in graduate education across medical, psychological, and healthcare occupations might promote their integration as future treatment options for those with SUD. Consideration of these issues today will likely ease the transition of these and other novel therapeutic techniques for SUD into widespread use moving forward.

Author details

William M. Meil*, William Farrell and Reem Satti
Department of Psychology, Indiana University of Pennsylvania,
Indiana, Pennsylvania, USA

*Address all correspondence to: meil@iup.edu

References

[1] Arria AM, McLellan TA. Evolution of concept - But not action - in addiction treatment. Substance Use Misuse. 2012; 47:1041-1048. DOI:10.3109/10826084.2012.663273

[2] Fleury M-JJ, Djouini A, Huỳnh C, Tremblay J, Ferland F, Menard JM, et al. Remission from substance use disorders: A systematic review and meta-analysis. Drug and Alcohol Dependence. 2016;168:293-306. DOI.org/10.1016/j.drugalcdep.2016.08.625

[3] Bahorik AL, Satre DD, Kline-Simon AH, Weisner CM, Campbell CI. Alcohol, cannabis, and opioid use disorders, and disease burden in an integrated healthcare system. Journal of Addiction Medicine. 2017; 1(1):3-9. DOI:10.1097/ADM.0000000000000260

[4] Substance Abuse and Mental Health Services Administration. (2020). Key substance use and mental health indicators in the United States: Results from the 2019 National Survey on Drug Use and Health (HHS Publication No. PEP20-07-01-001, NSDUH Series H-55). Rockville, MD: Center for Behavioral Health Statistics and Quality, Substance Abuse and Mental Health Services Administration. Retrieved from https://www.samhsa.gov/data/

[5] McLellan TA, Lewis DC, O'Brien CP, Kleber HD. Drug dependence, a chronic medical illness implication for treatment, insurance, and outcomes Evaluation. JAMA. 2000;284(13):1689-1695. DOI:10.1001/jama.284.13.1689

[6] Chung T, Maisto SA, Cornelius JR, Martin CS. Adolescents' alcohol and drug use trajectories in the year following treatment. J Stud Alcohol. 2004; 105-114. DOI: 10.15288/jsa.2004.65.105

[7] De Crescenzo F, Ciabattini M, Loreto D'Alò G, De Giorgi R, Del Giovane C, et al. Comparative efficacy and acceptability of psychosocial interventions for individuals with cocaine and amphetamine addiction: A systematic review and network meta-analysis. PLoS Med. 2018;15(12): e1002715. DOI.org/10.1371/journal.pmed.1002715

[8] Marel C, Mills KL, Slade T, Darke S, Ross J, Teesson M. Modelling long-term joint trajectories of heroin use and treatment utilisation: findings from the Australian treatment outcome study. E Clinical Medicine. 2019: DOI:https://doi.org/10.1016/j.eclinm.2019.07.01

[9] Timko C, Moos CR, Finney JW, Lesar MD. Long-term outcomes of alcohol use disorders: comparing untreated individuals with those in alcoholics anonymous and formal treatment. J Stud Alcohol. 2000;61(4):529-540. DOI:10.15288/jsa.2000.61.529

[10] Cranford JA, Krentzman AR, Mowbray O, Robinsonn EAR. Trajectories of alcohol use over time among adults with alcohol dependence. Addict Behavior. 2014;39(5):1006-1011. DOI: 10.1016/j.addbeh.2014.02.009

[11] Koob GF, Volkow ND. Neurobiology of addiction: a neurocircuitry analysis. The Lancet Psychiatry, 2016; 3(8):760-773. DOI.org/10.1016/S2215-0366(16)00104-8

[12] Nestler EJ, Lüscher C. The molecular basis of drug addiction: Linking epigenetic to synaptic and circuit mechanisms. Neuron. 2019;102:48-59. DOI.org/10.1016/j.neuron.2019.01.016

[13] Robison AJ, Nestler EJ. Transcriptional and epigenetic mechanisms of addiction Nature Reviews Neuroscience. 2011;12:623-637. DOI: 10.1038/nrn3111

[14] Advokat CD., Comtaty JE., Julien RM. Julien's Primer of Drug

Action. 14th ed. Worth publishers New York.

[15] Nichols DE. Hallucinogens. Pharmacological Reviews 2016; 68:264-355. Pharmacological Reviews DOI: https://doi.org/10.1124/pr.115.011478

[16] Geiger, HA, Wurst MG, Daniels RN. DARK classics in chemical neuroscience: Psilocybin. ACS Chemical Neuroscience. 2018;9:2438-2447. DOI: org/10.1021/acschemneuro.8b00186

[17] Morgan C, McAndrew A, Stevens T, Nutt D, Lawn W. Tripping up addiction: the use of psychedelic drugs in the treatment of problematic drug and alcohol use, Current Opinion in Behavioral Sciences. 2017;13:71-76. DOI.org/10.1016/j.cobeha.2016.10.009

[18] dos Santos RG, Osório FL, Crippa JAS, Riba J, Zuardi AW, et al. Antidepressive, anxiolytic, and antiaddictive effects of ayahuasca, psilocybin and lysergic acid diethylamide (LSD): a systematic review of clinical trials published in the last 25 years. Ther Adv Psychopharmacol. 2016;6(3):193-213. DOI:10.1177/2045125316638008

[19] Liester, MB, A review of lysergic acid diethylamide (LSD) in the treatment of addictions: historical perspectives and future prospects. Current Drug Abuse Reviews. 2014;7:146-156. DOI10.2174/1874473708666150107120522

[20] Grinspoon L, Bakalar JB. Psychedelic drugs reconsidered. NewYork: Lindesmith Center; 1997.

[21] Bogenschutz M, Forcehimes A. Development of a psychotherapeutic model for psilocybin-assisted treatment of alcoholism. Journal of Humanistic Psychology. 2017;57(4):389-414. DOI:10.1177/0022167816673493

[22] Hoffer A, Osmond H. The hallucinogens. New York: Academic Press; 1967.

[23] Fuentes JJ, Fonseca F, Elices M, Marré M, Torrens, M. Therapeutic use of LSD in psychiatry: A systematic review of randomized-controlled clinical trials. Front. Psychiatry. 2020;10. DOI.org/10.3389/fpsyt.2019.00943

[24] Nutt D. Psychedelic drugs-a new era in psychiatry? Review Dialogues Clin Neurosci. 2019;21(2):139-147. DOI: 10.31887/DCNS.2019.21.2/dnutt

[25] Dyck E. 'Hitting highs at rock bottom': LSD treatment for alcoholism, 1950-1970. Social History of Medicine, 2006;19(2): 313-329. DOI.org/10.1093/shm/hkl039

[26] Tanne JH. Humphry Osmond. BMJ. 2004; 328(7441): 713.

[27] Krebs TS, Johansen, PØ. Lysergic acid diethylamide (LSD) for alcoholism: meta-analysis of randomized controlled trials. J Psychopharmacol. 2012; 26:994-1002. DOI: 10.1177/0269881112439253

[28] Bas TH, Arnt AF, Schellekens MMM, Michel MM, Verheij J, et al. Psilocybin for treating substance use disorders? Expert Rev Neurother. 2017;17(2):203-212. DOI: 10.1080/14737175.2016.1220834

[29] From Marijuana To Mushrooms, Voters Want Drug Laws Eased [Internet]. 2020. Available from: https://www.npr.org/2020/11/04/931507602/from-marijuana-to-mushrooms-voters-want-drug-laws-eased [2020-11-04]

[30] Bogenschutz MP, Forcehimes AA, Pommy JA, Wilcox CE, Barbosa PCR, et al. Psilocybin-assisted treatment for alcohol dependence: a proof-of-concept study. J Psychopharmacol. 2015;29(3): 289-99. DOI:10.1177/0269881114565144

[31] Johnson MW, Garcia-Romeu A, Cosimano MP, Griffiths RR. Pilot study

of the 5-HT2AR agonist psilocybin in the treatment of tobacco addiction. J Psychopharmacol. 2014;28(11):983-92. Doi: 10.1177/0269881114548296

[32] Johnson MW, Garcia-Romeu A, Griffiths RR. Long-term follow-up of psilocybin-facilitated smoking cessation. Am J Drug Alcohol Abuse. 2017;43(1):55-60. DOI: 10.3109/00952990.2016.1170135

[33] Johnson MW, Griffiths RR, Hendricks PS, Henningfield JE. The abuse potential of medical psilocybin according to the 8 factors of the Controlled Substances Act. Neuropharmacology. 2018;142:143-166. DOI: 10.1016/j.neuropharm.2018.05.012

[34] Johnson MW, Griffiths RR. Potential Therapeutic Effects of Psilocybin. Neurotherapeutics. 2017;14(3):734-740. DOI: 10.1007/s13311-017-0542-y

[35] Zhou X, Qin B, Giovane CD, Pan J, Gentile S, et al. Efficacy and tolerability of antidepressants in the treatment of adolescents and young adults with depression and substance use disorders: a systematic review and meta-analysis. Addiction. 2015; 110(1):38-48. DOI: 10.1111/add.12698

[36] Tjagvad C, Clausen T, Handal M, kurtveit S. Benzodiazepine prescription for patients in treatment for drug use disorders: a nationwide cohort study in Denmark, 2000-2010. BMC Psychiatry. 2016;6:168. DOI: 10.1186/s12888-016-0881-y

[37] Streifel C, Servaty-Seib HL. Recovering from alcohol and other drug dependency: loss and spirituality in a 12-step context. Alcohol Treatment Quarterly. 27(2):184-198. DOI.org/10.1080/07347320902785558

[38] Wilson B, Bill W: My first 40 years. Center City, MN: Hazelden 2000

[39] Piderman KM, Schneekloth TD, Pankratz VS, Maloney SD, Altchuler SI. Spirituality in alcoholics during treatment. American Journal on Addictions. 2007; 16(3):232-237. DOI: 10.1080/10550490701375616

[40] Galanter M, Dermatis H, Bunt G, Williams C, Trujillo M, Steinke P. Assessment of spirituality and its relevance to addiction treatment. Journal of Substance Abuse Treatment. 2007;33(3):257-264. DOI: https://doi.org/10.1016/j.jsat.2006.06.014

[41] Garcia-Romeu A, Griffiths RR, Johnson MW. Psilocybin-occasioned mystical experiences in the treatment of tobacco addiction. Curr Drug Abuse Rev. 2015;7(3): 157-164. DOI: 10.2174/1874473708666150107121331

[42] Carhart-Harris RL, Erritzoe D, Williams T, Stone JM, Reed LJ, et al. Neural correlates of the psychedelic state as determined by fMRI studies with psilocybin. PNAS, 2012; 109 (6):2138-2143. DOI.org/10.1073/pnas.1119598109

[43] Carhart-Harris, RL, Muthukumaraswamy S, Roseman L, Kaelen M, Droog W, et al. Neural correlates of the LSD experience revealed by multimodal neuroimaging. PNAS, 2016;113 (17):4853-4858. DOI.org/10.1073/pnas.1518377113

[44] Lebedev A, Lövdén M, Rosenthal G, Feilding A, Nutt DJ, et al. Finding the self by losing the self: Neural correlates of ego-dissolution under psilocybin. Human Brain Mapping. 2015;36(8):3137-3153. DOI:10.1002/hbm.22833

[45] Bogenschutz MP. It's time to take psilocybin seriously as a possible treatment for substance use disorders. Am J Drug Alcohol Abuse. 2017; 43(1):4-6. DOI: 10.1080/00952990.2016.1200060

[46] Yaden DB, Yaden ME, Griffiths RR. Psychedelics in psychiatry-keeping the renaissance from going off the rails. JAMA Psychiatry. 2020; DOI: 10.1001/jamapsychiatry.2020.3672

[47] Tang X, Yang J, Wang W, Zeng Y, Li J, et al. Immunotherapy for treating methamphetamine, heroin and cocaine use disorders. Drug Discovery Today. 2020;25:610-619. DOI: 10.1016/j.drudis.2019.07.009

[48] Carrera MRA, Ashley JA, Parsons LH, et al. Suppression of psychoactive effects of cocaine by active immunization. Nature. 1995;378:727-730. DOI: 10.1038/378727a0

[49] Fox BS, Kantak KM, Edwards MA, et al. Efficacy of a therapeutic cocaine vaccine in rodent models. Nat Med. 1996;2:1129-1132. DOI: 10.1038/nm1096-1129

[50] Carrera MRA, Ashley JA, Zhou B, et al. Cocaine vaccines: Antibody protection against relapse in a rat model. Proceedings of the National Academy of Sciences. 2000;97:6202-6206. DOI: 10.1073/pnas.97.11.6202

[51] Kantak KM, Collins SL, Lipman EG, et al. Evaluation of anti-cocaine antibodies and a cocaine vaccine in a rat self-administration model. Psychopharmacology. 2000;148:251-262. DOI: 10.1007/s002130050049

[52] Kosten TR, Rosen M, Bond J, et al. Human therapeutic cocaine vaccine: safety and immunogenicity. Vaccine. 2002;20:1196-1204. DOI: 10.1016/S0264-410X(01)00425-X

[53] Martell BA, Mitchell E, Poling J, et al. Vaccine pharmacotherapy for the treatment of cocaine dependence. Biological Psychiatry. 2005;58: 158-164. DOI: 10.1016/j.biopsych.2005.04.032

[54] Haney M, Gunderson EW, Jiang H, et al. Cocaine-specific antibodies blunt the subjective effects of smoked cocaine in humans. Biological Psychiatry. 2010;67:59-65. DOI: 10.1016/j.biopsych.2009.08.031

[55] Martell BA, Orson FM, Poling J, et al. Cocaine vaccine for the treatment of cocaine dependence in methadone-maintained patients: A randomized, double-blind, placebo-controlled efficacy trial. Archives of General Psychiatry. 2009;66:1116-1123. DOI: 0.1001/archgenpsychiatry.2009.128

[56] Kosten TR, Domingo CB, Shorter D, et al. Vaccine for cocaine dependence: A randomized double-blind placebo-controlled efficacy trial. Drug and Alcohol Dependence. 2014;140: 42-47. DOI: 10.1016/j.drugalcdep.2014.04.003

[57] Koob G, J. Hicks M, Wee S, et al. Anti-cocaine vaccine based on coupling a cocaine analog to a disrupted adenovirus. CNSNDDT. 2011;10:899-904. DOI: 10.2174/187152711799219334

[58] Wee S, Hicks MJ, De BP, et al. Novel cocaine vaccine linked to a disrupted adenovirus gene transfer vector blocks cocaine psychostimulant and reinforcing effects. Neuropsychopharmacol. 2012;37:1083-1091. DOI: 10.1038/npp.2011.200

[59] Maoz A, Hicks MJ, Vallabhjosula S, et al. Adenovirus capsid-based anti-cocaine vaccine prevents cocaine from binding to the nonhuman primate CNS dopamine transporter. Neuropsychopharmacol. 2013;38:2170-2178. DOI: 10.1038/npp.2013.114

[60] Evans SM, Foltin RW, Hicks MJ, et al. Efficacy of an adenovirus-based anti-cocaine vaccine to reduce cocaine self-administration and reacquisition using a choice procedure in rhesus macaques. Pharmacology Biochemistry

and Behavior. 2016;150-151:76-86. DOI: 10.1016/j.pbb.2016.09.008

[61] Pentel PR, Malin DH, Ennifar S, et al. A nicotine conjugate vaccine reduces nicotine distribution to brain and attenuates its behavioral and cardiovascular effects in rats. Pharmacology Biochemistry and Behavior. 2000;65:191-198. DOI: 10.1016/S0091-3057(99)00206-3

[62] LeSage MG, Keyler DE, Hieda Y, et al. Effects of a nicotine conjugate vaccine on the acquisition and maintenance of nicotine self-administration in rats. Psychopharmacology. 2006;184:409-416. DOI: 10.1007/s00213-005-0027-2

[63] Esterlis I, Hannestad JO, Perkins E, et al. Effect of a nicotine vaccine on nicotine binding to β2*-nicotinic acetylcholine receptors in vivo in human tobacco smokers. Am J Psychiatry. 2013;170:399-407. DOI: 10.1176/appi.ajp.2012.12060793

[64] Hatsukami D, Rennard S, Jorenby D, et al. Safety and immunogenicity of a nicotine conjugate vaccine in current smokers. Clinical Pharmacology & Therapeutics. 2005;78:456-467. DOI: 10.1016/j.clpt.2005.08.007

[65] Hatsukami DK, Jorenby DE, Gonzales D, et al. Immunogenicity and smoking-cessation outcomes for a novel nicotine immunotherapeutic. Clin Pharmacol Ther. 2011;89:392-399. DOI: 10.1038/clpt.2010.317

[66] Fahim RE, Kessler PD, Kalnik MW. Therapeutic vaccines against tobacco addiction. Expert Review of Vaccines. 2013;12:333-342. DOI: 10.1586/ERV.13.13

[67] Hoogsteder PHJ, Kotz D, van Spiegel PI, et al. Efficacy of the nicotine vaccine 3′-AmNic-rEPA (NicVAX) co-administered with varenicline and counselling for smoking cessation: a randomized placebo-controlled trial. Addiction. 2014;109:1252-1259. DOI: 10.1111/add.12573

[68] Maurer P, Jennings GT, Willers J, et al. A therapeutic vaccine for nicotine dependence: preclinical efficacy, and phase I safety and immunogenicity. Eur J Immunol. 2005;35:2031-2040. DOI: 10.1002/eji.200526285

[69] Cornuz J, Zwahlen S, Jungi WF, et al. A vaccine against nicotine for smoking cessation: a randomized controlled trial. PLoS ONE. 2008;3:e2547. DOI:10.1371/journal.pone.0002547

[70] Fierce Biotech. Interim Analysis of an Ongoing Phase II Study With Nicotine Vaccine Shows Primary Endpoint Not Achieved [Internet]. 2009. Available from: https://www.fiercebiotech.com/biotech/interim-analysis-of-an-ongoing-phase-ii-study-nicotine-vaccine-shows-primary-endpoint-not [Accessed: 2020-11-17]

[71] Bremer PT, Schlosburg JE, Banks ML, et al. Development of a clinically viable heroin vaccine. J Am Chem Soc. 2017;139:8601-8611. DOI: 10.1021/jacs.7b03334

[72] Pravetoni M, Comer SD. Development of vaccines to treat opioid use disorders and reduce incidence of overdose. Neuropharmacology. 2019;158:107662. DOI: 10.1016/j.neuropharm.2019.06.001

[73] Pravetoni M, Pentel PR, Potter DN, et al. Effects of an oxycodone conjugate vaccine on oxycodone self-administration and oxycodone-induced brain gene expression in rats. PLoS ONE. 2014;9:e101807. DOI: 10.1371/journal.pone.0101807

[74] Raleigh MD, Baruffaldi F, Peterson SJ, et al. A fentanyl vaccine alters fentanyl distribution and protects

against fentanyl-induced effects in mice and rats. J Pharmacol Exp Ther. 2019;368:282-291. DOI: 10.1124/jpet.118.253674

[75] Bremer PT, Janda KD. Conjugate vaccine immunotherapy for substance use disorder. Pharmacol Rev. 2017;69:298-315. DOI: 10.1124/pr.117.013904

[76] Cornish KE, Harris AC, LeSage MG, et al. Combined active and passive immunization against nicotine: Minimizing monoclonal antibody requirements using a target antibody concentration strategy. International Immunopharmacology. 2011;11:1809-1815. DOI: 10.1016/j.intimp.2011.07.009

[77] Alzhrani RF, Xu H, Valdes SA, et al. Intranasal delivery of a nicotine vaccine candidate induces antibodies in mouse blood and lung mucosal secretions that specifically neutralize nicotine. Drug Development and Industrial Pharmacy. 2020;46:1656-1664. DOI: 10.1080/03639045.2020.1820033

[78] St John AL, Choi HW, Walker QD, et al. Novel mucosal adjuvant, mastoparan-7, improves cocaine vaccine efficacy. NPJ Vaccines. 2020;5:12. DOI: 10.1038/s41541-020-0161-1

[79] Hwang CS, Smith LC, Natori Y, et al. Improved admixture vaccine of fentanyl and heroin hapten immunoconjugates: Antinociceptive evaluation of fentanyl-contaminated heroin. ACS Omega. 2018;3:11537-11543. DOI: 10.1021/acsomega.8b01478

[80] Gorelick DA, Zangen A, George MS. Transcranial magnetic stimulation (TMS) in the treatment of substance addiction. Ann N Y Acad Sci. 2014;1327(1):79-93. DOI.org/10.1111/nyas.12479

[81] Hanlon CA, Dowdle LT, Henderson JS. Modulating neural circuits with transcranial magnetic stimulation: Implications for addiction treatment development. Pharmacological Reviews. 2018;70(3):661-683. DOI: DOI.org/10.1124/pr.116.013649

[82] Diana M, Raij T, Melis, M, Nummenmaa A, Leggio L, et al. Rehabilitating the addicted brain with transcranial magnetic stimulation. Nat Rev Neurosci. 2017; 18:685-693. DOI.org/10.1038/nrn.2017.113

[83] Salling M, Martinez, D. Brain stimulation in addiction. 2016. Neuropsychopharmacol. 41, 2798-2809; DOI.org/10.1038/npp.2016.80

[84] Noohi S, Amirsalari S. History, studies and specific uses of repetitive transcranial magnetic stimulation (rTMS) in treating epilepsy. Iran J Child Neurol. 2016;10(1):1-8.

[85] Liu X, Zhao X, Liu T, Liu Q, Tang L, et al. The effects of repetitive transcranial magnetic stimulation on cue-induced craving in male patients with heroin use disorder. EBioMedicine. 2020;56:102809. DOI: 10.1016/j.ebiom.2020.102809

[86] Su H, Liu Y, Yin D, Chen T, Li X, et al. Neuroplastic changes in resting-state functional connectivity after rTMS intervention for methamphetamine craving. Neuropharm. 2020;175:108177. DOI.org/10.1016/j.neuropharm.2020.108177

[87] Sahlem GL, Baker NL, George MS, Malcolm RJ, McRae-Clark AL. Repetitive transcranial magnetic stimulation (rTMS) administration to heavy cannabis users. Am J Drug Alcohol Abuse. 2018;44(1):47-55.DOI:10.1080/00952990.2017.1355920

[88] Mishra BR, Nizamie SH, Das B, Praharaj SK. Efficacy of repetitive transcranial magnetic stimulation in alcohol dependence: a sham-controlled study. Addiction. 2010;105(1):49-55. DOI: 10.1111/j.1360-0443.2009.02777.x

[89] Mishra BR, Praharaj SK, Katshu MZ, Sukanto Sarkar S, et al. Comparison of anticraving efficacy of right and left repetitive transcranial magnetic stimulation in alcohol dependence: A randomized double-blind study. J. Neuropsychiatry Clin Neurosci. 2015; DIO.org/10.1176/appi.neuropsych.13010013

[90] Herremans SC, Baeken C, Vanderbruggen N, Vanderhasselt MA, Zeeuws D, et al. No influence of one right-sided prefrontal HF-rTMS session on alcohol craving in recently detoxified alcohol-dependent patients: results of a naturalistic study. Drug Alcohol Depend. 2012;120(1-3):209-213. DOI: 10.1016/j.drugalcdep.2011.07.021

[91] Höppner J, Broese T, Wendler L, Berger C, Thome J Repetitive transcranial magnetic stimulation (rTMS) for treatment of alcohol dependence. World J Biol Psychiatry. 2011 Suppl 1:57-62. DOI: 10.3109/15622975.2011.598383

[92] Perini I, Kämpe R, Arlestig T, Karlsson H, Löfberg, A, et al. Repetitive transcranial magnetic stimulation targeting the insular cortex for reduction of heavy drinking in treatment-seeking alcohol-dependent subjects: a randomized controlled trial. Neuropsychopharm. 2020;45:842-850. DOI: 10.1038/s41386-019-0565-7

[93] Barr MS, Farzan F, Wing VC, George TP, Fitzgerald PB et al. Repetitive transcranial magnetic stimulation and drug addiction. Int Rev Psychiatry. 2011;(5):454-66. Doi: 10.3109/09540261.2011.618827

[94] Camprodon JA, Martínez-Raga J, Alonso-Alonso M, Mei-Chiung S, Pascual-Leone A. One session of high frequency repetitive transcranial magnetic stimulation (rTMS) to the right prefrontal cortex transiently reduces cocaine craving. Drug Alcohol Depend. 2007;86(1):91-4. DOI: 10.1016/j.drugalcdep.2006.06.002

[95] Terraneo A, Leggio L, Saladini M, Ermani M, Bonci A, et al. Transcranial magnetic stimulation of dorsolateral prefrontal cortex reduces cocaine use: A pilot study. Eur Neuropsychopharmacology. 2016;26(1):37-44. DOI: 10.1016/j.euroneuro.2015.11.011

[96] Pettorruso M, Martinotti G, Santacroce R, Montemitro C, Fanella F, et al. rTMS reduces psychopathological burden and cocaine consumption in treatment-seeking subjects with cocaine use disorder: An open label, feasibility study. Front Psychiatry. 2019;10:621. DOI: 10.3389/fpsyt.2019.00621

[97] Hanlon CA, Kearney-Ramos T, Dowdle LT, Hamilton S, DeVries W, et al. Developing repetitive transcranial magnetic stimulation (rTMS) as a treatment tool for cocaine use disorder: a series of six translational studies. Curr Behav Neurosci Rep. 2017;4(4):341-352. DOI: 10.1007/s40473-017-0135-4

[98] Amiaz R, Levy D, Vainiger D, Grunhaus L, Zangen A. Repeated high-frequency transcranial magnetic stimulation over the dorsolateral prefrontal cortex reduces cigarette craving and consumption. Addiction. 2009;104(4):653-60. DOI: 10.1111/j.1360-0443.2008.02448.x

[99] Dinur-Klein L, Dannon P, Hadar A, Rosenberg O, Roth Y, et al. Smoking cessation induced by deep repetitive transcranial magnetic stimulation of the prefrontal and insular cortices: a prospective, randomized controlled trial. Biol Psychiatry. 2014;76(9):742-9. DOI: 10.1016/j.biopsych.2014.05.020

[100] Hauer L, Scarano GI, Brigo F, Golaszewski S, Lochner P, et al. Effects of repetitive transcranial magnetic stimulation on nicotine consumption and craving: A systematic review. Psychiatry Res. 2019;281:112562. DOI: 10.1016/j.psychres.2019.112562